F

Conceiving Healthy Babies

This is a must-read for any couple struggling to get pregnant and start a family. Heartfully honest, the author shares her own deeply personal story as she explores the depth of the problems surrounding fertilty – or lack of it. After endless amounts of experience and research – and two successful pregnancies – this woman who was tagged "infertile" has a whole lot to say on the subject. This a wise, truthful empowering book, and offers some of the best advice I've seen on the subject of creating healthy thriving babies. May *Building Healthy Babies* find its way into the hands and heart of every woman and man who needs to read it.

—Rosemary Gladstar, herbalist and author

It's been said that genius is focus. If this is so, and I suspect it is, there is true genius revealed in this book. Dawn Combs' conversation about building healthy babies has documents the path of a devoted warrior. Dismissing the deluded conclusions of medical authorities that her re-productive system was "broken," Dawn and her husband, using natural methods, rekindled balance in their bodies and conceived a healthy child. And a second one. Congratulations! Herein is a vivid testament that our health is natural and both men and women have options when necessary to revive and experience it.

—James Green, herbalist and author, *The Male Herbal* and *The Herbal Medicine-Maker's Handbook*

Conceiving Healthy Babies is a guide to living well along with being a guide to healing fertility issues. The focus on preconception care is the right approach to creating ad raising healthy children. As an integrative pedi-atrician whose practice focuses on whole food nutrition and keeping the gut healthy, Dawn's book resonates with my philosophy of care for my pa-tients and their families. *Conceiving Healthy Babies* provides a roadmap for couples and families to healthfully navigate preconception, pregnancy and lactation and ultimately the raising of the healthiest child possible.

—Dhanu Sant, MD, WholeKids Pediatrics

I am so excited about this book. I can't wait to get it into the hands of our clients. It is clear, concise and informative, and this information is immeasurably needed in a medical environment where infertility is treated as a one-treatment-fits-all issue, rather than as a multifaceted and individualized wellness issue. I especially like the reccurring message that each person has their own best formula for healthy balance and listening to your body is the key to finding yours. Thank you for this gift to childbearing women.

—Nina McIndoe, CPM, Executive Director,
Center for Humane Options in Childbirth Experiences

This is a wonderful book and a welcome addition to any herbal or natural birthing library.

—Stephen Harrod Buhner, award-winning author,
Herbal Antibiotics and *Plant Intelligence and the Imaginal Realm*

Couples who find themselves frustrated when navigating fertility options in our modern system will find an exhale of relief in Dawn Combs' *Conceiving Healthy Babies*. This brilliant new book offers straightforward, practical advice on natural methods for fertility support from a place of personal experience. Couples will find reassurance in her guidance on nutrition, herbs, and plant-based solutions for building a healthy baby. The time-honored teachings reintroduced through this book find modern relevance through pragmatic and thoughtful recommendations on how to weave them into daily practice. Every couple struggling to conceive should read this book.

—Emily Ruff, herbalist and director,
Florida School of Holistic Living and Florida Herbal Conference

Conceiving Healthy Babies is written with the knowledge of understanding. First of all, understanding what it is like to be told by a broken "healthcare" system that one is broken. Secondly, the understanding that comes from taking control of one's own health in order to regain the balance that is our birthright. And finally, the understanding that comes from having an academic AND working knowledge of the herbs grown on her own biodynamic family farm. Dawn Combs is a teacher and a healer in the truest sense of these words.

—Dr. Kathryn M. Bennett, DC, Worthington Optimal Wellness

CONCEIVING HEALTHY BABIES

AN HERBAL GUIDE to SUPPORT PRECONCEPTION, PREGNANCY and LACTATION

Dawn Combs

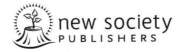

new society
PUBLISHERS

Cover design by Diane McIntosh.
All images © iStock (Newborn: hannamonika; Red Raspberry Leaf: anna1311;
Dandelion: UroshPetrovic; Gingko leaves: Tihis; Hops: nndemidchick)

Printed in Canada.

New Society Publishers acknowledges the financial support of the Government of
Canada through the Canada Book Fund (CBF) for our publishing activities.

Paperback ISBN: 978-0-86571-780-0

Ebook ISBN: 978-1-55092-574-6

Inquiries regarding requests to reprint all or part of *Conceiving Healthy Babies* should be
addressed to New Society Publishers at the address below.

To order directly from the publishers, please call toll-free (North America)
1-800-567-6772, or order online at www.newsociety.com

Any other inquiries can be directed by mail to:

New Society Publishers
P.O. Box 189, Gabriola Island, BC V0R 1X0, Canada
(250) 247-9737

New Society Publishers' mission is to publish books that contribute in fundamental ways
to building an ecologically sustainable and just society, and to do so with the least possible
impact on the environment, in a manner that models this vision. We are committed to
doing this not just through education, but through action. The interior pages of our bound
books are printed on Forest Stewardship Council®-registered acid-free paper that is **100%
post-consumer recycled** (100% old growth forest-free), processed chlorine-free, and
printed with vegetable-based, low-VOC inks, with covers produced using FSC®-registered
stock. New Society also works to reduce its carbon footprint, and purchases carbon offsets
based on an annual audit to ensure a carbon neutral footprint. For further information, or to
browse our full list of books and purchase securely, visit our website at: www.newsociety.com

Library and Archives Canada Cataloguing in Publication

Combs, Dawn, author
      Conceiving healthy babies : an herbal guide to support
preconception, pregnancy and lactation / Dawn Combs.

Includes bibliographical references and index.
Issued in print and electronic formats.
ISBN 978-0-86571-780-0 (pbk.).--ISBN 978-1-55092-574-6 (ebook)

      1. Pregnancy--Nutritional aspects--Popular works. 2. Lactation--Nutritional
aspects--Popular works. 3. Preconception care--Popular works. 4. Fertility, Human--
Nutritional aspects--Popular works. 5. Herbs--Theraputic use--Popular works. I. Title.
RG559.C57 2014   618.2'42   C2014-904449-6
                                                          C2014-904450-X

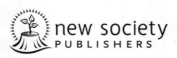

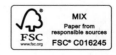

This book is dedicated to every couple who struggles at any point in their journey to hold a beautiful, healthy child in their arms. To all of you who are made to feel like a number in a hopeless, voiceless and powerless system … may you see there is light and hope in returning to our "roots" and reconnecting to the small quiet voice within. May you be inspired by our personal story.

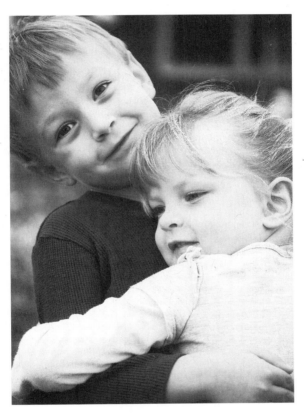

Sometimes great struggle is worth the reward.

© Rachael Brugger

Contents

Acknowledgments xi

Preface xiii

Foreword by Carson Combs xvii

Introduction 1

A Journey to Family 5
  Our Infertility Story 5
  Preparing Traditional Whole Foods 14
  Asking the Herbs for Help... 16
  My First Pregnancy... 19
  My First Birth.. 20
  Nursing Troubles 24
  My Own Formula 29
  My Second Birth 33
  Choosing a Path 36

Strategies for Building a Healthy Baby.................................. 39
  Herbal Therapies for Fertility 39
  Herbal Therapies for Your Partner.................................... 44
  Foods for Preconception... 47

The Mental Component in Fertility.. 53
Alternative Therapies.. 54
Breast Health and Building Your Baby...................................... 56
Preconception and Pregnancy.. 60
Foods for Pregnancy and Lactation 64
Chiropractic and Low Milk Supply 70
Supplemental Feeding Equipment 71
Mental Component in Breastfeeding.. 73
The Concept of Nursing Through 75

General Herb Use... 81

Determining the Quality of Herbs 83
Sustainable Suppliers.. 85
Standardized Method versus the Simplers Method................... 87

Whole versus Isolated Constituents:
The Side Effects of Ethnobotany....................................... 89
A Word About Supplements 92
Homeopathics 93
Essential Oils 94
Flower Essences... 95
General Herbal Components to Watch....................................... 95
Cleansing and Detoxing 98
Prescription, OTC and Illegal Drugs.. 103
A Final Word.. 104

Healthy Baby Herbal Reference Guide............................ 107

Using the Herbal Guide 107

Foods and Supplements 297

Afterword 313

Further Reading... 317

Notes.. 319

Glossary 327

Appendices

    Appendix A: Whole-Food/Whole-Plant Resources.............. 331

    Appendix B: Baby Formulas 335

    Appendix C: Breast Massage Techniques 339

    Appendix D: Child Dosage Table 343

    Appendix E: United Plant Savers................................. 345

    Appendix F: Comfrey: Poison or Panacea?................. 347

    Appendix G: Gluten-Free Lactation Cookies 349

    Appendix H: Build a Baby Worksheet................................ 351

Index 358

About the Author 375

Acknowledgments

MY THANKS GO TO MY MOTHER AND FATHER, who taught me that all things are possible with hard work and determination. Thanks for encouraging me to not only have dreams, but to fearlessly chase them as well.

To my husband, Carson, who walked with me on this path, who held my hand, fought with me through infertility and who is a loving partner and father. Thank you for allowing me to attain my dreams so I have room to dream new ones. I love you.

To Rosemary Gladstar, who planted the seed and began my personal relationship with the plants. I will forever be grateful to you for sharing your spirit and gifts with me so that I could share them with others.

To Nina McIndoe and Kelley Daniel, who delivered both my children at home in a safe and loving environment. Thank you for delivering me into the experience of motherhood in my chosen way. You both handled the surprises and challenges my deliveries presented with amazing calm and skill. I feel privileged to have you as part of our birth story.

To the plants, who teach me daily about myself while they reveal more of the wisdom they are anxious to share with a needy humanity — I am in awe.

To my children, Jacy and Aidan, thank you for entering our lives. You are what my soul craved most. Thank you for being patient while I wrote this book.

A word of thanks must also go to the following people: Scott Steedman, my editor; the hugely supportive and hardworking staff at New Society Publishers; Ingrid Witvoet; all of the staff at CHOICE Midwives; Sally Fallon Morell, for her baby formula recipe; Dr. Alison Hazelbaker; Vanessa Prentice, Janet, Brooke Sackenheim, Erica Powell, Dr. Donald Lateiner, and Scott and Julie Wood for their encouragement and friendship.

Preface

THE PERSONAL STORY I SHARE IN THESE PAGES is intended to be part inspiration and part cautionary tale. I learned many lessons as I worked through my own infertility, pregnancy and difficulties with breastfeeding. I found things that worked very well for me and learned things I wish I'd known long before I started. I hope that my personal story and my analysis of these lessons learned will give women more information to form their own plans for building a healthy baby.

While writing this book, I have revisited every emotion and every bit of research I did from the beginning of my journey. It has been illuminating in my personal life and in my farm business. As we have grown as a farm, our regular customers have watched me get hugely pregnant, carry around infants and chase toddlers. Through it all we have brought the kids along to farmers' markets and festivals. A few times, passersby have commented that we should have a babysitter. I didn't recognize at the time why I had such a visceral, negative internal reaction to this. Now I understand. Our farm business is our kids. I worked in corporate America until about a year after we bought our land. When I "retired" it was in anticipation of getting pregnant. I had the grand plan that I would start a cute little farm market booth, we would get pregnant, and I would have a small business that would keep me active and contributing while allowing me to raise our kids at home. Then I was smacked with the reality that I couldn't have children. As I meditated with the land each day during this struggle, I asked that I be given the opportunity to raise a child in the green. I envisioned that child deeply steeped in knowledge of the plants and in sync with the natural world. I have been given that precious opportunity with not one, but two children. They are part of our contract with our land and part of what we are building for the future of our community.

As I look over the many products I make on our farm today, they all came about during, and because of, my struggle through infertility, pregnancy and lactation. The first thing I did was to chuck out of our medicine cabinet my cosmetics and beauty preparations. Making our own cleaning supplies, medicinal preparations and skin care products was a way to remove the synthetic from our bodies. These were products that I then wanted to share with my community. When we moved on to preparing whole and traditional foods, it was important to share that as well. Our children are the reason behind what we do. To leave them at home with a sitter while we do the business of our farm has never felt right to me. I think I knew subconsiously that their presence was just as important as the honey spreads that sat on the table we were standing behind at the farmer's market. Our journey to meet them is an amazing story that I am now proud to share with my community and beyond.

This book is a practical herbal for preconception, pregnancy and lactation enclosed in a personal journey through all of these stages. There are four main things I learned along the way that I wish to convey to readers.

A Comprehensive Approach to Building Babies

A baby is built from preconception all the way through lactation. It is one continuous arc. Until we recognize this fact we will continue to have difficulty with fertility, we will have children who are born with nutritional deficiencies and, worse, we will continue to see increasing difficulties with the breastfeeding relationship.

Our alternative practitioners need to begin to build a framework in which they communicate with one another (general practitioner to midwife, midwife to lactation consultant) and pass along information. The ideal would be that a lactation consultant could see the history of the mother and child before her all the way back to preconception, so she can begin to understand the origins of any problems.

Know Yourself and Know Your Health

As women, and as couples, must take back our power and our voice. We must begin to know our bodies and how they interact with the natural rhythms of the Earth. Until we reclaim this inner knowing we are powerless and dependent on someone else. We all need a health care team of professionals to act as consultants but, when it comes right down to it, the one who lives in the body is the expert on what goes on there.

Fertility is Connected to Whole Food and Healthy Digestion

To be fertile, we must base our diet on whole, nutrient-dense foods. Fertility is where it all begins, and it is not enough to just be "able" to have children. Both partners need to be fortified with good nutrition before conception, and both mother and child need to be well nourished throughout pregnancy and nursing.

Good nutrition is not found in the latest diet or the bottom of a supplement bottle. It is found in whole, nutrient-dense foods that are traditionally prepared. We can no longer eat adulterated, synthetic food and try to make up for it with vitamin pills. We need the nutrition available to us in organic or biodynamic foods, grown, raised and prepared properly — this is the basis for sustainable health for ourselves and our families.

There are many "right" ways to eat; it all depends on what is specifically right for your body. There are absolutes when it comes to the health of our digestion, which I will argue is the key to abundant health. By caring for digestion first, above any legalistic dietary stipulation or fad, we can allow for a great diversity in eating habits.

During the time we are trying to conceive or grow our babies there are some guidelines that I believe are universal — we need to lower our sugar intake, increase good sources of protein and eat good, whole fats and more non-starchy vegetables.

Focus on the Whole Plant

We need to be aware of what we are doing when we take plant medicine down to its chemical components. Our drugs are either based on or modeled from these building blocks from the plant world. Using the plants in this fashion guarantees nutritional deficiency and negative side effects. Vitamin supplements are largely based on substances that cannot be absorbed by the human body. If we went back to using whole plants in their original form we could save ourselves a lot of trouble and money. Further, the plants have more to offer us — in the form of spiritual, emotional and physical medicine — than just the sum of their parts.

It is my hope that, if you are a birthworker, you are reading this book as a guide to help your clients safely use whole-food and whole-plant healing. So many books tell us that an herb is dangerous, but do not say why. I believe that every woman should make her own decision. To do that, she needs to know the reason behind the caution. Not every caution applies to every woman or her baby. It is my hope that, having all the information, each woman can consult with her health care team and make a better decision as to what is right for her unique situation.

Foreword

by Carson Combs (husband, partner and biggest fan)

ABSOLUTE HORROR. That was the look I received from practically everyone I told that Dawn and I were going to have a home birth for our first child Aidan. Little did they know the amount of research and months of planning that had gone into having a child in the safety and comfort of our own home. Ironically, Dawn probably saw the same look of horror on my face the first time she broached the subject. Like every other major life decision in our marriage, she had to apply a great deal of salesmanship to make me comfortable with the idea of having a child at home.

I grew up in rural Northwest Ohio, where babies are born in hospitals, the menu includes an epidural and a C-section, newborns are vaccinated, boys are circumcised and people just do what the doctor orders by swallowing a pill. Based on my upbringing, I would have liked to take the easy way out and pass Dawn off to a team of doctors, but I knew my wife all too well. I recognized the train wreck that would lie ahead if she had to give birth in a sterile hospital environment surrounded by bright lights and masks. What Dawn taught me is that our health choices, our life changes and our fertility options should arise from knowledge and informed individual choice. I've been fortunate enough to marry someone whose very nature is to boldly question the status quo and tirelessly seek out her own truth.

Looking back, it was really Dawn who did most of the work. She searched online and studied medical research, evaluated options and the pros and cons and found out what we would need to go through to do a home birth and raise a child naturally. After the initial shock wore off, I gradually came around to the idea that we were indeed headed down the right path ... but it was always Dawn who persevered and tirelessly struggled to ensure that we would wind up where we needed to be.

Despite being probably some of the most well-read and informed future parents you could ever meet, there was no way we could anticipate the struggles that would lie ahead after the arrival of our first child. After such a long journey to even conceive, the battles we then faced with breastfeeding and weight problems were no match for one person alone. Sticking to our established goals and principles and pursuing the use of homemade baby formula highlighted the amazing lengths to which Dawn was able to push herself and not give up ... even when I was silently tempted to buckle under the strain.

Our arduous journey to children began a few years back. By chance, I met a beautiful, extremely intelligent woman at a local restaurant who for the first time made me stop on a dime. At the time, I knew she had gone to Ohio Wesleyan, studied botany and the classics and traveled abroad to study in the Galapagos. She was an obsessive reader, devouring books at a scary pace, and always interested in new topics. The completion of nearly eight years of undergraduate and post-graduate study had left me with a far lower appreciation for extracurricular reading. We married a year to the day after we first met, but little did I know that these tiny facts about Dawn would alter our lives forever.

Dawn had worked in web support for a Fortune 500 banking institution, and I was a city planner living in the Columbus, Ohio area. Unfortunately, I wanted to live in an historic downtown neighborhood and Dawn preferred a hundred acres in North Dakota. That also should have been a clue to my future. Our solution was to compromise somewhere in the middle.

Probably similar to most married couples, after purchasing a new home, our focus quickly became the "how many" and "when" of children. This was a topic we had actually discussed while we were dating. As a married man, I knew kids were in the future, but was not completely invested in the idea right then. As newlyweds, we enjoyed the good income and open evenings. I also liked being able to spend weekends watching football with limited interruptions. With rings on our fingers, we decided to just let nature take its course, assuming that kids would soon follow.

After months and months of no results, "nature" quickly turned into a roller coaster when we found out that conceiving children would be difficult. We mutually decided to pursue non-invasive options and started down the path of fertility treatments. While Dawn's studies made me more aware each day of herbal alternatives and other alternatives to Western medicine, insurance made it easy to invest in just one more treatment of clomid or another test, despite the resulting mood swings and what we knew about Dawn's cycles. Today, I'm embarrassed at how far I was willing to nudge Dawn before I finally snapped to and realized we had gone more than far enough.

Test tubes and science were not options for us. To explore our own fertility alternatives, we realized that we needed to make many significant life changes. These alterations in medicine, lifestyle and eating mirrored the growth and development of Dawn's herbal knowledge and our farm business. While I was somewhat hesitant, as a partner I committed to the changes we felt were necessary to achieve what other medical options had not obtained. Dawn's growing herbal expertise also helped increase our comfort level.

Like most people, I had always equated illness and health issues to an immediate trip to the local doctor's office. My culture had ingrained in me to not ask questions and to do what the doctor ordered. But my relationship with Dawn has taught me to step back and evaluate injuries and symptoms more calmly, while considering appropriate options. Today in our household, Western medicine is reserved for truly serious conditions and emergencies, and the pursuit of whole-plant and whole-food health with herbs has become our primary focus.

Dawn's never-ending tea brewing and cycle charting became agonizing to watch. There were mornings when I audibly groaned as her first waking thought was to grab a thermometer and fill out a chart. At many points, I was willing to just let things go, telling myself that maybe focusing on our growing farm was meant to be.

As my energies shifted toward the farm, Dawn revealed that she was interested in adoption. We weren't so far removed from being newly married, so I sought to support her wherever possible. She had mentioned the idea previously, but I had always dismissed it as a passing comment that would go away. The day I found that she had researched tax breaks, work benefits and countries for adoption, a little voice inside of me angrily awakened. I just could not accept the idea that my future child would not be of our own making. While I applaud anyone who could make that kind of life choice, for me it just did not resonate. Maybe this was the turning point that pushed me to help Dawn in her search for solutions.

Leaving her stressful job was a first major step toward pursuing children. I was always the conservative one who hesitated to consider new ideas. To Dawn's frustration, I generally created debate and played the devil's advocate, but would eventually take the long road to agree with her point of view. Not long after the adoption discussion and upheaval at her office, we decided that she needed a significant life change. While leaving her job greatly reduced Dawn's stress level, the change left me with uneasiness and an added weight.

Self-diagnosis and herbal options were starting points on our own journey toward conception, but ridding our home of common household cleaners unsettled things extremely. Being a neat freak, the idea of purging our home of cleaners and personal care items was more than I could take. How could baking soda, white vinegar and a few other supplies do the job? Despite all of my foot-dragging, however, Dawn never strayed course in eliminating elements from our daily lives that might hinder our chances.

The changes we were making in our personal lives also transformed how we were developing the farm around us. It made sense that if we were dealing with environmental factors and chemicals in our health, the bees on our honey farm should be given the same consideration. Thus began our efforts to research and implement alternative, chemical-free practices to improve bee health and reduce our increasingly disappointing winter losses. These efforts led us to develop sustainable beekeeping methods that we now teach to others on the farm.

As Dawn's constant thirst for knowledge grew, her herbal studies at Sage Mountain with Rosemary Gladstar further transformed our farm toward a truly medicinal purpose. While most herbalists focus on infusing herbs to create teas and tinctures, Dawn quickly saw the connection between medicinal herbs and a perfectly sweet delivery system: our honey. Our plain honey sales at local markets evolved into a line of herbal-infused honeys that emphasized the health benefits of raw honey and herbs together as a culinary medium.

Living just miles from the headquarters of the world's largest marketer of chemical lawn and garden products in an area dominated by conventional farming and Western medicine, Dawn has used the farm and her studies to blaze a trail in an area of the country largely devoid of herbal options. From the very beginning of her studies, Dawn has emphasized our farm as a medium for teaching and has sought to disseminate knowledge to those who seek information. I've always been amazed at her ability to speak to crowds on herbal topics with little preparation, making the technical and complicated easy to understand. It's as if she becomes a conduit of herbal knowledge.

Dawn's initial honey infusions received national press and local notoriety, but our farm products have since been transformed as our lives have also evolved. Parenthood led her to develop herbal honey spreads as a way to get our children to take herbal medicine through food. As homesteaders, the products she formulated for our personal use as part of this struggle have also resonated with local customers. After eight years of hard work to build a farm from the ground up, each week brings us more and more people who try herbal products for the first time and return to report success and life-changing improvements.

Dawn's relentless pursuit of new books to read eventually led us to Hippocrates' famous quote, "Let your food be your medicine, and your medicine your food." If we were going to have any chance of changing our childless outcome, we also had to consider our food choices in addition to alternative medicines and a chemical-free farm. Of all the upheavals in our lives, food changes have been for me the most difficult to implement. I've always liked to eat what I wanted and was frankly very resistant. At the time, it seemed as though every aspect of my life was being disrupted, so working outside the home in an office environment provided a means to rebel like a teenager during lunchtime.

The purging of our pantry at home to remove processed foods almost put me over the edge, but still Dawn persisted and I reluctantly moved toward the center. Today we eat primarily organics, grow much of our own food, soak and sprout grains, make our own flour and sourdough and create our own raw dairy products when our milk is available. Dawn's pursuit of food knowledge has rubbed off, and given time I have slowly changed my eating habits. Many of my favorite foods and restaurants have been forever ruined by the changes that have occurred to my palette over the last few years. Like everyone, we're not perfect, and there are times when we feel like we're "too tired to cook." Today, however, we fully understand the impacts of the food choices we make that are not so healthy.

Much like with medicine, I previously went through life with very little understanding of what goes into the products on a store shelf and what information is being hidden from consumers. Fortunately for me, I had a partner who constantly looked beyond symptoms and considered the larger picture ... from why her body's cycle wasn't functioning like a medical textbook's proverbial clock, to how our medicines, food choices and household products all combined to create a canvas that perhaps would not accept paint.

Looking at the WHOLE picture has become a different way of thinking that developed through our fertility experience with food and plants. That larger way of thinking has been expressed on our farm through the sustainable methods and biodynamic principles that we utilize in our beekeeping, animal husbandry and herbal agriculture. Our experiences have taught us to strongly believe that the soil is the foundation for good health. As we employ our farming techniques to naturally nurture the soil, it gives our plants more complete nutrition for use by both us and our bees. Good health should not come from treating symptoms by spraying a chemical, but by understanding that weeds serve to tell us to look deeper for an underlying nutritional deficiency in the soil that is hindering balance. Dawn's long and continuing journey into herbalism, food and farming has taught me that finding balance in our lives and our bodies is the ultimate goal. If only we would stop chasing symptoms with a pill or a quick fix and listen to what our bodies are telling us, miracles like our two are possible.

Introduction

THIS BOOK IS BASED ON MY PERSONAL JOURNEY that began in a struggle with infertility, moved through a successful pregnancy, endured challenges in lactation and celebrated a final surprise pregnancy. People often ask how I studied to become who I am today. My parents raised their own fruits and vegetables, and we lived in a rural area. I was raised to be a good steward of the land and to be respectful with our resources. I took animals and sewing and cooking projects to the Madison County and Ohio State fairs as part of a 4-H club. I went on to earn a BA in botany from Ohio Wesleyan University focusing on the phytochemical constituents in plants and how we use them for medicine. This led me to seek out and apprentice with Rosemary Gladstar.

I consider myself to be both an ethnobotanist and a homestead herbalist. I live on a working medicinal herb farm, consult on the use of herbs in my community and teach in the Mockingbird Meadows Eclectic Herbal Institute. We farm here using biodynamic principles that further deepen our relationship to the land and the plants and animals that grow here. I spend a lot of time working with and listening to the plants. In the end you can read a lot of books about the chemical constituents of plants, but until you have cultivated a personal relationship with them, watched them grow and listened to their ancient voices, you can never know even a fraction of what they have to share with us. I don't believe you should find my book informative or useful because of any letters after my name. I did not write this book in the sterile light of academia. I lived this book. I am speaking to you as a mother who has personally experienced what it takes to reconnect with real food, nature's cycles and the herbs to heal her body.

I have tried hard to speak for the herbs that most needed to be included and to speak for them honestly and fairly. There are many herbs that get a bad name because of a problem with one chemical in their makeup. We must return to using these plants in their whole form. When we isolate components to make supplements or allopathic drugs we change their action in the body. We create "side effects" because the components are no longer acting in concert with the other chemicals within the plant upon which they depend. We need to return to using our herbs with respect rather than fear.

I have shared the food that worked for me; I believe in nutrient-dense, traditional foods and farm-fresh products as the best way to build a healthy baby, before conception, in the womb and at the breast. This book is not a "diet plan." You must evaluate what I did in light of the work you are doing to know your own body. Most importantly, any eating style that we use to build our babies needs to be based on whole, nutrient-dense foods. Cultures the world over have found ways to do that based on what their environment provided. No one had access to all the food we do today. The only absolute is in the need to choose real and whole instead of artificial to address the nutrient requirements of our bodies. The specific foods that can do that are as varied as the cultures that enjoy them. The arguments over which superfood must be eaten by everyone for optimal health can remain in academia. In real life, what matters is what food is right for you alone.

This book is meant for any couple on their individual path. For some, the hormonal balance needed for fertility, pregnancy and lactation comes easily ... for others it can be difficult and heartwrenching. It is my intention that all couples, regardless of their situation, including those seeking to adopt, will find this book useful. All of our paths are similar in that we wish to nourish our children the best way we know how.

I am passionate about the idea of building a baby from preconception all the way through lactation. We do not build a baby only during the nine months of gestation. If you have not found this book until the latter parts of your pregnancy or during lactation and didn't do all the things I suggest, please don't feel like it is too late to make positive changes! In a perfect world we would all follow the arguments set forth in this book. In the real world, many of us begin to change our own body's makeup only when we begin researching what we want for our children. Often that is after we've already had one child or are already well into a pregnancy. Always remember that we do the best we can with the information we have at the time.

I would like to see this book used as a tool for change in our child-rearing conversations, not as a weapon to be wielded against mothers by themselves or those around them. This book is also meant for the birthworker and lactation consultant professional, and it is my hope that it is easy to use in a clinical setting.

I believe that the path to fertility is troublesome in our current society. I believe couples can reclaim their hope, voice and power through natural methods to rebalance for fertility.

I believe that we have disconnected ourselves from the entire birthing process by dismantling and devaluing the continuity from preconception to pregnancy to lactation. We do not honor the nutritional preparation it takes to create a baby and are therefore seeing more and more need for medical intervention in the pregnancy and lactation stages of our children's lives. As a result, we are also seeing more and more mental and physical disease as our children grow independently of our wombs.

I believe that breast milk is best, as you will read in my personal story. That said, my experience taught me that sometimes, exclusive breastfeeding is not possible in the way we envisioned. There is no reason for women who struggle with this to feel less-than, and there is no reason they should be left without nutrient-dense options simply because they aren't able to exclusively nurse. I hope I can encourage many of you who struggle to continue to nurse as you wanted while supplementing in a way that is supportive of that goal.

I invite you to disagree with, question and challenge all that I have to say. In the end, we are all experts only in our own life experience.

This is my journey; may you have much success and joy in yours.

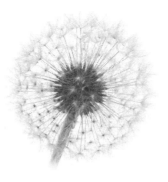

A Journey to Family

Our Infertility Story

WHEN I WAS YOUNG I HAD MY LIFE ALL PLANNED OUT. I would get married by my early twenties to someone I had dated for more than a year. We would spend at least five years as just the two of us before deciding to get pregnant, which would be easy, and I would have my multiple children in close succession before I was thirty. Then real life happened. I was married at the age of twenty-eight to someone I had known exactly a year on the night of our wedding. Within a year I saw thirty creeping up fast and decided that a career change was in order and we needed to think about having our first child. It was then that I hit the proverbial brick wall.

I had never had what would be called "regular" cycles. They came and went as they saw fit. Sometimes a month or more would go by without a cycle. I never really had cramping or heavy bleeding and was never all that inconvenienced by my period. I realized that this could present a problem and began asking the conventional gynecologist that I saw at the time if there were ways to "make me more regular." She asked me how long we had been trying; it had been three months.

This conversation with my doctor was to be a pretty big moment in my journey to conception; she diagnosed me with infertility. I was stunned and couldn't believe that a brief three months was sufficient for such a life-altering diagnosis, but she was quite certain. With my irregular cycles and lack of pregnancy in three months, I fit the criteria. It was time to take some blood samples and start me on Clomid. Clomid, she explained, would help my body to function normally. I did a few cycles on it before I was back in the office. I still wasn't seeing the 28-day cycle. Time seemed to stretch for an eternity from the start of one bleed to the next. When I next went in I asked my gynecologist, "Will Clomid make my body fit into the 28-day cycle ideal, or will Clomid help my body to regulate to its own rhythmn — a day length that represents a normal cycle for me?" Her answer was a little fuzzy, but the gist was that it would make me fit into the 28-day "normal" box.

Clearly my body was not responding to the new directive, and since it was so stubborn, we would add Premarin to force my cycle to start, and then each time the Clomid did not work we would increase the dose. We started with 50 mg and by the time we stopped we had moved up to 150 mg. During all this time, there were still very few cycles. The Premarin just managed to make me CRAZY. I had never before felt so out of control. We had to take a break from this treatment.

As the last of the drugs left my system, it was clear to both my husband and me that neither Clomid nor Premarin was a good solution to our problem. I began to do my own research and about that time discovered a book called *Taking Charge of Your Fertility*. I started charting my temperatures and cervical fluid. Armed with this new information, I went looking for a different doctor's office. I had heard from friends about a local practice that included midwives. Unfortunately, the midwives were merely extensions of the doctors, and the story was the same. This time I had a year or more of charts to show the doctors. The response when I brought out my notebook was discouraging. In every instance, the doctors thought it was "cute" that I thought I could know something about my body. They all insisted that my problem was a lack of ovulation, but I felt I had proof that I *was* ovulating. While I was studying my own body I was slowly getting back in touch with my inner voice.

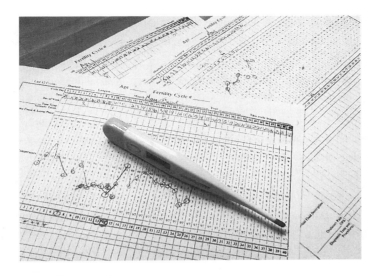

The fertility medicine industry in our country feeds on the hope of couples but quickly renders them voiceless and powerless. My experience gave me the feeling that I was to listen and blindly follow doctor's orders as we walked through a standard protocol that never varies. There was never any indication that we were on a team, that my input was valued or that questions were welcome. I came to the conclusion that many of the technologies available in this industry are just a stab in the dark or a roll of the dice. If the medication or procedure is successful, it gets written into the store of data they are collecting. In my opinion, none of the procedures have been satisfactorily tested for long-term repercussions. Many of them appear to have very little basis in how the female body actually works. I often felt that the doctors I encountered knew they were throwing random darts at the dartboard. Asking logical and informed questions simply threatened to uncover how little they knew about my particular issue. The truth is that the current fertility medicine industry is particularly talented at addressing structural issues that prevent conception. Western medicine is extremely well suited to performing surgeries and procedures. Unfortunately, it is less in the know when it comes to the "unexplained infertility" that plagues most couples.

We did not have any structural problems. So when these new doctors set aside my charting research and announced we would start on a new course of Clomid, my inner voice rebelled. I felt I had ample proof that I was ovulating. Unfortunately, I was not yet confident in my own wisdom, so I again decided to go along with the doctor. To take responsibility for believing what I thought I knew meant that I could be wrong. I could be passing up my only chance to have a child — something I desperately wanted. So, once again, we followed the protocol prescribed by this practice. I did the blood testing, took the Clomid and even began to do injectable hormones. We had ultrasounds of my fallopian tubes and ovaries. For my husband, the bonding act of creating a new life together had degenerated into using a plastic cup, nervously watching injections and hoping that each stressful doctor's visit would be the last. It also meant that each morning my first attention and thoughts went to a thermometer and a chart instead of the man lying next to me. We practically lived in the doctor's office, and sex became as mechanistic and procedural as our medical care.

During this time with the new doctors I began to use herbs that promoted ovulation. We decided to stop using the Clomid because of the side effects, and I began looking for natural options. We always had been against unnatural medical interventions and saw the initial round of Clomid as just "dipping our toes in the water." It is incredibly easy to lose yourself in these therapies as you grow more desperate to have a child. When you suppress your inner voice, give up power to medical professionals and place your hopes in unexplained technology, it is easy to be pulled in and enticed. We definitely compromised our beliefs chasing the next "possibility." We fell into the trap of believing that the next pill or injection might be the one that worked. Not to mention, that when we had invested so much to come to this point, we felt almost an obligation to keep moving until we had results. One day we found ourselves sitting across the desk from our doctor and he was telling us that I was "broken." They had done all they could do to try to get my body to "work," he claimed, and the next step was in vitro fertilization (IVF). At that moment my husband and I simultaneously woke up.

IVF was a step too far. Until that time, each step was a small progression that seemed minor. One small drug led to another. Once I had accepted those drugs into my system, one small technology was introduced and then another more invasive one was brought in when I'd accepted the idea of intervention. The further along the spectrum we went without succeeding, the more desperate we became. Suddenly the things we were *never* going to do seemed like the very thing we *had to do*. We were being shipped to the next doctor's office. The build-a-baby technology was in levels as well. We would again start at the lowest level of loss of control and move to greater loss of self. Eventually, we would progress to technology that no longer involved making a baby with either my eggs or Carson's sperm. At this point, having a baby would no longer resemble anything we set out to accomplish in the first place.

The office visit where we were told that I was "broken" and couldn't be fixed was the point at which our roller coaster ride came to an abrupt stop. We both wanted a baby, but we still had enough wits about us not to go against what we personally believed. Instead I went home, mourned and tried to accept the idea that we would never have children. I spent a lot of time on adoption websites. My growing desire to have a child transformed into considerations of tax credits and employee reimbursements to adopt a child from a foreign country. I was convinced that we needed to consider adoption, but Carson struggled with the idea. As our thought processes continued to diverge, the pursuit of a child grew more and more tension-filled.

One day, as I sat researching, that small quiet voice inside me spoke up again. Before I knew it, I was back in my dresser drawer ripping out charts. When my husband came into the bedroom that afternoon, I had my charted cycles for almost two years spread out side by side on the floor. I was in the middle crouched on them like a feverish animal. "None of those doctors ever listened to me," I said. "Look at these charts! Every single one of the them shows an ovulation." All of the therapies that I'd endured for more than two years had been aimed at forcing my body to ovulate. In front of me was proof that two years of tribulation had not been necessary. The worst part was that I had known it all along. *I* hadn't listened to me either! I had even gone so far as to spend time doing herbal therapies to encourage ovulation. I had ignored my intuition to such an extent that even when I was trying to do things naturally, it was still within the frame of a Western diagnosis.

It was time to start all over again. I threw out all the medication. I rejected the notion that I didn't ovulate, and I released everything I had been told. Then I sat down with my charts and looked at them with fresh eyes. My cycles were long, usually trending at about 35 to 36 days. That wasn't optimal, because it reduced the number of chances I had to get pregnant in a given year. I let go of the 28-day cycle and focused on *my* body's unique rhythm. It looked like I was having long ovulatory phases and then ovulating on day 25! So I wasn't usually ovulating until the typical time in a cycle when most women were starting to bleed. The doctors could not possibly have seen "proper" hormone levels in my blood because they tested at inappropriate times in my cycle. No one had ever asked me what my bleeding was like. No one asked me if I had any cramping, or when. These were simple questions that would have told them what my issue was if they had known what the answers meant.

When I analyzed all the clues while looking at my charts, it was obvious that my luteal phase, after ovulation and before the start of my next cycle, was too short. My shortened luteal phase indicated that my progesterone levels were insufficient. Ironically, all the therapies I'd received up to this point focused on increasing my estrogen levels. Increased estrogen levels through drugs and food were driving down progesterone levels in the body. All the time I was being "treated" with Western medicine, my body was actually getting further out of balance!

Now I had a sense of direction. I created a protocol for myself involving two different herbal tea formulations and a few additions and corrections to my diet.

My charts did not reveal a progesterone deficiency through my temperature readings alone. One of the main reasons the Western medicine model can throw stones at the idea of charting your fertility, called the Fertility Awareness Method, is in characterizing it as "the rhythm method." Today there are even applications for your wireless technology that will help you monitor your cycles. Unfortunately, many of the applications and the rhythm method are neither reliable nor helpful. The Fertility Awareness Method not only monitors your temperature but also your cervical fluid (and if you decide to take it a step further, your cervix position as well). When I monitored both my temperature and my cervical fluid I had solid evidence of my hormonal levels that did not require multiple blood draws.

More telling even than my short luteal phase was the fact that each month's bleeding began and ended with dark brown discharge. My frustration mounted as I began to study how the female body works. Why on earth are we not telling our children what balance looks like? Every health class I attended on the human reproductive system preached a 28-day cycle with ovulation on day 14 and your choice of pad or tampon. As I researched, I grew more convinced that we need to be talking about what balance looks like and throw out the 28-day model. Balance is red blood, not too much and not too little, without the appearance of clotting from the first day of bleeding to the end. A balanced cycle should have around five days of bleeding and a luteal phase that lasts between 12 and 14 days.

Because my mother had been taught the same things I learned in public school, our similar cycles gave me the false idea that everything I experienced was normal. I later came to understand that when a woman is pregnant with a girl, she carries her daughter and her granddaughter in her womb. A developing female fetus has all the eggs she will produce in her lifetime, and therefore all the pregnancies she will carry, in utero.[1] I believe it is in this way that we "inherit" a propensity for hormonal balance, and our starting nutritional deficiencies, from our mothers and sometimes even our grandmothers.

I became angry as I realized that my cycles had sent signals of imbalance since puberty. How much of my struggle in infertility could have been prevented if I had known I needed to work toward balance eighteen years earlier?

It is progesterone that controls the shedding of the uterine lining each month, and the brown blood shows up in a cycle as a result of low progesterone levels. Without sufficient progesterone to fully flush the lining, some of it remains. During the next month's bleeding, that old blood begins to seep out along with the new lining and the uterus is never fully cleansed. As our uterus is one of the organs of elimination, it is part of our body's ability to properly detoxify each month. When the lining is not completely purged, old blood and toxins build up, creating a potentially dangerous situation. The uterus is never really cleansed, so the situation is ripe for infections and abnormal cell growth. Many women will see this brown blood disappear when they have a baby. The uterus is effectively a clean slate at this point, having just birthed an intact lining: the placenta. These women will almost certainly see the brown blood appear again in short order if they have not corrected the underlying issues that lead to progesterone imbalance.

Now that I understood the situation, it was vital that I get my system balanced and working properly. This was not just because I wanted a baby, but also because I wanted to be vital and to preserve my own health well into old age. I had to make my health and balance the first priority and hope that when I got there my body would be ready to carry another life.

I began by purging my bathroom cabinet. In the drawers were my beloved nail polishes, hair gel, mousse, body butters and facial miracle creams. My body was struggling to remove toxicity, and my liver was weakened and clogged. I decided I needed to remove all of the toxic soup to which I was purposely subjecting it. I began to use my herbal knowledge to experiment more in the kitchen to create fresh, natural replacements for my favorite products.

Next I turned my attention to the first-aid cupboard, where I had taken for granted my use of so many over-the-counter medications.

As I pulled out the bottles and jars I really *looked* at them for the first time. I read the labels and was shocked at what I had put into my body. My husband had been less than thrilled when I packed up all my expensive bubble baths and body creams that were birthday, Christmas and anniversary presents, but now he positively rebelled. We reached a truce when I agreed to place everything into a box and carry it to the garage. I spent hours in the kitchen creating herbal replacements for everything we commonly used. Everything from indigestion to headaches to diarrhea got a new, updated herbal solution. I cataloged all of my new creations in an old recipe box with instructions on how to use everything. The compromise in the garage sat untouched for over a year before it was finally properly trashed.

I spent so much time in the kitchen that I began to notice our cleaning supplies. Our house was filled to the brim with things to clean the floor, sanitize the bathroom, spray on the furniture and scrub the dishes and clothes. This was the hardest change for my husband, who is at heart a very clean person. The cleaning supplies were very important to him and, therefore, the most difficult thing to relinquish. I bought several books, a lot of supplies and a whole lot of essential oils before he was convinced to let go of everything in his stash of chemicals. Now our most common cleaning supplies are white vinegar, castille soap, baking soda, soap nuts and essential oils.

While all the cleaning supplies were being purged, our food also began to change. I'm a big bookworm, and I love to research. I actually have a bit of a book problem and have been known to hide a new purchase in between older books on the shelves in my home. A lot of these new books were related to aphrodisiac foods, foods to increase fertility and so on. There is a lot of misinformation when it comes to food in general and food for fertility in particular. The bottom line I took away was this: Eat whole foods that are as close to their original form as possible. Instead of drinking orange juice, we eat an orange. We eat organic corn instead of processed corn (high-fructose corn syrup, xantham gum or Lauryl glucoside).

Ingredients to Eliminate while Building a Baby

- High Fructose Corn Syrup (HFCS)
- Hydrogenated Oils
- Unfermented Soy
- Processed Sugars
- Processed Flours
- Fat-Free or Reduced Fat
- "Diet" Anything
- GMOs
- Caffeine

When you start thinking about new food choices, there are also foods you need to remove from your diet. I went through our cupboards, refrigerator and freezer and disposed of everything man-made, processed or otherwise unpronounceable.

With very little in the house left to eat, we next had to go out and fill up our pantry with real food. We began to focus on buying ingredients rather than prepared foods. For us, this meant grass-fed organic meats, organic cheeses and a raw milk herdshare, organic breads and bread products, organic dry beans and organic fruits and vegetables. It is many years since, and we now buy organic grain instead of bread products. There are some great resources I've included to help you learn to prepare traditional foods in Appendix A.

Preparing Traditional Whole Foods

I want to say a few things about the journey to traditional whole foods preparation from personal experience. I live what I believe to be the "gold standard" in food these days. I wake up in the morning, grind my grain fresh, feed my sourdough starter and put a bread recipe out to soak along with some beans to have for dinner the next night. Meanwhile, I'm finishing up a batch of water kefir on the side counter and pulling a batch of homemade sourdough English muffins out of the oven for breakfast. There is always some raw, fermented goodie on the table and we freely use bitters in our meals or before them. My kids enjoy a homemade, raw-milk kefir smoothie with organic fruit, raw honey, raw pollen and coconut oil. We follow that in a few minutes with our fermented cod liver oil and finish breakfast while Carson goes out to milk the cow.

I want to clarify that this is where I am *today*. I started out several years ago popping two blueberry pastries in the toaster and heading off to work, where I would microwave lunch and pick up some take-out for dinner on the way home. The difference is profound. I can tell you that I feel like a completely different — and better — me these days. I can also tell you without any reservation or hesitation that there have been enough failures to fill two lifetimes as we've traveled between these two scenarios. I have killed more sourdough than I have made successfully. I have mercilessly and ruthlessly killed kefir cultures, ruined dinners, burned roasts and turned out loaves of bread that could have been used as weapons. If you read someone's blog or book and it looks like they have it all together in the food department, it is probably not a lie. But don't get discouraged and think you can never get there, so why try? Behind every one of us who has unlearned the American food culture is a graveyard of once-beautiful living cultures and ingredients that never had a fighting chance. My lesson has been to keep trying and find people in the community who are either ahead of you in this change or who can struggle, laugh and cry along with you.

Along with the omissions and changes to our diet, there were a lot of additions. Carson and I both added fermented cod liver oil capsules. We began to eat organic chicken liver once a week. We ate all the fat and skin on our organic, pastured meats as well as full-fat raw milk and full-fat yogurt. We ate a lot more steamed or sautéed green leafy veggies. We began soaking our grains before we cooked them and added in a pinch of naturally fermented vegetables or fruits with each meal. If you get one thing from this book, understand that the digestive system and liver are more important than you were ever told before. They are the root of how we handle sugars, how our immune system works, how we detoxify our bodies, how we stay sane and how our hormones act. If you get your digestion (and that of your unborn infant or growing child) right, most everything else will fall into line.

Asking the Herbs for Help

With our food heading in the right direction and my household cleansed of unnecessary toxins, I was ready to ask the herbs for help. I decided to use tea for this work. Tea as a therapy does not work for everyone. Some people don't enjoy it, for starters, and even if they do, it can become tedious to make it all the time. Drinking a therapeutic tea three times a day for months is a huge undertaking that many people abandon if they aren't strongly committed. So always choose the therapy that is most appropriate for your needs. I chose tea because I recognized in myself the tendency to always run on to the next thing. There wasn't a lot of standing still or sitting with myself. Maybe that allowed me to avoid looking at things I didn't want to see. At any rate, making tea every day was a way to begin folding in a habit of creating time for myself.

I did use some shortcuts that everyone should know about. When you are making a tea for therapeutic use, it is best to make it in a "batch" rather than cup by cup. I always make at least a quart at a time. A mason jar is your best friend when you are making simple infusions. Just put your tea in the bottom of the jar and add boiling water. After putting on a lid, let it sit for at least fifteen minutes or even overnight. Strain it into a thermos and you are set for the day. When you make decoctions (simmering the herbs and water together on the stovetop for 15–20 minutes) you are working with stronger stuff such as bark, roots and nuts. You can often use the same herbs two or three times, straining the tea into a pitcher each time for storage in the refrigerator. This way you can make several days' worth of tea in one session rather than a cup at a time.

For my herbal program, I switched between two teas. My Tonic Tea was an infusion that I used in the ovulatory phase of my cycle.

This tea is made up of herbs that are nourishing and tonic for the reproductive organs. It also contains support for overworked adrenals (licorice root) and the stressed liver and kidneys (dandelion leaf). Motherwort was an important addition here because of its work in helping to regulate cycles. In retrospect, it would have been nice to have added yarrow to this mix to help move out the old blood that remained in my cycle. I wasn't as familiar with yarrow (*Achillea mille-folium*) at the time, so I didn't know to reach out for its help.

Tonic Tea

2 parts raspberry leaf (*Rubus idaeus*)
1 part nettle (*Urtica dioica*)
1 part alfalfa (*Medicago sativa*)
2 parts peppermint (*Mentha piperita*)
1 part dandelion leaf (*Taraxacum officinale*)
1 part licorice root (*Glycyrrhiza glabra*)
1 part motherwort leaf (*Leonurus cardiaca*)

The second tea I used was my least favorite. I called it my Barky Rooty Tea. I started drinking it each month from the time just after I had ovulated up until I started bleeding. These herbs are stronger, deeper and more robust in nature. They are hormonal balancers with a special nudge on the side of progesterone. By using only the progesterone supporters in the luteal phase of my cycle I was using the herbs in a new way. Practitioners often suggest using these progesterone-stimulating herbs throughout the cycle, and it would not be harmful to do so. However, by using them only in the part of my cycle where I felt I needed this support, I was showing my body how the natural rythym should be established. It wasn't appropriate to introduce higher levels of progesterone in the ovulatory phase, so I didn't do so.

I chose wild yam root (*Dioscorea villosa*) for my Barky Rooty Blend because of its added abilities to improve a congested liver. This tea is spicy and earthy in flavor, and it was dedication alone that kept me at it when I first started. Some of these plants are great dyers, and I had spots on my carpet and sofa to prove it.

It seemed I was always curled up drinking this tea. The herbs quickly caused me to crave them. Their grounded energy called to me as they worked themselves deep into the buried and entrenched dysfunction to which my body stubbornly held. Many of these herbs reach deep into the soil, bringing up nutrition and releasing toxicity that is bound and otherwise unavailable in the subsoil. As I took them into my own body, I came to understand the nature of these plants much more deeply than just a superficial understanding of phyto-chemicals. These plants heal the soil and the communities in which they grow in the same way that they heal us. Only by knowing my medicine in its living form was I able to grasp this information.

It is interesting to note that most of the herbs that are important for female balancing are forest dwellers that thrive in cool, moist environments. Often when women are imbalanced, it is because we have become too hot and dry. This greater awareness of the plants that were helping me to heal convinced me that I wanted to create a plant sanctuary where everyone could have the opportunity to "meet" their medicine. Our active observations of the plants teach us more about the medicines they contain than we can ever know taking a disconnected supplement from the store.

Barky Rooty Tea

3 parts wild yam root (*Dioscorea villosa*)

2 parts licorice root (*Glycyrrhiza glabra*)

4 parts sassafrass root (*Sassafrass albidum*)

1 part vitex (*Vitex agnus-castus*)

½ part dong quai (*Angelica sinensis*)

1 part ginger root (*Zingiber officinale*)

1 part cinnamon (*Cinnamomum zeylanicum*)

¼ part orange peel (*Citrus sinensis*)

I switched back to my Tonic Tea when I began bleeding, or I mixed a separate batch of Barky Rooty without the dong quai to keep drinking. Dong quai can encourage inappropriate bleeding, so you shouldn't drink it on a therapeutic level while menstruating.

Since I was no longer working with a doctor's office, I didn't have access to blood testing to watch my progress. Instead I charted my temperatures and my cervical fluid religiously. Slowly, I began to see results. My cycles began to shorten overall, and within a year's time my luteal phase moved to an appropriate 12 days. I was pregnant shortly thereafter.

My First Pregnancy

My first pregnancy ended at 8 weeks. I'll never know if my recovering (but perhaps still insufficient) progesterone levels had anything to do with this; I do know that there was no heartbeat at the 8-week ultrasound, and the baby had stopped growing some time before. I suspect that the fault was not my hormone levels but a simple misstep in the genetic code. Many pregnancies end at this early stage because of the kindness of Mother Nature. One tiny thing at 5 weeks becomes many major things at full term.

A baby that ceases to develop can often be a mercy for everyone, but I was devastated at the ultrasound. I had worked so hard to allow my body to do this. If I had cared to ask any of the many doctors we had worked with years before, they would have said it was a miracle that I was pregnant at all. I had time to mourn, therefore, before I was awakened in the night with the contractions that would end my pregnancy. My miscarriage was an amazing, awe-inspiring and empowering experience. I spent the night riding out the powerful contractions in our bathtub. At one point, as I ran some more hot water, Carson got up and came to check on me. When I told him what was happening, he calmly asked me if we should go to the hospital.

Carson had, in the past, been very comfortable with Western medicine. But his small, quiet voice grew during our journey as well. When I told him things were fine, he accepted it and merely stripped off his clothes to climb into the tub with me. That night was amazing for our relationship. We drew closer than we had ever been before. We both watched as my body did this wondrous work. The power of the female body to care for itself when no one gets in the way was awe-inspiring.

In the morning I did not need medical intervention as an ultrasound proved that my uterus was clean. The final parting shot from our soon-to-be-former doctor came as he prepared me for examination. I explained to him that I knew everything was out because I had had contractions until I had passed a large mass. I described how for the next hour or so I continued to have painful contractions until I passed another small mass. After that, I told him that I was able to sleep peacefully without any pain. His lack of true understanding of a non-medicalized woman's body was laughingly obvious. He insisted that I needed an ultrasound because what I was describing "doesn't tell me anything about the state of your uterus. Those weren't contractions," he said. "Those were just cramps."

My First Birth

Before too many more months went by, I was pregnant again. I didn't look forward to the 8-week ultrasound, but everything progressed normally. We found a group of midwives practicing locally who were experienced at delivering babies at home. They valued the small quiet voice inside both my husband and me. My confidence in my body, my intuition and my husband had been tested and had grown. I went into the delivery of my first child having had a preview of sorts, but also with appropriate respect for the amazing thing my body is able to do when it's in balance.

Aidan's birth was an example of a delivery that would have been a nightmare had it taken place in a hospital environment. There are many women who get very nervous at the first contraction and relax once they reach the confines of a hospital room. I am *not* one of those women. Given my relationship with doctors in the past, I knew that a trip to the hospital would cause me to tense up, become nervous and defensive and ultimately act out in terror. None of that is conducive to a successful birth. It was very obvious to both of us that I needed to give birth at home.

The night I went into labor, we did not wonder and we did not have any false alarms. I already knew what I would be feeling because of my earlier miscarriage. As I felt the early contractions, we pulled up a timer on our laptop and began to time. We started this process at around 4:30 a.m.

Given our busy life running a farm and working full-time, Carson had not really figured out how to put the birthing tub together. There were a few hours where I watched the timer while monitoring an increasingly flustered husband as he figured out the lining, the thermostat and the garden hose we had brought inside. Eventually, warm water filled the tub and I climbed in. It was a hot summer evening in June, and the frogs on the pond outside our window filled the room with their music. Candlelight flickered low as I floated in the water. This was how I had envisioned this birth. When my miscarriage occurred, I had instinctively gone to our bathtub. It was clear that this environment was most comforting for me.

We rode out most of the night like this. We alternated between listening to the frogs and CDs on the stereo until the contractions started picking up. We decided to call our midwives at about 6 a.m. Soon my mother, midwives Nina and Kelley, Carson and I were waiting in the quiet of our bedroom as my contractions came and went. At about 9 a.m, Nina and Kelley suggested that we check my cervix to see if I had progressed. They almost didn't want to tell me that nothing was happening, but told me 0.5 centimeter to make me feel better; I was not really dilated at all. They determined that our baby was probably not going to arrive until the next day, and decided to head home and come back when things began to progress. As they headed toward the door, both midwives suggested we put on some movies and try to relax to slow things down until I was really ready to give birth. To say I was disappointed puts it mildly. As they walked out the door, Carson and I began to pour a small glass of wine and I downed a few droppers of valerian (*Valeriana officinalis*) tincture to relax.

I had prepared a number of tinctures as part of my birth kit: a skullcap (*Scutellaria lateriflora*) tincture for pain, a valerian tincture for muscle relaxation and pain, a blue cohosh (*Caulophyllum thalictroides*)/black cohosh (*Cimicifuga racemosa*) tincture in the event that labor stalled and a witch hazel (*Hamamelis virginiana*)/motherwort tincture for excessive bleeding. I also made raspberry leaf ice cubes to assist with contractions.

As the midwives headed out the door, my mother fatefully pulled them aside. She told them before they left that her labor with me had been very similar, up until the last few minutes when she dilated quickly and the doctor almost didn't get there in time. Within minutes (just enough time for their cars to disappear out of sight) everything changed drastically. I had never gotten out of the birthing tub because I was comfortable there. My contractions quickly came on hard, and were back to back with no time to breathe in between. My birth plan was for a water birth, but I kept things loose to allow myself to be in the moment. It is so important to accept that you just don't know what you will want or need in that situation and to be ready to "go with it." Against my plans, I got out of the tub as my contractions intensified. I went to the bed and lay on my side. All I could do was scream when the contractions intensified until they overlapped one another. My poor husband was with me, and our plan had been that my mom would remain in the kitchen until after the birth. I screamed and screamed, pleading with him to take me to the hospital. I even used our code word!

Carson smiled nervously and listened as he held my hand. He went to the living room to pace and wring his hands. He had the car keys in his hand and was heading to the bedroom when my mom stepped in. "She's asking for everything she said she never wanted," he told her: "She says she wants pain medication and a hospital."

My mom had the cooler head and became the birth advocate that every woman needs in this situation. I was under the misconception that since my midwives had said I wasn't dilating, this was just unrelated pain. I decided that I couldn't do this level of pain for nothing.

My mom sat next to me as Carson called the midwives. She assured me that the contractions and the intense pain were absolutely from dilation. So many first-time mothers are confused and frightened by the level of pain that it takes to birth a child. My birth experience explains why it is so important to have advocates who will listen — really listen to you and the situation. My mother knew that I did not want a hospital. She knew that I did not want to take medication. She also was able to assess the situation and see that I did not need to give these things up; that I was not in danger. And quite honestly, there was no way they could have gotten me into the car or transported me anyway!

You cannot enter a birthing situation with the idea that you will wait and see what you think about medication. If you do, you have already decided to take it. The bottom line is that if you do the research and make a firm decision against medical intervention, you need to surround yourself with people who understand that intention. If I had been in a hospital, I am convinced I would have been medicated and received a C-section.

I spent so much time waiting for our midwives to return — trying not to push as my body wanted — that I was soon exhausted. Waiting seemed like an eternity, and I finally told Carson to go get our birthing manual to deliver the baby! As he flipped through the manual in a panic, the midwives arrived just in time to help me push. We started in the birthing tub, but I was so tired I could not get enough leverage to push hard. Nina and Kelley quickly grabbed their birthing stool and after a couple pushes, Aidan was born. He was 10 pounds 4 ounces, and both of us were a bit worse for wear. I essentially went from zero to pushing in under an hour. This type of intensity in a birth is hard on mom and baby, and I would later come to learn how it can also affect the nursing relationship.

Aidan and I got into bed shortly after he was born. After he had caught his breath, we nursed for the first time. Nina and Kelley would later tell us that they were very close to transferring us to the hospital because of his breathing. Amid the exhaustion of such a crazy birth,

I was never worried. In some way I knew that he was fine and would recover if given some time. We delayed cutting the umbilical cord for about an hour and a half to allow for all his blood to return to his body and to give us time for bonding. This was a great help in his recovery from such a rushed birth. Climbing into my own bed with a cocktail of chlorophyll-laced water and a small toast of champagne with my mom, dad, husband and new baby was a great end to my first birth experience.

Nursing Troubles

For all of my teen years and most of my adult years, I hated my breasts. I felt they were too small and made me decidedly less womanly and attractive. I don't think it's a coincidence that when I finally settled down and began the reproductive phase of my life they went on strike. As women, we are culturally programmed to focus a lot of critical attention on perceived bodily imperfections. All of this negative energy has to go somewhere. I struggled to conceive due to a hormonal imbalance, and then when I'd finally learned to love my small breasts — breasts that allowed me to play hockey, football and volleyball, breasts that allowed me to comfortably run a few amazing triathlons — when at last I appreciated them for all they were and all they had given me, they left me high and dry.

Oh, I know it's not funny to those of us who struggle with a low milk supply. But looking back, you have to appreciate the irony in my case. Breastfeeding difficulties can have many causes. I suspect that I tend to have a low supply naturally. It also appears that during my first pregnancy I did not develop the glandular tissue that I should have in response to the hormonal cues in my body; whether that is evidence of a further imbalance that I hadn't yet addressed or just my genetic inheritance, I will never know. What I do know is that my firstborn, my son Aidan, also contributed to our difficult breastfeeding relationship.

When he was born I was probably more informed than your average mother, but still missing so much information! I immediately had him checked to ensure he was not tongue-tied and was relieved to find that he was not. After that, I assumed that all I needed to be successful at breastfeeding was patience, proper technique and determination. I was horribly wrong. Aidan seemed to have a good latch. When you put your finger in his mouth he'd practically take your fingernail off, so we felt we could also check off the box next to "good suck."

Aidan was born at home into a comfortable environment, but his birth was still a little traumatic. My active labor had been so intense and so fast. He had traveled down the birth canal so quickly that he hadn't fully purged the liquid from his lungs and he wasn't breathing as well as he should have. He also had the cord wrapped twice around his neck to further complicate things. After masterfully unwinding the cord, the midwives gave him some oxygen while he lay on my chest for a bit and got his blood supply back from the placenta. He recovered pretty quickly and seemed to latch on shortly thereafter without any trouble.

Our nursing problems started almost immediately. I had read about what was normal for a healthy baby and was looking for the correct number of wet diapers and watching for the "black tar" to appear. For the first day, Aidan had the appropriate amount of wet diapers. Soon they began to be less wet, and more and more yellow. Within a day or two they had progressed to where we were seeing a faint pink stain in the middle of his diaper.

We knew something wasn't right and began our search for help. Aidan cried constantly. He was never satisfied after eating and never ate for very long. He pulled back from my breast and fussed, tossing his head around. When he would get really angry he would go stiff and bend backward in my arms. He was really strong and if I wasn't ready for this, I would almost drop him.

We took him to our family physician within the first few days. I also scheduled him with our chiropractor, thinking something may have been out of alignment because of the fast birth. We had him checked over in our postnatal midwife appointments and took him to see someone who advertised herself as a cranial-sacral therapist. I interpreted the message as he was fine, to be patient, and that it was normal for some babies not to have bowel movements

Everyone looked at his suck and his latch, but no one saw any cause for alarm. Aidan continued to lose weight. He grew gaunt and cried and struggled less. Our physician began to schedule weekly weight checks to monitor him. As he was a big baby (10 pounds, 4 ounces) to begin with, I was still hearing that weight loss was common at first for a breastfed baby and not to be alarmed. My motherly intuition was screaming at this point, and I kept doing the rounds of any health practitioner I could find to look at him. Finally, our family physician felt we needed to begin using a supplement. She was very supportive of breastfeeding and we were lucky to find a doctor like her. She felt that supplementation might just be needed to get him going in the right direction ... just a little. It was clear to me that something had to be done. I was heartbroken, and completely invested in breast milk only. We were in an emergency situation when we finally broke down and bought some organic formula. While my husband sat and gave Aidan his first bottle at about 4 weeks, I sat on the sofa and cried.

All this time, my midwives had been suggesting I talk to a local lactation consultant. I had called several times and got voicemail but hadn't left a message. I suspect I was hesitant because my breasts had always been such a source of anxiety and low self-esteem. I'm a pretty independent person and always want to feel like I can do things myself. So it's probably pride and old wounds that had kept me from leaving messages. When we were forced to give Aidan formula I swallowed any hesitation and set up an appointment. During this first 4 weeks of struggling to find an answer, I had had very little sleep and had literally been nursing almost 24 hours a day. I just lay on the couch with Aidan at the breast all day, most of the time skin to skin. What a blessing he was born in the summer! If he wasn't feeding, he was generally crying ... he rarely slept. I kept thinking that the problem was with my supply and that my milk just wasn't coming in. I was taking a milk-promoting tincture; I drank galactagogue tea; I ate milk-producing foods; I drank a ton of water; I nursed and waited.

The fact that I nursed constantly is probably what kept Aidan's systems functioning. I couldn't see how bad he was beginning to look, but I see pictures from that time now and am shocked.

The first thing my new lactation consultant had me do was sit and nurse. Because her skill set was so specialized, she immediately saw that Aidan was not latching on properly; she could also tell by the way he worked his mouth and the way he grasped the nipple that he was not sucking properly. What we had all thought was a strong suck turned out to be tension. Aidan had developed so much tension in his throat that he was unable to swallow correctly, creating a blockage of sorts. In retrospect, this tension could have originated from the cord wrap, or from the tube used to help suction his lungs shortly after birth. His full body rigidity and arching back were strong indications that we hadn't recognized. His palate was also pinched, narrow and high, making it difficult for him to align the nipple for a proper suck. The tension in his throat made it nearly impossible for his tongue to thrust forward in its proper nursing position.

My lactation consultant began working to correct Aidan's suck by feeding him with a finger feeder and performing cranial-sacral therapy on his palate while he ate. He responded quickly to the work she did, but many visits were necessary before she was able to completely work through his tension and rigidity and get him to nurse properly. I began nursing him at home with the finger feeder taped to my nipple for supplemental feeding between appointments and he slowly climbed back out of the hole.

I still had one problem: the supplement. I was well aware of the dangers of formula: contamination; inappropriate or incomplete nutrient levels; increased incidence of SIDS and degenerative diseases such as diabetes; developmental changes and hormonal alterations, just to name a few.[2,3] In the end, I only gave Aidan less than a week of commercial organic formula as I ventured into uncharted (and as I later discovered, very controversial) waters by making my own!

I would be remiss if I didn't mention another great option: a breast milk bank. However, federal standards require that breast milk in banks be pasteurized. I have not seen any studies to show what kind of damage this process may do, but knowing what happens with cow and goat milk does not make me comfortable. Borrowing breast milk from someone I did not know outside the breast milk bank sys-tem did not work for me either, and I didn't have any close friends who were nursing at the time, but this may be the right choice for many other women. Those who need that type of support can find a network of women who are willing to share their breast milk supply through local midwives' offices or La Leche chapters.

When I studied to become an herbalist, I was introduced to the book *Nourishing Traditions* and read it cover to cover. I remembered reading about homemade baby formula, so I got the cookbook off the shelf. Making my own formula gave me quality control: I could be sure the food going into my baby's body was fresh, organic and as nutritionally balanced as I could make it. Beyond my firm conviction that breast milk was the best I could provide for my son, I also wanted to bond and have the feeling that I was providing his nourishment. Making the food myself with the best of ingredients gave me that same feeling, and I needed that emotionally.

While I believe that I most likely would not have had enough milk for him anyway, the fact that we were not in sync during the first few critical days of our breastfeeding relationship made things worse. (Those first few days are critical in setting up your future sup-ply.) Because Aidan wasn't demanding it, my body wasn't working to make milk — it was, in essence, shutting down the factory. At the one-month point we found I was producing only between one and a half and two ounces a day! It was going to be hard work to increase my supply, and it was never going to be all he needed. The great thing about breast milk, though, is that even if you can't supply enough for all your baby's needs, they will still benefit from whatever they receive. It doesn't have to be an all-or-nothing situation!

It was clear that I would probably always be supplementing more ounces than I was providing in breast milk. I had too many things going against me, from the disjointed start to a lack of glandular development. For that reason, it was very important to me that I was giving him the next best thing. I now tell anyone who will listen that regardless of whether you are breastfeeding or planning to give formula from a bottle, it is imperative that you involve a lactation consultant in your birth plans. Aidan would have had the problems he had taking in food even if I was using a bottle exclusively.

One of my midwives recently told me that when she was young they didn't have all the commercial formulas now available; bottle-fed babies were given a mixture of evaporated milk and karo syrup. In some ways we have come a long way. Bottlefeeding should be and can be the exception rather than the rule. When the mother does need to supplement, she should continue breastfeeding *while* supplementing if she produces any milk at all. Unfortunately, most couples do not know there are whole-food alternatives. The commercial formulas are all too prevalent, incredibly easy to access and readily available when such a need arises. Aside from the many problems I have already mentioned, they encourage a disconnect from whole-food and whole-plant health from the earliest conceivable moments in life.

My Own Formula

Had I not had trouble breastfeeding, I never would have considered a supplement of any kind. I was desperate to provide what I knew to be the best for my babies. The recipe I used included healthy fats, a proper balance of milk sugar to protein and the necessary nutrients to best mimic the high quality of breast milk. (See Appendix B.) I took the recipe to my lactation consultant when I began making it to see what she thought. I was shocked when she told me I was the first mother she'd seen making her own formula. I couldn't believe no one had shown her the recipe before. While I made the supplement, she and I worked tirelessly to, if not increase my own milk supply, at least ensure that I continued to steadily make the same amount.

Anytime you talk about feeding babies, it sets off a firestorm. Talking about milk, let alone raw milk, in conjunction with that same issue encourages people to go to a very dark place. Recently, a representative for the Virginia Department of Agriculture and Consumer Services, on the public record, equated giving raw milk to children to having them assassinated. I can only speak from my own personal experience. For me, breast milk will always be the best thing to feed babies.

I want to stress that if you suspect you or your baby is having difficulties with breastfeeding, *never* self diagnose. *Never* decide to start giving your baby something other than breast milk without consulting a lactation professional. While homemade formula can be the right answer for some, others often face issues that are easy to correct. As soon as you begin to introduce something other than breast milk, you change the nursing relationship in terms of supply and even your baby's mouth structure, depending on how you feed. It is further important to note that without the help of a consultant, you can permanently affect your child's gut flora. The repercussions of this can be seen all around us in the many diseases that plague our population. The gut flora of your baby is the foundation on which their immune system will be built. It is critical that this foundation be rock solid. Be sure you exhaust all possibilities of feeding your baby exclusively with breast milk before you look at a supplement, even one as high quality as the one I used.

In my observation, those who strongly oppose discussing alternative ways of feeding babies worry that this will somehow deter women from breastfeeding altogether. It is a valid concern to be ever vigilant about the message that breast milk is the best possible food for our babies. We truly need to find ways to entrench breastfeeding as the rule and supplementation as the exception in human society. We simply cannot lose sight of what we tell women who have trouble breastfeeding, and we cannot deny access to a clean, safe, organic supplement option to those women. Instead, we need to be supportive of every woman's individual need. If she can't breastfeed at all for some health reason (such as a mastectomy), then we need to support her emotional desire to "make" her baby's food. If a woman has a low supply, then let's find a way to support the breastfeeding that she can do for as long as she can do it while giving her a safe supplement.

Making something you will be feeding to your infant is pretty nerve-racking! I had long understood the reasons for consuming raw milk over pasteurized. At the time I began making formula I was using a lightly pasteurized, non-homogenized milk from a local organic grass-fed dairy. There are those who are opposed to a milk-based formula because it's not a good idea for the infant's digestive system to ingest cow's milk. This is a legitimate concern — when the milk is pasteurized. For this formula it is important to first ferment pasteurized milk into kefir or piima. Fermentation adds back some of the active cultures and makes it safer and easier to digest for your baby. I found when using kefir grains with pasteurized milk that they do not multiply as well and die more quickly than with raw milk. If you are using pasteurized milk, you will need to replenish your grains more often.

I had never fermented milk before I started this. The first few times I set milk out on the counter for twenty hours, my husband was more than a little hesitant about the idea. We both eventually got used to the process of making our own formula, and it became second nature. I continued to use only the finger feeder at the breast, eventually working up to two feeders taped together as he grew. This was a pain in the rear, I'll admit, but I was stubbornly focused on ensuring Aidan's immune system had its best start.

Our focus on Aidan's immune system was foundational to every other decision we were making for him. We had decided to raise a healthy child who could operate independently of the medical system. This involves developing an immune system strong enough to fight off most infection and disease on its own. Our subsequent choice not to vaccinate was inextricably linked with the need to breastfeed. In fact, it was the same decision.

We did not opt out of vaccines because of a growing mistrust of Western medicine or because it was trendy. It is our strongly held belief that vaccinations cripple the immune system, fundamentally changing the bacterial environment in the body. Breastfeeding, in contrast, builds the immune system and creates proper gut flora. When we found I couldn't exclusively breastfeed, a whole-food, nutrient-dense supplement was the next best thing. It fits in with a holistic philosophy like ours because, while not optimal, it still provides a strong foundation for immune system and gut health.

When we chose not to vaccinate, we didn't think that we were going to be transported through time to a place where bacteria and viruses do not exist. We don't seek to prevent any exposure to bacteria or germs. We don't assume that because we feed our children good food they will never get sick — that any illness is a failure of our grand experiment. Instead, we assume the responsibility that they may get sick from time to time. In a greater sense we seek to protect our child's intact abilities to interact properly with the world instead. We prepare for how we will treat our family if we are hit with the dreaded childhood illnesses and work to strengthen a natural immune system that can protect the body for a lifetime. Our philosophy to breastfeed, to avoid commercial supplements, synthetic foods and vaccines and to treat our family with whole plants and whole foods for common ailments comes from the wholistic belief in allowing the immune system to develop and operate as intended.

Many independent studies and incidental parental observations support our beliefs. That said, the medical establishment firmly denies these connection and to date claim to have found no evidence in clinical study. We decided not to wait for them to produce a study that proves what we know to be true.

If you decide to make your own supplement, as I did, prepare for a variety of reactions. Many people are very comfortable with the FDA standards for safety; others are not. I have encountered people who think making your own formula is tantamount to child abuse and the authorities should be involved. To be fair, I feel a similar horror about commercial formula. Some feel they don't have the time to make their own or worry that it's not cost effective. What's more important than ensuring that your child has a strong immune system to build on for the rest of their life? Even if it does cost a little more, think of all the savings in early childhood doctor visits, allergy medications and so on. In the end, it is actually slightly cheaper to make your own formula in this way than it is to buy commercial formula. Aidan is thriving, he is an average weight for his age and highly active and intelligent. In his two and a half years, and now Jacy's one year, my children have each had one fever (probably teething) and one cold. We have never been to the doctor for anything other than a well-child visit. Most of my friends with kids have a much different tale to tell. I'm satisfied that continuing to breastfeed and adding in homemade formula was the right thing to do.

My Second Birth

When I became pregnant with Jacy, I was still nursing Aidan. He was ten months old. We had ceased making a supplement because he was eating solid food, though he exclusively ate breast milk when he wasn't at the table. Within a month he had lost interest in nursing, probably due to the change my pregnancy had caused in my milk. I had hoped to nurse him for two years, but he made his own decision.

For some time I had pushed my husband to get goats so that we would have a home supply of raw milk. When I discovered I was pregnant, I thought back over all the issues we had had with Aidan. I had learned those lessons and arranged to see a lactation consultant right after the birth. I also made sure I had a raw milk source to make supplement in the event I needed it again and vowed to do a better job with my nutrition while she was gestating. I finally made a good enough case and we got our first milking goat about four months before my due date. From that point on, I was drinking fresh raw milk.

I was speaking one day to a reporter who was interviewing me about our farm. She asked me what I was doing with the milk from our goats. I smiled and said, "That's our home milk supply." She was quite taken aback: "How does your doctor feel about the fact that you're drinking raw milk while you're pregnant?" she asked. It hadn't occurred to me that my doctor would think anything about it; I wasn't concerned about myself or my baby. In fact, I was looking forward to the health benefits drinking clean, raw milk during pregnancy would bring me. It was only later that I fully understood what drinking that milk would do for *her*.

My daughter Jacy was born at home, just like her brother, and just like him her umbilical cord was wrapped around her neck. It was a much calmer birth, I managed the pain better and stayed in the birthing tub this time. While she came quite quickly through the birth canal, she was born into the water. She latched on immediately and we could hear her swallow. When we went to see our lactation consultant, we found that her suck and latch were perfect.

The Case for an Appropriate Diet

Animal feed experiments show that many changes besides bone growth take place when cooked foods are used. One extensive study, involving 900 cats over a period of 10 years, was done by F.M. Pottenger, Jr., M.D. Cats receiving raw meat and raw milk reproduced normally from one generation to the next. All kittens showed the same good bone structure, were able to nurse, were resistant to infections and parasites and behaved in a predictable manner. From generation to generation they maintained regular broad faces with adequeate nasal cavitites, broad dental arches and regular dentition with firm, pink membranes and no evidence of infection.

Cats receiving cooked meat presented quite a different picture. Abortion was about 25 percent in the first generation and 70 percent in the second generation. Deliveries were difficult, many cats dying in labor. Mortality rates of the kittens were high, frequently due to the failure of the mother to lactate, or the kittens being too frail to nurse. The kittens did not have the homogeneity of those cats fed on raw foods. Instead, each kitten was different in skeletal pattern.

In the second generation the kittens had irregularities in the skull and longer, narrower faces; the teeth did not erupt at the regular time; and diseases of the gums developed. By the third generation the bones were ☞

very fine with scarcely enough structure to hold the skull together. The teeth were smaller and more irregular. Some mothers steadily declined in health, dying from some obscure tissue exhaustion about three months after delivery.

The cooked-meat-fed cats were irritable, the females dangerous to handle, and the males more docile often to the point of being unaggressive. Sex interest was slack or perverted; and skin lesions, allergies and intestinal parasites became progressively worse from one generation to the next. Pneumonia, diarrhea, osteomyelitis, arthritis and many other degenerative conditions familiar in human medicine were observed. The kittens of the third generation were so degenerated that none lived beyond the sixth month, thus terminating the strain.

At autopsy the cooked-meat-fed females frequently were found to have ovarian atrophy and uterine congestion, and the males showed failure in the development of active sperm. Organs showed signs of degenerative disease. Bones were longer but smaller in diameter and had less calcium. In the third generation some had bones as soft as rubber — a true condition of osteogenesis.[4]

A dentist named Weston Price traveled the world making observations on the relationship between mouth structure and cavities and the introduction of the Western diet. He noted that societies that were still eating a traditional diet filled with nutrient-dense whole foods not only had no cavities, but also that their children were born with a palate that was wide enough to accommodate all their teeth without crowding. Putting my two children side by side, there is a difference in their ability to breastfeed that's related to their palates. Aidan's was pinched, narrow and high while Jacy's was wide and low. Interestingly enough, I was drinking clean, raw milk with a focus on a nutrient-dense diet during Jacy's gestation but not for Aidan's.

This change in diet and the corresponding difference in the palate structure reinforced my belief that diet during pregnancy is very important. As a society, we make sure that our pregnant women take prenatal vitamins, but beyond that, what are we suggesting for optimal health? How are we building our babies?

Choosing a Path

Our journey to become a family has been one of enormous growth. What a crime that it took reaching my mid-thirties to reclaim my own inner voice. We, like so many others, externalized our health and gave power to someone in a white lab coat.

The plants are ready and waiting to help us, but as a society we somehow aren't listening or can't hear. I think in my own case, I had become disconnected from nature and her rhythms. This happened in a variety of ways: eating a commercial diet filled with non-food and food-like substances; spending most of my time in manmade structures under artificial light; sleeping little and not spending enough time outside. I had become a disconnected, sick and imbalanced person. My life was like a speeding car that I wasn't steering.

To achieve balance and fertility, I had to put my hands back on the wheel, take responsibility and make my own decisions. By reconnecting to whole-plant and whole-food medicine (throwing out the chemicals and synthetics) my body was able to regain good digestive health. Removing toxic buildup in my liver also helped my hormones to balance and begin to function normally.

Reaching out to the plants for help takes commitment. Herbal therapies are aimed at balance, not "cure." The difference in language is important. To me, "cure" implies something external that will return you to health. Balance, on the other hand, requires our active participation. It takes commitment to use an herb three or four times a day for many months. It takes faith in your partnership with nature to see an end goal far in the future, while not expecting instant gratification and success. We all need a little more faith in our bodies and in nature; both are perfect systems when we don't interfere.

Reconnecting to this faith in ourselves and nature requires a return to real food. Changing our diet and stepping away from the mainstream way of eating can be quite an undertaking. There are many great eating styles out there: Weston-Price, paleo, eating for your blood type, ayurveda, grain-free, gluten-free and more. Many of us who start down this path do so because we are trying to address a health issue and have realized one key fact: food is both the problem and the solution.

There is no need to adhere strictly to any of these diets simply because someone you know had success eating that way. You may not be comfortable with raw milk, but that shouldn't discourage you from eating "real" food. You may feel your best when you have eliminated all grains, while your friend or family member may not feel good without them. It is very trendy right now to eat a vegetarian or vegan diet. I would caution anyone looking to conceive and grow a baby that this is not the time to miss out on the important nutrition we only get from meat. These diets may be right for some people, but it takes a *lot* of work and research to know what supplements are required for optimal health. What is most important is that you listen to how your individual body reacts to each food and begin to craft the diet that works best for you and your digestion, within a nutrient-dense, traditionally prepared, whole-foods model.

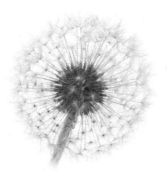

Strategies for Building a Healthy Baby

Herbal Therapies for Fertility

OUR MODELS IN NATURE CONTRAST SHARPLY with the way we currently live our lives. In nature, you must have roots before branches. The tree focuses on healthy roots before anything else. If transplanted, it might drop its leaves to put energy into first building healthy roots. It certainly would never focus energy to produce fruit unless all was right within itself.

Reproduction is an important function in the plant world, but if a plant is imbalanced you might see it die all the way back to the roots, store its energy and try again next year when it is healthy. We are acting contrary to our teachers in nature when we try to not just create branches but produce fruit before our roots are strong and our trunk is whole. We need to take care of ourselves first before we can properly nurture someone else.

When you discover that you are struggling to have a baby, minutes start to matter. With such a busy life, it can feel as though there just isn't enough time to slow down and fix your own issues, whether mental or physical. Many women pack these imbalances up in a box and set them aside so they won't interfere with the more important goal at hand. Unfortunately, our bodies don't operate that way. We cannot compartmentalize dysfunction because we are complex systems. We must be whole and balanced in order to foster a new life that is whole and balanced. Some women may be able to conceive despite imbalance, but why be in such a rush? It is important to know how safe the many allopathic medications one might take while building a baby are, but quite honestly, this becomes a non-issue if we slow down and heal our imbalances before we try to conceive.

As a child I learned a song about a wise man and a foolish man. The foolish man built his house upon the sand and it washed away during a rainstorm. The wise man built his house upon the rock and his house withstood the storm. What a great metaphor for how to build a new life. Build your baby's foundation on the solid bedrock of your fully nourished and healthy body. It is much more complex than the difference between being foolish and wise. No woman wishes to provide a shaky foundation for her child, and it doesn't happen because she is foolish. We are building shaky foundations because our culture is not properly supporting us to create solid ones.

Giving your baby the best chance in life is so much more than taking prenatal vitamins and feeding with breast milk. Without a strong foundation, your baby can be born with structural weaknesses in such areas as the immune or digestive system. These weaknesses can be addressed, but it is much more difficult to do so *after* a child is born.

The following few chapters detail how I began building that solid foundation in my life and how I achieved balance in my own body to make it possible to conceive. Once my body balanced, it stayed balanced. In fact, after all the work to conceive the first time, our second pregnancy was a complete surprise. Today my cycle is still "in balance," and while I am no longer trying to conceive, I monitor this as an indicator of my overall health.

Through most of our journey, I was still learning to make my health and vitality a priority. I hope that my story demonstrates that balance is possible, and that a diagnosis of infertility can be overcome with time and patience. It requires a committment to eating whole foods, working through emotional problems and reaching out to whole-plant medicine for hormonal balance. Above all it requires a mindset that will make the health and balance of your own body a priority, in the belief that a beautiful, nutritionally complete baby will follow. My specific plan may not be anything like yours, but let it serve as a framework from which to create *your* plan to overcome *your* specific imbalance or disease.

Achieving whole-plant and whole-food health is a process worth the time and energy. It takes time to shift the paradigm for how we conceive and grow babies, and until we do, we will continue to have high rates of infertility. Our children are sicker than ever before. For the first time, their life expectancy will not surpass that of their parents.[5] Until we start building our babies in a body that is fully healthy prior to conception, we will continue to select for a weakened human population primed and ready for degenerative conditions and diseases.

First and foremost, I recommend that every woman I consult with begin charting her temperatures and cervical fluid. Our bodies are very complex. The mistake of the allopathic model relating to fertility is to assume that any issues lie in a lack of ovulation. In my opinion, lack of ovulation is fairly rare. According to the American Pregnancy Association, one third of fertility problems are due to male issues, one third are due to women's issues with the rest unexplained. It is believed that the most common cause of infertility, coming in at approximately 25 percent of cases, is a problem with ovulation.[6] This last figure is an estimate for which I cannot find any basis. Perhaps the 25 percent represents the women who were found to respond to the current fertility drug protocol. They would be the very women who did in fact have an ovulation issue. The 20 percent of "unexplained" fertility problems may easier to explain than the medical establishment realizes.

Our conventional food system creates such an overabundance of estrogen in the body (from sources such as pasteurized milk products, soy and conventional meats) that it seems unlikely that many women have low levels of estrogen. Here at the farm, I meet with more women who have low levels of progesterone as a result of diet

and/or inherited imbalance. It may be that I am seeing only the out-
liers. One could make the argument that I see a disproportionate
number of women who have not been helped by conventional medicine — those who, like me, have been labeled "broken." At any rate, I
cannot shake the conviction that progesterone levels should be looked
at more closely in conjunction with individual charting for those who
are more comfortable within the allopathic model.

Above all, it is important to get an individual picture of what is
going on in your body before you seek treatment. Would you am-
putate a leg because your foot hurts? You'd probably want to have
an X-ray at the very least. We all have different reasons for our imbalances, so understanding the cause of the problem should precede
treatment, especially when that treatment is "one-size-fits-all."

Charting cycles provides another important benefit. The allopathic fertility model serves to "other" the body. Rather than plugging
in and learning all about ourselves, we are encouraged to distance
ourselves even more and to rely on what I call "external knowing" (relying on someone else) to solve the problem. This model continues
into pregnancy, when a medical professional controls the proceed-
ings rather than allowing the body to function as it was designed.
Charting demonstrates to couples that we can know our bodies. Men
can understand their partners and help them stay in balance. Women
too can understand their bodies and then begin to predict their cycles.

We must begin to discuss balance rather than what is "normal."
There is no universal "normal" when it comes to women's bodies. Just
as the fashion industry has established a stereotypical vision of the
female figure that is not typical, most women do not operate on an
idealized 28-day cycle. The trick is to understand what "balance" looks
like for *you*. Once you do that, you can better understand when you
are heading into imbalance. You have a better handle on your overall
health, as well as an understanding of how your individual reproductive health works.

By charting, you can become intimately aware of the ebb and
flow of hormones, fluids, emotions and fertility that make up your

monthly cycles. This is a tool that can help you identify patterns in heavy bleeding, spotting, heavy cramping or mood swings. By becoming acquainted with your own body you can find your balance and learn what it takes to keep it.

In a simplistic way, I view progesterone and estrogen as a tee-ter-totter. When the estrogen side goes up too high the progesterone side drops low, and vice versa. The key to reproductive health is balance. Using herbs and making dietary changes can be a very simple solution to allow your body to rebalance naturally.

Often women who have difficulty finding hormonal balance are experiencing a congested liver. The liver is one of the body's filters. When there are too many toxins attempting to go through it at once, it becomes clogged. The liver cleans the blood and is responsible for:

+ Contributing to the regulation of blood glucose levels
+ Storing the fat-soluble vitamins A, E, D, K and B_{12} and the minerals iron and copper
+ Making bile to aid the digestion of fats
+ Metabolizing proteins
+ Balancing hormones by filtering exogenous estrogen, corticosteroids and steroids from the blood stream
+ Filtering toxins, drugs, foreign molecules and chemicals out of the bloodstream.

All of the blood that runs through our body is filtered through our liver. A strong liver therefore has the ability to strengthen and enliven every other body system as it performs more functions than any other single organ. In traditional Chinese medicine it is considered the "seat of life" and is believed to house the soul.

Symptoms of PMS and infertility, as well as imbalances associated with the kidneys, heart, skin, respiratory system and urinary tract, can often be traced back to a "clogged" liver. For this reason, it is always appropriate to work toward a decongested liver as part of any herbal therapy associated with the reproductive system.

Many herbs are available to us for this purpose. Called "alteratives," they include sassafrass (*Sassafrass albidum*), yellow dock root (*Rumex crispus*), dandelion root and leaf (*Taraxacum officinale*), nettles (*Urtica dioica*) and burdock root (*Arctium lappa*). Many of the herbs for the liver are roots, which by their very nature reach deep into the soil just as they reach to the depths of our imbalance. With any liver therapy it is also helpful to focus on an alkalizing diet and bitter foods that stimulate a healthy digestion. You will find more information on these herbs as well as many others that can be used in a gentle way to help the liver heal in the Healthy Baby Herbal Reference Guide at the end of this book.

Herbal Strategies for Your Partner

Balaced fertility isn't just about the female body. We have lost sight of the fact that a baby is made of two contributing cells. We value the quality of the egg and the health of the woman as the vessel in which it grows so highly that we forget the quality of the sperm, which is one half of the equation. It just isn't enough to have only one parent be fully nourished at the time of conception. Diet informs the health of the sperm as much as it does the ovum. Healthy sperm not only provide a better chance at conception, but they contribute to a balanced nutritional start for a healthy baby. This is why it is so important that both the man and the woman take the time to address their nutritional deficiencies and health imbalances before trying to get pregnant.

When a couple begins to research their issues with conception, both partners are tested. In many cases a hormonal imbalance in the female is the cause. In cases where there is an issue with sperm motility, quality or count, herbal therapies can be just as effective for men as they are for women. In too many instances, couples who find there is a reproductive imbalance with the male partner give up on their efforts to have a child. It doesn't necessarily have to be that way. It can be more difficult for a man to seek help in this area, but if both partners are equally committed to having a child this can be overcome.

Regardless of who has the primary imbalance, both members of the couple are affected and both must work on their diet together to obtain optimal health.

Diet, environmental factors and stress can wreak havoc on a man's body and cause disruptions that can impact fertility. The overconsumption of estrogenic foods does not solely affect women. Men, too, have a delicate interplay of hormones in their body that becomes imbalanced with high levels of estrogen or insulin. Lifestyle has a big role to play in many imbalances when it comes to reproduction for men. Long hours at work, dissatisfaction and depression over a job and large amounts of time sitting can all cause emotional and physical damage to the body's delicate hormonal balance. Smoking is another big contributor to fertility problems in men, just as it is in women. It has been shown that smoking contributes to impotence and that one in four male smokers has poor circulation to their penis compared to only one in twelve non-smokers.[7]

Many prescription and over-the-counter drugs also contribute to a prevalence of impotence, both long term and temporary. There is generally very little mention of this side effect and many men tend to be unaware. Sugar levels (both high and low) and insulin in the blood, causing irritation and inflammation are also big factors in what could be considered an epidemic of impotence in the United States. The Massachusetts Male Aging Study reported an average rate of impotence in men aged 40 to 70 of 52 percent.[8] This rate increased incrementally each year after age 40. There are now reports of rising rates in even younger men.

While the endocrine system is clearly very important in this discussion, it is critical to address any stressors on the nervous and circulatory systems. Just as women can suffer from congestion in their pelvic region, so too can men. Congestion and/or improper circulation can lead to a much more visible situation for men, of course, as it often results in erectile dysfunction. The drugs prescribed for sexual dysfunction have painful and sometimes dangerous side effects. The good news is that there are safer herbal alternatives.

We aren't so different in the end as we would like to believe. At 10 weeks development, in utero, a male and a female fetus have identical reproductive structures. From there on in, the analogous structures diverge dramatically. There is evidence that these organs and glands, while they no longer look exactly the same, retain similarities of function.

The prostate is analogous to the uterus in some theories, the breasts in another. All of these organs, as will be discussed later, have sensitivities to the negative energies of others and the feelings we harbor about ourselves.

The testicles and the ovaries are similar. They are both controlled by the pituitary gland and both produce testosterone and estrogen, though in different concentrations in the male or female body. If a male experiences trauma to his testicles, he feels the pain in the same area of the body where the ovaries are located in the female and, incidentally, where the testicles were located in the male prior to birth.

Erectile tissue is found in both the male and the female around the genitals and in breast tissue. The penis and clitoris both have a glans and a foreskin. Finally, the scrotum is analogous to the labia.

When you begin to see the similarities in our reproductive structures, you can read the typical herbal differently. Most herbals are focused on how herbs affect the female body. This is most likely because most of the herbal wisdom keepers in our culture have been women, treating women. Thus, when you come upon an herb that has benefits for the pituitary gland in women, you can deduce that it will act upon the pituitary gland in men. You can further assume that the herb will act upon the testicles and help with the balance of testosterone and estrogen in the male body. While we cannot treat men as women (men tend to need more yang, or hot energy, while women need more yin, cool energy), we can begin to see how some of the same herbs can be used to treat both sexes. There are some issues that often get attributed only to men that are beginning to affect women as well. Low libido is just such a dysfunction that we must address equally for both partners for fertility to be enhanced.

The Healthy Baby Herbal Reference Guide in this book has many herbs that are useful in treating both men and women for general issues, but specific fertility notes for men are called out separately. There is no reason why male reproductive and endocrine imbalances cannot be addressed with both diet and herbs.

Foods for Preconception

Whole, nutrient-dense foods are imperative in conceiving and growing a healthy baby. Eating in preconception is very similar to eating during pregnancy, but there are some differences as you attempt to boost your fertility in preconception. Aside from the fun aphrodisiac foods, there are some things that can help focus your body on the work to come.

Superfoods

Some foods are particularly high in nutrients or phytochemical properties and are great additions to your regular diet. Yams, walnuts, bee pollen, spirulina and maca are just some examples of "superfoods" that pack the greatest punch.

Grass-fed Organic Meats

Grass-fed organic meats with their fat are especially important now as our meat supply becomes more tainted with antibiotics and unhealthy proportions of omega-3 and omega-6 due to improper feeding.[9] Our reproductive health requires plenty of high-quality protein to function optimally. Those who don't eat meat must supplement vitamin B_{12}, zinc and iron because the absorbable forms of these nutrients are primarily found in meat. Use whole foods and whole herbs as much as possible for substitutions to ensure the body can adequately absorb the needed nutrients.

Proper Fats

If you aren't getting these, the body doesn't have what it requires to make hormones. You must have fats in your diet to get pregnant.

Good fats that will support a healthy pregnancy include coconut oil, grass-fed meats, butterfat and soaked seeds and nuts.

Organ Meats

Want to get that all-important dose of folic acid? Forget the pricey supplements and go for grass-fed organic liver! Along with vitamins B$_{12}$ and D, zinc and iron, it has 200 percent of the recommended daily allowance (RDA) of folic acid. For those who can't stand the taste or texture of liver, I often suggest adding it to bone broths in the last hour or so. This infuses the broth with the nutrition of liver but doesn't require chewing. You may also choose to source a high-quality desiccated liver capsule.

Essential Fatty Acids

Omega-3 in particular is great at helping to regulate hormones, increase cervical mucus and promote ovulation. EFAs can be found in salmon, flax seeds, soaked and sprouted walnuts, sardines, halibut, snapper, shrimp and scallops.

Cod Liver Oil with High-Vitamin Butter Oil

Cod liver oil is a great source of vitamins A and D, which are very important in the fertility of mom and dad. They are the precursors to many other biological functions, including the absorption of other water-soluble vitamins and minerals. It contains docosaheaxaenoic acid (DHA) and eicosapentaenoic acid (EPA). Altogether, this superfood is very important in contributing to proper brain function, eyesight and proper synthesis of the omega-3 and omega-6 fatty acids. Unfortunately, cod liver oil on its own is not very effective. It is best taken with a butterfat of some kind so that its nutrition can be absorbed.

Bitters

Bitters come in all forms. You can buy a bottle of "bitters" that are created much like a tincture. You may even see one at your favorite bar next to the liquors. In the American diet you won't find many of them on the menu, unfortunately. Foods like dandelion greens and bitter melon stimulate a part of our tongue most people aren't aware of. Nope, not the sour receptor: the bitter receptor. When stimulated, this receptor signals to our liver and gallbladder that it is time to produce bile. This is why salads at the beginning of a meal were once made up of bitter greens. They served a purpose before they became piles of sweet iceberg lettuce with a cream dressing. Without this re-action we don't produce enough digestive juices, our food doesn't get digested properly, we don't absorb nutrition and our health suffers. Why do I list it as a superfood? A lazy liver stops filtering properly. A lazy digestive system stops absorbing nutrition and eliminating waste properly. We become deficient and toxic very quickly without the bitter taste and most of us have been conditioned to avoid it at all costs.

Zinc

Zinc is a very important nutrient for both our immune system and for balancing hormones. Proper levels of zinc will help heal wounds and are needed for proper growth and devlopment. Soaked, raw pumpkin seeds are one of the best ways to get your zinc because it is a heat-sensitive nutrient. Zinc is also found in liver, oysters, sesame seeds, yogurt, shrimp and venison.

Magnesium

Magnesium is a very important nutrient in our bodies for every-thing from the proper functioning of the nervous system to heart and circulatory health. If you are a woman who believes herself to be deficient in progesterone it is even more important. Proper levels of magnesium are needed to maintain proper levels of progesterone in the body. A handful of soaked, raw, organic almonds each day would cover both your need for magnesium and the all-important Vitamin E. You might also supplement your magnesium levels with a steady supply of properly prepared bone broth.

Calcium

Another important nutrient to be concerned with before conception is calcium. As we all know by now, calcium is important for bone health. It is also critical for our endocrine and reproductive systems. Without a sufficient level of usable calcium in the body it is difficult to maintain hormonal balance. Calcium deficiency can also cause menstrual difficulties. Supplementing with calcium can be problematic and controversial. Many of the supplements on the market are made from things the body cannot digest, so you are better off adding some of the calcium superfoods to your diet in preconception, such as seaweed or fermented or raw milk products.

Whole Grains

While whole grains are generally promoted as healthy, they should be soaked, sprouted or soured only! Unless grains are prepared properly, they still contain all the protective mechanisms designed to ensure survival for the seed.

Each seed that drops from a plant is wrapped in a seed coat that protects the seed from germinating at the wrong time (such as the dead of winter) and dying. The seed coat dissolves only when conditions are right for germination, usually when it is warm and wet. The protective mechanisms (often called anti-nutrients) within the seed coat include phytic acids, enzyme inhibitors, and proteins (gluten and others) in their whole, and hard-to-digest, state. By preparing our grains properly, the difficult parts of the grain can be neutralized and pre-digested to protect us from inflammation, irritation and nutrient loss.

Most traditional cultures soaked, sprouted or soured their grains. Elimination of this important step in cooking is resulting in rampant levels of digestive disorders and other degenerative diseases. The USDA food plate suggests that the American eater should focus on whole grains as a healthy choice. Unfortunately, without education on how to prepare these grains properly, this advice causes more harm than good. Increasingly, people are choosing a completely grain-free diet instead.

Unfortunately, the seed coat is not the only issue with grain. Most consumers buy bags of flour rather than the grain itself, not knowing that flour should be fresh ground and/or stored in the freezer to avoid rancidity. Further, today's grains are highly contaminated with GMOs; they must be organic to have any chance of avoiding this contamination.

Along with including higher levels of these foods in your diet, it is important to lower your intake of sugar and things that the body reads as sugar. Keep in mind that insulin is a hormone. All of our hormones need to be in balance for us to operate at our optimal level, especially when it comes to fertility. An abundance of insulin in the bloodstream will lead to inflammation and high blood sugar.

Now that I have frightened you with all the "rules," I want to give you something very simple to tie it all together. Superfoods are important when we talk about fertility because conception is a time when our body should feel like it is getting the fat of the land. The messages

Bone Broths

Much different than the soup stock you may be accustomed to, bone broth incorporates an acid to help release valuable minerals. For every quart of water you add to your bones you can generally expect to add ¼ cup of apple cider vinegar, wine, kombucha or citrus juice. Bone broths are essential to gut health and a key component to addressing digestive disorders such as "leaky gut." These magical soup bases can be eaten all on their own with a bit of seasoning, used as basic soup stocks or to cook rice or vegetables. The acid releases minerals such as calcium, potassium and magnesium as well as the all-important gelatin. This is why a good bone broth becomes solid after a night in the refrigerator. Gelatin is so important to healing our digestive system. It is a common treatment in many degenerative diseases that have inflammation at their root.[10] In a food culture that routinely buys pre-packaged cuts of meat in the supermarket, we are discarding the most nutritious and readily digestible portion of our meats — the bones!

we send our body when we want to become pregnant should be about abundance, luxury and plenty. There is definitely a whole host of nutrients, fats, proteins and the like that are very important. But please hear this — if you follow all the rules but don't have a properly fired digestion *you will not* absorb most of what you feed your body.

It is very important to understand why we need to properly prepare our dairy, nuts, seeds and grains. This is *not* because the body *can't* digest them — it is because they slow down digestion. Our digestion needs to run like the coal burner of a steam engine. Food needs to go in and be completely burnt down so that the digestive system can access the nutrition trapped inside. If your digestive fire has gone out (by years of eating too much ice and sugar, not enough bitters or things that slow down digestion or reduce digestive juices) you do not burn down your food properly. Your liver and gallbladder become flaccid with a lack of exercise because you are no longer making calls to them to produce digestive juices (bile). You no longer absorb the nutrition from your food, and transit time from one end of your digestion to the other is either stopped (chronic constipation) or sped up (chronic diarrhea).

So the take-away is to know the rules but not run your life by them. Be aware that you don't want to eat very much improperly prepared grain in a given day because it will slow down your digestion and depress all of your other body systems. Too much pasteurized cheese? The same story. Chew slowly, and don't drink water with your meals except for the occasional sip. Don't eat on the run. Create your diet with a heavy handful of superfoods and the things your body can digest easily. Don't stress about the things that creep into your diet that don't match the ideal, just keep them to a minimum each day and watch your body for signs that you are over-indulging.

Unfortunately, I see a lot of women after they have tried almost everything under the sun to have a baby. They have often spent countless hours and lots of money before being flushed out of the medical system as hopeless cases. Unless they have a structural issue, even these women can achieve balance. The downside is that by this point they are often beginning to feel the pressure of their age. You read about it everywhere. There is supposed to be a ticking time bomb on your eggs once you get past thirty-five. It can be a pretty hard sell when I start talking about an herbal therapy plan that involves slow and steady change toward balance for a year or more. When you desperately want a child, any amount of waiting can seem like an eternity, but having a child that is healthy, fully nourished and vital is worth it!

Taking the time to rebalance your body not only gives your child the best chance at a healthy life, it protects your health as a parent. The very imbalances that lead to infertility can follow you into menopause and cause difficulties. It is my strong belief that these same imbalances contribute to many of the cancers we see in later adulthood as well. I have supported many women as they decided that the medical fertility treatment route was the best choice for them. When that is the case, it is important to understand that there are herbal therapies that can support health during that process. In the end, if you do get pregnant, you need to be ready to go back and do the work you skipped over. These hormonal imbalances often show up again after pregnancy in the form of lactation issues and post-partum depression or anxiety.

Taking the time to rebalance for fertility pays off. The premier nutrition that you work into your diet and that of your partner will also prolong your years of prime fertility and offset the arbitrary timelines of medical science.

The Mental Component in Fertility

So many of the women I talk to about hormonal balance and fertility issues, in particular, have some sort of deeply buried emotional issue. In some ways, I believe women are taught to do this. "Don't dwell on that ... focus on the positives in your life." "That's the past, you won't be defined by it ... move on." Unfortunately, the truth is very different from the public's prescription for a cheery self.

Our bodies are powerfully connected to our minds. Think what a potent message an unexpressed thought like, "I'd never be able to live through a miscarriage" can be to our reproductive organs. Our bodies powerfully protect us from what we fear. What the mind believes, the body achieves. What are you telling your body?

There are many ways to move beyond the mental traps we set for ourselves. Identifying where we get stuck in a negative cycle is a good place to start. Ritualizing the release of past emotion is something I highly recommend. Take the case, for example, of the woman who already has a child but is having trouble conceiving again. Perhaps there are physical issues, but in talking with this woman it comes out that her first child was born in a hospital and the experience of becoming a new mother was so traumatic that she has not yet dealt with her feelings about it. Since coming home from the hospital she has decided to put a brave face on things and focus on the fact that she has a healthy baby. Unfortunately, until she deals with the pain, anger and disappointment that are hiding behind that decision, her body may ultimately protect her from experiencing another birth.

It can be very helpful to actively ritualize letting go of the negativity attached to this birth. Perhaps she goes to a quiet place with a few items that remind her of the loss of power she experienced. There she may pray, sing, burn incense, journal or any number of other meaningful actions as she physically releases these muscle memories and emotions from her body. She may choose to burn or bury the items to symbolize that she is resolving these feelings and then moving on, fully integrating the experience and not allowing it to fester in denial. Ritual is a powerful way to shine light in the darkness. It has been used for centuries in religion as a way to make feelings and beliefs tangible and to celebrate or vanquish them.

What are you holding inside? What are you waiting to face? Never be fooled into thinking that the clock is ticking and you will deal with emotional issues after you get pregnant ... you may find the thing standing in your way is you.

Alternative Therapies

Diet and herbs alone can help to make some amazing changes in our overall health. But other therapies can be helpful as well. Because of our lifestyle, many of us spend long hours in a seated position. We sit in our cars or at a desk for most of our day. This alone can cause stagnation of energy, lymphatic fluids, digestive fluids and blood in our pelvic region. Other factors that can cause this stagnation include low kidney qi, "stuck" emotions, a tipped uterus or injury. If we are not getting proper blood flow to our primary organs of reproduction we are going to have a plethora of problems, including such things as decreased cervical fluid.

To address the "stuck" energy or bloodflow it can be very helpful to see a chiropractor and/or an acupuncturist. A chiropractor can ensure that you do not have any misalignments that could be pinching nerves or impeding blood flow. This is particularly important as the nervous system is intimately linked to the delicate interplay involved in the proper production and release of many of our hormones. Acupuncturists can address stagnation due to low qi and emotions. They work on the nervous system as well, reconnecting the energetic pathway by which the nerves communicate throughout the body. If you have never understood all the talk about "energy" in the body, go see an acupuncturist. When you stand up after a treatment and feel how the body is supposed to communicate, you will be hooked.

There are energy workers who can also help with emotional memories that are stuck in our muscles, or deficiencies in our chakras. An example of energy work is reiki. There are reiki practitioners in a variety of fields, from yoga to massage. You can often benefit more deeply from someone who has this secondary talent. Massage is a great example. Massage should be a part of your maintenance plan for good health for its impact on (among other things) the immune, reproductive, muscular and skeletal systems. If you can find a massage therapist who is also trained in reiki, you are in for a real treat.

Yoga, tai chi and qigong are great examples of movement practice that can connect your spiritual and physical bodies. They are a great way to slow down and begin the journey of learning about your body in a very personal way.

There are very simple herbal therapies that are also helpful for pelvic congestion and "stuck" energy. The sitz bath has long been associated with post-natal recuperation. Both men and women can benefit from the therapeutic application of alternating hot and cold. This creates a sort of natural pump action in our pelvic region that can release tensions and congestion and allow blood to flow properly. Sitz baths can be used in any kind of infertility, hemmorhoids or a tendency to bloat. The other therapy I use often is a poultice of warming or invigorating herbs. Herbs such as ginger or pennyroyal can be warmed and placed over the pelvic area under a heating pad to encourage the release of congestion and maintain proper blood flow.

Finally, I want to mention the practice of earthing and how it can apply to the work of rebalancing for fertility. Very simply, this is the act of "grounding" ourselves to the negative ions produced by the Earth. Spending as much time as possible touching the ground with your bare skin is beneficial for whole body health. This is often the reason behind the city dweller's instinctual need to go to the park and walk through the grass in bare feet.

As we seek to bring our cycles and hormones more in balance, a special form of earthing can be useful. Our bodies are meant to be in tune with the cycles of the moon. The moon has a special affinity for the waters in a woman's body. A great first step to rebalancing is in finding ways to reconnect with the moon and her cycles. Whenever the weather cooperates, be sure to spend some time outside each night, barefoot under the moon as it waxes and wanes. This earthing practice will greatly support all the other work you are doing to gain your optimal level of fertility.

Breast Health and Building your Baby

Throughout the Herbal Reference section of this book you will find tips for treating specific physical problems with our breasts. Preparing our bodies to carry a child involves balancing for robust health and healing issues that arise naturally. One of the most common things we can address with our breasts is fibrocystic breast lumps. Some women live with these as a fact of life. They can often be painful, and can also cause anxiety over the possibility of a cancer diagnosis. They can even hide lumps that may actually prove worrisome. Women who ingest a lot of caffeine (in the form of pop, chocolate or coffee) are more likely to suffer from them. By changing their dietary habits, however, many women can rebalance their bodies and eliminate the condition.

If we are attempting to change the way we look at our bodies in a complete arc from preconception to lactation, we must take a closer look at our breast health in preconception. Some women struggle in lactation when they belatedly realize they have (or are diagnosed with) issues such as inverted nipples or hypoplastic breasts, also known as insufficient glandular tissue (IGT). Inverted nipples or other nipple malformations are usually more obvious, though they too require work to correct ahead of time. IGT is caused by improper glandular development in puberty. It cannot be identified merely by looking at breast size: women who suffer from it may have large or small breasts. If you are struggling with hormonal imbalances, particularly if you have had lifelong progesterone deficiencies, you might want to take a look at this possibility. There are, of course, many drugs now being prescribed for it. If you wish to avoid taking synthetic progesterone or medication while pregnant or nursing, it is critical that you focus on a balanced, properly functioning endocrine system prior to pregnancy. If you have any reason to suspect that your breasts have developed differently, it is important that you meet with a birthcare practitioner who is trained in prenatal breast assessment, looking for markers associated with insufficient glandular development. The lack of development can occur in varying degrees. You may have no trouble feeding your child or you may not be able to breastfeed at all. Knowing this in advance will allow you to make dietary and herbal changes to encourage glandular development, and/or support what breastfeeding you will be able to do. It is also important information to take to the lactation consultant you will involve in your birth plan. Be sure to seek one out who is experienced in working with women with low milk supply.

Some of the physical problems that women see with their breasts arise from the mental and emotional space. When it comes to our fertility, we may have work to do in mending our relationship with our breasts. In the latter phases of writing this book I attended a women's shamanism weekend. When I arrived on Friday, I had been suffering for more than a year with a fatty tumor that sat on top of one of my vertebrae. When I returned home on Monday, the tumor was gone. Some of the weekend focused on emotions that I had been holding onto, while some of the time was spent in physical cleansing and massage. I believe both of them impacted the change I experienced.

Our emotions are strong energies that can become trapped in our tissues if we don't have strategies to move them out. Talk therapy, reiki, massage, acupuncture, exercise, yoga, dance … all are great ways to help our tissues release strong emotion, and there are many more. When we hold onto emotions in our tissues, they turn into constrictions and disease. I was suffering from a benign, fatty tumor called a lipoma, a hard pocket of fat that had accumulated in a specific area because of some sort of constriction, blockage or congestion. This fat would normally have settled out through my tissues and either been metabolized properly … or run down to join its friends on my thighs! For some reason, it was stuck. I did not put it together at the time, but this tumor was situated right over the vertebrae where my bra would normally have fastened. I had given up wearing a bra several years before this thing developed, so I knew that clothing hadn't contributed to the problem. I highly recommend giving up your bra. If you are too buxom to go without, at the very least give up the underwires. Our breast tissue is part of the lymphatic system. When we constrict the flow of toxins through our lymphatic system, we're asking for problems.

At any rate, that weekend I dealt with some pretty deep emotions I hadn't been aware I was holding on to. I believe that unclinched the tissues that were holding that fat pocket captive.

One of the highlights for me was meeting Rocio Alarçon a well-known ethnopharmacologist, ethnobotanist and shaman from

Ecuador. Rocio shared with our group a technique for cleansing and massaging our breasts. In America, our typical breast massage is a self-exam for the purpose of identifying lumps. The intimacy and appreciation for our breasts has been replaced by a purposeful focus on the medical. Rocio introduced us to the concept that women need to cleanse their breasts of the energy they receive. She stressed that we need to do this when we are intimate with our partners, and most especially when we nurse.

This traditional method is a combination of cleansing the breasts and massaging to move our lymphatic system. It requires a partner, which may be part of the medicine. When she taught us, our partners were our women friends. Being naked in front of a community of women is not something we do in our culture. We tend to feel judged by other women, and that judgement turns internal and becomes a constant voice supporting our feelings of inadequacy. When you are naked in the presence of a community of women, small or large, you find that we are all beautiful in our own ways. We subject our young women and ourselves to images of one particular type of woman, an airbrushed ideal of female perfection. If we were naked in women's community more often, we could teach young girls that breasts come in all shapes and sizes ... that it's OK to be soft ... that we all have cellulite. Community like this would also help young girls to differentiate between problems with their own development and different individual rates of growth. Discovering at this stage that a lack of development was caused by a hormonal imbalance would make it easy to remedy, as opposed to later in life when a woman would like to breastfeed.

Women's community that embraced different body shapes could so easily silence the negative voice in our heads and begin to release many of the emotions that we hold in our tissues. Too many women are carrying breast, ovarian and uterine cancer. What kinds of emotions are we locking inside only to see them manifest physically later in life?

When we have problems with our breasts, whether it be lumps, mastitis, blocked milk ducts and so on, we look solely to the nipple and fatty tissue that we call our breasts. Rocio's massage technique could easily be used as an alternative treatment for many of these common problems that carry symptoms of "stuck" energy or lymphatic fluid. By expanding our concept of "breast tissue" to include the areas around the back, following our bra and under the arms, we could trade a prescription for massage.

I gradually came to realize that my lipoma had formed only after my emotional and difficult nursing experience. It wasn't until I finally resolved my feelings of betrayal toward my breasts that the tissue relaxed enough to let go of the energy stored where the tumor had been. We must be very careful of the emotions we harbor within ourselves. It is better to let go of negative emotions before they transform into a tumor, benign or otherwise.

Given my personal experience, I believe we could use this therapy (see Appendix C) weekly with great results. Do you have a daughter or a good girlfriend who would help you with this massage? How about your partner? My husband helps me. It is a loving thing he is doing for me, but he can benefit in the same way I do, from a lymphatic health standpoint. For massage therapists or birthworkers, the technique could provide a new avenue for care.

As you begin your fertility journey, why not start a new relationship with your breasts? Learn to love them just as they are. Appreciate them for what they can do for you. Let go of the negative energy that you and others have sent their way. Anticipate a rewarding nursing relationship with your child to come.

Preconception and Pregnancy

My birth story taught me that building a baby does not begin at conception. Technically, it begins at least six months, and some would argue one year, earlier; I would contend that often it involves even more time than that. This depends on how much toxicity you have in your tissues, and how nourished you are at the time you begin to plan for a family. There is no better rule of thumb than to say that your journey toward parenthood would optimally move into pregnancy only when your own body is completely balanced, detoxed and nourished.

As women, we are the soil in which our children grow. Many of us have lived a contemporary lifestyle filled with additives, dyes, chemicals and metals while taking "safe" over-the-counter drugs and prescriptions. The truth is that this is not a safe or healthy foundation on which to build your family. We build our babies out of the flesh, bones and blood that we have at the time of conception. You wouldn't plant a garden in undernourished soil without adding good compost, cleaning up debris and (if you suspected toxic dumping) having the soil tested. Why would you give more consideration to a corn seed than your child?

Couples today have the great freedom to pursue a high-powered career and put family off until later. Many of us have taken full advantage of that. Keep in mind that if you want to have it all, you will have to do some work in the transitions from one phase to another. I had an extremely demanding corporate career. I worked odd hours and endured heavy stress, always waiting for the phone to ring, even in my sleep. This changed my internal rhythms and definitely affected both my hormones and my eating habits. I needed a number of years to recover before I was ready to carry a child. If we don't build our bodies before conception, we are choosing to build a baby that will require more work after birth to achieve full health and balance.

We ignore, or simply aren't aware of, the need to rebalance our bodies and care for ourselves because we have been socially conditioned that nutrition for our baby starts at conception. We are told that as long as we start taking a prenatal vitamin and a folic acid supplement when we find out we're pregnant, that will be sufficient. It is true that we can positively impact our growing child by eating healthy and supplementing wisely during pregnancy. It is also true that we can be caught off-guard with a pregnancy and not be as fully healthy as we would like. Not ever pregnancy can be perectly planned. It is ideal to have a healthy diet during preconception, but if you didn't, by no means should you just give up and eat poorly.

Why wait until conception if you don't have to? I believe relying solely on what you can do during pregnancy is a cultural "rationalization." Many women tell themselves that their individual health is not important; they can just make up the difference with vitamins. This rationalization allows us to play fast and loose with the future health of our society.

In traditional societies, an engagement period was not just a time to go to parties and plan a wedding. It was a time to focus heavily on the nourishment that would build a strong fertility in both partners. It was a time to begin building the type of baby the community wanted to have as a contributing member in the future. As both the young man and woman began to prepare for marriage, they were given the best cuts of meat. They were given the fat of the land and the choicest bits of organ meat. Often an engagement was timed in order to take advantage of the rainy season when grass-fed dairy was most plentiful. The young couple was fed on grass-fed butter, milk and fermented dairy products to ensure that all the building blocks were there for the healthiest baby possible.

Contrast that to today's preparation for a baby in our society. It is now very common for couples to wait several years into their union to begin trying for a baby. Often these early years of marriage involve a lot of birth control medication for the woman. When it is time to begin trying for a baby, only the woman's health is addressed. She must now contend with a liver that is clogged and hormones that are imbalanced from years of suppression. If she is lucky enough to bounce back quickly from this situation, she is creating a baby on a foundation that is unstable at best.

We are currently setting our children on a life path fraught with health problems. Autism, allergies and their ilk are common in our society. Autistic spectrum disorders alone are growing by 10–17 percent annually.[11] We are building children on a poorly nourished foundation. When they are born, their livers are still forming. It is unfair and unconscionable to force them to filter toxins from momma that could be avoided.

The liver is responsible for filtering toxins such as pesticides, exogenous estrogens and prescription and over-the-counter drugs. When it is clogged it does not filter properly and our blood becomes "dirty." This dirty blood circulates throughout the body and during pregnancy much of this toxicity crosses the placental barrier. While the liver of the fetus is not fully functional before birth, it does function enough to filter its own blood supply. By attempting to filter the toxins passed from the mother's body, the fetus begins to experience stress on the liver. Further, anything that your baby is not able to filter can remain resident in the tissues of their body ... waiting to be filtered after birth.

Drugs and vaccinations, added during or shortly after birth, put added stress on a brand new liver. Although science has not definitively proven that these interventions are the cause of many of the inflammatory childhood diseases we see today (such as arthritis, diabetes, autism and allergies), I believe they are contributors. Being exposed to vaccinations or prescription drugs alone may not tip a child into the autistic spectrum. Instead it is the addition of the toxicity that accompanies them to an already stressed and newly developing liver that creates congestion and begins a cascade of disease within your baby's body. A congested liver can lead to hormonal imbalances, improper digestion, overactive histamine reactions and more. The gut flora in a developing body is also damaged when vaccines, antibiotics and food toxins are introduced early on. The digestive tract is an important source of both physical and mental health, and can become highly inflamed if important strains of bacteria are absent or there is an overgrowth of the wrong types of bacteria.[12,13]

We cannot eliminate all toxins while we are preparing to carry or are carrying a baby. We cannot live in a bubble. The good news is that our liver is a powerful organ fully capable of protecting us from reasonable amounts of daily toxins. The trick is to help it by avoiding as many toxins as possible. We must be mindful from the time we enter preconception all the way through our nursing relationship to eat foods that are chemical, heavy metal, pesticide and antibiotic free. We can evaluate the medications we take and eliminate, reduce or find better alternatives wherever we can. We can avoid BPA, phthalates, microwaved food, chemical cleaners, paints and other neurotoxins. We *are* what we eat, touch and breathe in ... and the children we grow in our womb and feed at our breasts are also made up of these things.

Foods for Pregnancy and Lactation

Traditional societies prepared men and women for conception in advance with the best of the best in their diet. Often the only advice given these days is to start taking a folic acid supplement. During my pregnancy I was even told (not by my midwives of course) that it didn't matter what I ate because the baby would take what it needed out of my body's tissues. That is partially true, but misguided at best. First, the nutrition must be in your tissues, a situation that is predicated on the fact that you are eating a healthy preconception diet. Second, the baby may take what it needs from your tissues, but where does that leave your health after the birth? In what state does that leave your body when you make demands on it to nurse?

There is a better way. If you look at the body as a pantry, you'd want to stock all the shelves with the necessities before you invite someone (a growing baby, in this case) over for dinner. It is never too late to start eating a proper diet for this purpose, whether you are getting ready for pregnancy, six months along or already nursing. It's important to nourish your body so that you have everything you need as well as proper nutrition to pass along. I was definitely not eating like this when I was pregnant with my son, but followed a lot of these guidelines during my second pregnancy, and there was definitely a difference in their palates and nursing abilities. There was also a difference in food sensitivity: Aidan was sensitive to eggs for a time and Jacy never had that problem.

If you have come upon this book after you are well into a pregnancy and haven't been eating very well, I would suggest you start with the preconception dietary suggestions I made earlier. If you have been following along on your own or with this book and are wondering what to focus on nutrionally for a pregnancy, I suggest taking a fermented cod liver oil supplement. This one small thing each day can contribute to the proper amounts of vitamin A, vitamin D and elongated omega-3 fatty acids. Not only are these nutrients present, but they are in a form that is readily absorbed. Vitamin A is the precursor to our body's anti-inflammatory process and and we need it to absorb most minerals and water-soluble vitamins. Vitamin D is difficult to get from food so many people are deficient. You will receive the same nutrition in regular cod liver oil. The difference is that you will need to take less of the fermented cod liver oil due to its concentrated nature.

If you find yourself still deficient in vitamin D after taking cod liver oil for a while, ask your health care team to check your blood levels of magnesium. Magnesium is an important precursor to vitamin D absorption and many Americans have low levels. Supplementing for magnesium and calcium becomes easy with the regular addition of bone broths to your diet. This robust soup stock is made with an acid to pull out valuable vitamins, minerals and gelatin and can be sipped on its own or used to cook vegetables, rice and soups. You will find more information on how to make this all-important food item in the earlier section on Foods for Preconception.

Elongated omega-3 fatty acids are important to balance out the onslaught of omega-6 fatty acids that are in our food supply due to an overabundance of vegetable oils. An imbalance of omega-3 and omega-6 in the body can lead to high levels of inflammation and can contribute to degenerative diseases and infertility. While your diet is coming into better balance, a cod liver oil supplement can help bridge this gap.

I take a high-vitamin butter oil combined with fermented cod liver oil non-gelatin capsule from Green Pastures. I found the capsules easier to take than the liquid. The combination capsule also saves time, as otherwise you must always ensure you're taking your cod liver oil with a fat, which you need to allow your body to properly absorb vitamin A. A good morning breakfast consisting of an egg fried in butter in a cast-iron pan would be a great companion to a daily dose of regular cod liver oil.

Good sources of protein are important — remember, protein is a builder. This is important from preconception on, but don't forget that you are still doing heavy lifting while nursing. It is easy to lose sight of the fact that while you are no longer "building" your baby inside the womb, you are continuing to build and grow them while they nurse. Remember that grass-fed, antibiotic-free meats are all important here when you are looking for protein sources. Other protein sources such as beans and nuts must be soaked before you eat them. If you eat these without preparing them properly they will inhibit your ability to absorb valuable vitamins and minerals, reduce your digestive function and cause irritation and inflammation, which is the enemy of fertility. While we're on the subject, it is best to soak, sprout or sour your grains as well, for the same reasons.

Digestion is always the focus of a healthy, balanced system. One of the best tips for encouraging proper digestion at each meal is to eat something lacto-fermented or raw. Lacto-fermented foods are made with living bacteria, not vinegar. They add to your healthy gut flora and are so delicious and easy to make! They are also packed with the feel-good B vitamins.

Lacto-Fermented Honey Mustard

½ cup mustard powder

3 Tbsp whey

2 Tbsp fresh lemon juice

4 Tbsp chopped fresh dill

4 Tbsp raw honey

1 tsp sea salt

Stir all ingredients together in a small bowl. Pour into a pint jar. Cover tightly with an airtight lid and leave your mustard on the counter for about three days. At the end of the fermentation time, move it into the refrigerator and it's ready to use. This will last several months.

Finally, on the subject of milk, get out there and read about it! Make up your own mind. You will find that there are many camps on this one. There are some who feel that milk is not appropriate for humans after they are weaned from breast milk. You will also find some that believe worrying about antibiotics in conventional milk is silly. I land somewhere in the middle. I believe raw milk is appropriate for our bodies when it is organic, grass-fed and clean, and I believe you should avoid milk altogether if you only use pasteurized.

It is vital to get your raw milk from a cow (or goat) that is grass-fed and free of confinement, antibiotics and chemical hormones, and essential that you or your farmer handle the milk in the correct manner. Like any product we consume, milk can become contaminated and unsafe for us to drink. There is a vast difference between the milk from a cow that roams freely and feeds on pasture and the milk from a cow that lives in confinement with many others and is fed antibiotics and grain. No one who recommends raw milk as a health food would ever advise you to get it from the latter cow, or from a supplier who is preparing their milk exclusively for pasteurization.

Under the conditions mentioned, raw milk is a complete food source that has everything in it our bodies require for proper digestion. In fact, pasteurization destroys the very enzymes needed to digest lactose, along with beneficial bacteria, living enzymes and valuable vitamins like C, B_6 and B_{12}.[14] That said, some people's genetic makeup makes it it hard for them to digest lactose and even more people have trouble with casein. Lactose and casein are two of the most difficult food compounds for the human body to digest when not broken down first, as happens in the lacto-fermentation process by which we make many of these delicious milk products. People with sensitivities to these milk components are best served by eating fermented raw dairy such as kefir or buttermilk, because fermenting makes milk more digestible. If you are opposed to raw milk, it is best to avoid dairy altogether. Pasteurized, homogenized dairy is an irritant that feeds the inflammatory response in our bodies. High inflammation will not help at any time while you are building a healthy baby and will certainly affect your overall health and theirs in the long run. There are a number of ways to get your calcium intake other than dairy, my favorite among them being any kind of seaweed!

As with any herbal protocol or new way of eating, there are some food products that are best avoided. Here are a few items you will not want to add to your body or that of your growing child.

High Fructose Corn Syrup (HFCS)

This cheap food additive is in more than you think! Go through your pantry, refrigerator and freezer. It is highly refined and mainly made of genetically modified organism (GMO) corn, and then there is the problem of the fructose itself. While fructose is a natural part of sucrose, it is the harmful part. It can cause degenerative diseases like diabetes, repress liver function and negatively affect the metabolism of growing children. While there are many reasons to avoid this product, the biggest one is that anything that represses our liver function can contribute to hormonal imbalance and therefore has to go. Here at our farm, we eschew the conventional beekeeping practice of feeding this substance to our bees … why then would we feed it to ourselves?

Hydrogenated Oils

The process to create these oils that remain solid at room temperature involves chemical changes that are toxic to the human body. These *trans* fats become part of your body's cells and have been shown to lead to many of the current degenerative diseases. The oils most often used are soy, corn, cottonseed and canola, all of which are often GMO and go rancid very easily when extracted. The inflammation hydrogenated oils produce can contribute to imbalanced hormones and problems with reproduction.

Unfermented Soy

Soy in any form other than fermented and organic should be avoided. Fermented soy includes miso, tamari, natto, tempeh and bean paste. This is a topic for another book — and there are already some good ones out there — but suffice to say that unfermented soy is highly estrogenic and a danger to all humans in any stage of their development. Foods such as soy milk, soy protein powders, soy meat replacements and tofu should be consumed only in very small amounts very occasionally, and must be organic. Conventional soy is one of the most genetically modified crops to date. It is difficult to minimize the amount of soy we eat unless we pay very close attention to labels. Soy is found in almost all processed or prepared foods and may masquerade as hydrolyzed vegetable protein, soy protein isolate or simply vegetable oil on the label. Unfermented soy can cause hormonal imbalance, suppressed thyroid function, nutritional deficiencies and digestive issues.[15,16,17] Evidence suggests that it also can contribute to the formation of breast, thyroid and prostate cancers. Under no circumstances should it be fed to an infant. On our farm, we avoid unfermented soy as much as possible. Because we consume many of the products that our animals provide to us, we also do not feed it to our farm animals.

Processed Sugars

Processed and refined sugars and grains should be greatly reduced if not eliminated from the diet. This includes pasteurized fruit juices and soda. A high concentration of sugar increases the amount of insulin in the bloodstream and can be a major contributor to hormonal imbalance.

Low Fat, Reduced Fat and Anything "Diet"

Fat is very important for fertility. Usually when a food product (such as yogurt) brags about being low fat it has actually had the healthy fat removed; moreover, most of these products contain high levels of sugar and many involve chemical adulterants or heavy metals in their production processes as well. None of this is helpful at any time while you are building a baby.

Genetically Modified Organisms (GMOs)

Lab tests have found that animals eating GMO diets can no longer reproduce naturally by the third generation.[18] There are no laws in the United States that govern the labeling of GMOs but most of the rest of the modern world has banned them in their food. In the US they are not labeled and have not been tested for safety in the human population for any length of time. Our current population is the test pool. Though there are many health issues that are anecdotally trace-able to GMO emergence, the medical community has yet to agree. The only way to be sure you are not eating these toxic subtances is to eat organic or biodynamic or to know your farmer. On the horizon is the specter of the ultimate modified organism, the "clone." To be clear, lab-created food is not a good choice for building your baby.

Caffeine

Cafeine is very hard on our adrenal glands, which we need for hor-monal balance. Further, if you are having any insufficiency issues with estrogen, caffeine can have a drying effect on your cervical fluid. If you are pregnant or nursing it may have negative effects on your child.[19] It is best to find ways to replace your morning coffee before you begin building a baby.

Eating for pregnancy and lactation is a very important job. We need to remember that what we put in our bodies is so much more than fuel. It is the building material that makes up both ourselves and the babies we grow and feed. When you make any of these changes, always think of replacing a food rather than denying yourself. Instead of "taking away" your favorite coffee drink or chocolate bar, replace it with something just as delicious that is healthy, like a hot cinnamon tea. You will quickly find that eating for two might not only get your baby off to a good start but enrich your life as well.

Chiropractic and Low Milk Supply

I didn't suffer from post-partum depression; instead I endured post-partum anxiety. It constantly amazes me how I repeatedly fail to see the connection between the health of my nervous system and symptoms of imbalance. As I sat in my marathon nursing sessions, I struggled to find just the right position that gave my children support while being comfortable for me. This involved multiple chairs, pillows, boppies — you name it, I tried it. At some point in all of this, as I sat buried under a child, unable to do the things I was dying to get done, I started to notice my anxiety levels were really high. Next I noticed that when I sat to nurse I would get heart palpitations. Of course the anxiety fed the heart palpitations, and vice versa.

I suffered with cold sweats for a day or so while I wondered how my children would grow up without me, because I was obviously dying. And then it finally occurred to me that after all the stress of a very hard labor, I might just have something out of place. Sure enough, when I went to see my chiropractor, he told me that heart palpitations are a common occurrence when there is a subluxation in the upper cervical or mid-thoracic areas. In a recent discussion with him, he further elaborated that this is the area feeding the nerves associated with enabling sufficient breast milk supply. I suffered from just such a misalignment and struggled with supply with both my children. This is a great illustration of why you need to have multiple caregivers on your health care team. A chiropractor, massage therapist, acupuncturist, midwife/OB/gynecologist, general practitioner and herbalist would be great. In a perfect world you would make sure that all these experts were able to talk about your case so you could get the best benefit of all their care!

Supplemental Feeding Equipment

To continue breastfeeding while I supplemented, I needed the right equipment. I could, of course, have used a bottle, but constantly switching back and forth between the bottle and the breast can cause nipple confusion at best. There are actually more serious consequences. Breastfeeding is important for more than just nourishment. The physical action of sucking at the breast is very different from sucking on a bottle. Bottle feeding changes the coordination required to feed at the breast and can impair the proper development of the jaw, sinus cavity and hard palate. It can also impair future teeth placement and impact a proper swallow mechanism. Studies are now showing that the prevalence of dangerous sleep disorders in infancy and adulthood can be lowered by breastfeeding.[20,21] So it is important, not just that your baby receives your breast milk, but also that he or she actively breastfeeds to receive it.

If I had merely fed with a bottle and occasionally nursed my children, my already meager supply would have vanished quite quickly. To ensure that I could continue to nurse and provide supplemental feeding at the breast I used a supplemental feeding device. There are several different options on the market (see Appendix A for a list), but they all contain a bottle of some sort that connects to very fine tubing. The tubing is taped to the nipple and when the device is turned on a child can get both breast milk and supplement, or supplement alone.

One of these devices could also help an adopting mother who hopes to kickstart lactation, or who would like to provide the structural benefit to breastfeeding while forging a bond. If you are hoping to stimulate a milk flow without having given birth, be sure to take special note of the herbs in this book that are labeled as galactagogues (milk stimulators). Goat's rue (*Galega officinalis*) is a standout herb for this purpose and can help to develop glandular tissue as well as promote a good milk supply. Also be sure to reach out to your local La Leche League for advice and support in feeding your adopted little one.

For me, this device was a lifesaver. My babies continued to stimulate my milk production, receive whatever valuable milk I could produce and develop their facial structures properly. I had a bit of trouble due to the thickness of my homemade formula, but I often found it just needed a bit of warming in my hand to prevent clogging in the tiny tube.

You may wonder at the convenience factor of making formula, filling a finger feeder and taping it to your breast every time you need to feed your child. I can only respond that you get used to the routine. I knew what I needed to give my children and this was the way to do it, so I just did it. Having a support system is key. Be sure that you have a lactation consultant in your health care team. Get support from your partner, a friend and/or family members. This is a big help — especially when you could use a third hand! You can also reach out to a local La Leche group. They are always willing to help with tips and encouragement to keep going. Breastfeeding isn't always easy and or instinctual. Unfortunately, as we get further and further from a traditional diet, our children are increasingly being born with a mouth structure that cannot nurse properly without expert intervention. We will continue to need help from qualified consultants and the courage to forge ahead and do what is best for our children, even when it's difficult or inconvenient.

The Mental Component in Breastfeeding

Women who wish to breastfeed should be aware that we have officially lost the connection to our bodies and our cultural heritage that would enable most of us to nurse effortlessly from the start. Nursing definitely requires consulting with an expert, but it also takes determination and hard work. Just as there is a transitional phase in a natural birth, there is one in nursing. In birth, this transition is often the signal for a midwife that it is almost time to push; it is the point at which many women feel that they just can't go on anymore. A good midwife or doula will tell her client that the shaking her body is doing and the mental fatigue she is feeling are signs that she is near the end of labor. In nursing, the transition period comes at about the third or fourth day when your milk hasn't come in yet. There is a similar feeling of anxiety, a feeling that you can't possibly go on. Usually this is around the time that milk production begins and colostrum tapers off. Women need to be prepared for this anxious period when they will be tempted by their own feelings and by well-meaning advice from others. Suggestions to "just give the baby some formula" or that "maybe you can't produce enough milk and it would be better to use formula" often creep in right at this time of desperation. Gather around yourself a team of professionals and a supportive community of women who can talk you through this second transition phase just as the midwife does in labor.

I began my nursing experience thinking that the baby did all the work. Everything I read gave me the impression that as long as I was in the correct posture and had made the correct latch, the baby's sucking would bring down my milk. It finally occurred to me one day that there was one vital piece missing. I was focused on the television but had noticed that my daughter was struggling, pulling away and "bouncing" on the nipple and kicking and pushing on my breast. This had happened before and I had always just assumed I wasn't producing from that side and should go get some supplement. This time, though, I had a new thought. What if I concentrated on letting my milk go? I had read books that suggested you find a quiet spot to "focus on feeding your baby," but no one had ever addressed why this was important to the letdown reflex.

The only comparison I can find is the sensation we get when we focus to release for urination. It is a voluntary release that had to happen for me to allow the muscles to relax and let the flow occur. We take this type of focus for granted once we have completed our childhood potty training; we know we cannot urinate while consciously telling our body not to go. It's a very subtle bit of control, of which most of us as adults are unaware. There are internal muscles that must be relaxed for urine to flow freely from the body. This is so in the breast as well. There is a similar bit of conscious "letting down" that must be exercised. Our bodies are, of course, made to produce and release milk without our active participation. Unfortunately, a woman who is stressed or preoccupied may involuntarily fight against this natural mechanism. I noticed that as soon as I concentrated on letting go of my milk, my daughter immediately quieted down and stayed latched, and I began to hear her swallowing.

My husband sees a parallel to this process in his relationship with our cow at milking time. Very often, she is so excited to see the hay he's put out for her that she forgets what she's in the milking stand to do. Occasionally he has to tap her hindquarters or yell to get her attention before she remembers to relax and let her milk down for him.

We can take all the herbs ever suggested in a book and eat all the right foods, and our children can latch and suck properly, but we can still have difficulties with nursing. If we don't consciously relax to let the milk down to our baby, our nursing relationship will never be as full and successful as it could be. I once heard a quote that I follow in my day-to-day life: "What the mind believes the body achieves." Those of us who believe that we will never have enough milk and do not therefore focus on letting our supply down will certainly prove ourselves correct.

The Concept of Nursing Through

Maintaining your own optimal health, with an emphasis on diet while nursing, is the best way to ensure the health and immune strength of your infant. In an ideal world, your child receives "perfect" nutrition as a by-product of you doing the same. Unfortunately, we aren't all perfect. Though we try our best, our diet is often less than optimal. But it is important to note that you *must* eat properly for breastfeeding, to provide the best benefit to your baby. If "you are what you eat," the same is true for your nursing infant. If you take the time to be fully healthy before getting pregnant, including removing any stored toxicity from your body, you will be less likely to pass on these unintended extras, and can also increase the quality of your breast milk. Breast milk and the process of breastfeeding are always best. It is important, however, to be aware that contaminants *can* pass through breast milk, which is the reason you definitely want to clean up your "internal" environment while avoiding external risks such as heavy pollution and paint fumes.

Even if you breastfeed, your child will occasionally get a good immune system workout from a passing cold or that seasonal flu that's been going around. Illnesses can actually be beneficial in developing a strong immune system for your child. During those times, herbs that can help alleviate symptoms and shorten the duration of illness are available *through* your breast milk.

The nutrients we get from our food and the medicines we take wind up in our blood plasma, where they nourish cells or fight disease. Our blood is made up of what we eat and what our liver sheds into our intestinal tract. Because of today's eating habits, many of us have damaged our digestion and developed a condition called "leaky gut" syndrome. This, in effect, means that our intestinal walls have become porous and we are leaking more substances — sugar, undigested proteins, and so on — into our plasma than what is good for the body. Most of us are clogging our livers with toxins, food-like substances and hormones, making it difficult or impossible for our liver to break down the toxicity it is intended to filter. When the liver ceases to synthesize poisons such as allergenic proteins or exogenous estrogen, they pass through unaltered into the intestine, where they are often absorbed into our blood plasma. Anything floating around in our plasma, good or bad, is fair game for our body to transfer across the placenta[22,23] or into the alveoli in our breasts to be used in producing milk.[24]

Although we can pass on iron, calcium and good fats through nursing, our children may also receive alkaloids, volatile oils and minute amounts of some drugs in our breast milk. The amount passed depends on molecular weight, lipid solubility and pH. [25,26,27] Reference guides on prescription drugs and nursing list the levels of each drug that cross the breast milk barrier and then draw conclusions about relative safety based on the presence of either acceptable (in the reviewer's opinion) or absent reactions in the infant. An infant's exposure to perhaps 1 to 2 percent of the maternal dose is generally regarded as relatively safe (10 percent is the top limit in most cases) except in specifically contraindicated pharmaceuticals.[28,29]

Instead of looking at the amount of an individual drug the infant is exposed to, we need to look at the cumulative effect of a number of different substances. Also, while we may not be seeing a direct impact from an individual drug, I think it is shortsighted to think it is necessarily "safe" for breastfeeding. A developing liver will be impacted by the need to filter these chemicals out of the bloodstream of a tiny body regardless of serum concentration, possibly without exhibiting any symptoms at the time. If the mother is passing along multiple drugs and chemicals, we must be concerned with the impact the ensuing toxicity may have on the infant's liver, digestive system and immune system.

Knowing that we can affect our baby negatively through our breast milk is not the only way to look at this relationship. Allopathic practitioners usually hand a mile-long list of herbs to avoid to their pregnant or nursing patients. This list was created because most of these herbs will readily cross the placental barrier and some will cross the breast milk barrier. Also, most doctors are not comfortable with their knowledge of herbs, so they err on the side of caution and advise their patients to just avoid them all.

I believe we need to start looking at herbs with respect rather than fear. Instead of avoiding them all to be safe, we need to spread the knowledge of how to use them responsibly. If we know that what we eat passes into our plasma and much of it becomes available in our breast milk, we can use that very system to increase the healthy effects for our baby. In fact, we can use the same herbs with which we treat ourselves to gently and simply give relief to our babies when they suffer from minor ailments. Each and every herb hasn't been studied to determine how much it passes through into breast milk. These studies should be done; in the meantime, when we use herbs in their whole form, they may be considered a whole food. We know that nutritional factors and flavors pass through into breast milk from whole foods, and also have much written and anecdotal history from women who have used herbs in their whole form to favorably affect their nursing children. Until such time as we have more research, we need to approach herbs with the mindset that there are benefits as well as risks to using them in the breastfeeding relationship. We should take in this information, consult with our health care advisors, and then watch our babies carefully, armed with our motherly intuition.

There are some special considerations to keep in mind when using herbs to either direct dose or to nurse through. When discussing how much and how often to give an herb, the first thing to understand is whether the issue is chronic or acute. A chronic issue is something an individual has been struggling with for a long time; examples include eczema, diabetes and arthritis. These issues are deeply rooted and have taken a long time to develop. Therefore, they take longer to treat and do not respond as quickly. The goal is to maintain a constant level of the herb within the bloodstream for an extended period of time.

An acute issue is something that arises quickly, often because of sudden injury or body system abuse. Acute issues range from colic to headaches caused by too much sun. With these issues, you are typically aiming at a fast response to treatment. The issue may be tied to a deeper imbalance, and you may move on to treat that next, but for right now you are reducing discomfort caused by the symptom. Treating acute issues calls for smaller doses at more frequent intervals because you want the body to respond quickly.

For the purpose of nursing through, a chronic dosage would not require any change in the nursing routine. You would simply choose your preferred herbal medicine and use it as directed. For an acute situation with your baby, it can be helpful to offer the breast more often until symptoms subside. If you are a nurse-on-demand mommy, you may find yourself doing this anyway as you will most likely be nursing to soothe your baby.

In the extremely rare situation requiring that you stop breastfeeding, direct dosing may be required. If you have frozen breast milk available or are comfortable getting some from a breast milk bank or a friend, it would be great to add these dosages to a small amount of breast milk. See Appendix D for an expanded childhood dosage

When Nursing An Herb Through
(Mother Ingesting and Baby Nursing)

Tea	
Chronic dosage	3–4 cups per day
Acute dosage	¼ cup, every 20–30 minutes
Tincture	
Chronic dosage	½–1 tsp (30–60 drops), 3–4 times per day
Acute dosage	⅛–¼ tsp (7–15 drops), every 20–30 minutes

chart. These are all general guidelines. You should always take your child's age, weight, overall constitution, the nature of their illness and the strength of the herbs being used into account to make your final decision on dosage. If your infant needs to be directly dosed for some reason, here are some general guidelines for a child under one year old:

When Administering Directly to Baby

Tea	
Chronic dosage	2 tsp, 3 times per day
Acute dosage	½ tsp, every 20–30 minutes
Tincture	
Chronic dosage	Age ≤3 months 2 drops
	Age 3–6 months 3 drops
	Age 6–9 months 4 drops
	Age 9–12 months 5 drops
Acute dosage	Not advised, as the size of the dosage required would be too small to measure at home. Consider teas or homeopathic options instead.

Expanded from Rosemary Gladstar's Herbal Home Study Course.
(See Further Reading page 317.)

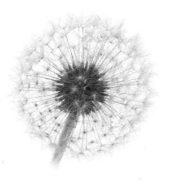

General Herb Use

T HERE ARE MANY DIFFERENT WAYS that you can use our plant allies for health and remedy. The form you choose should be the form that you find easiest to take. My personal preference is to use herbs in their most "food-like" state, so I generally start with teas.

Always start slowly and watch for changes, keeping in mind any known health issues. Treating a generally healthy adult or child for basic issues is one thing. But if herbs are being considered for a disease and there is a special need or known allergy involved, always check with an experienced herbal practitioner for any possible contraindications.

When using herbs for health, always ensure that you know the Latin (botanical) name of the plant in question. In this book each herb is listed first by its common name followed by its Latin name in parentheses, such as dandelion (*Taraxacum officinale*).

It is extremely important that you never buy an herb strictly on the basis of its common name. If any retailer or herbal source does not list both the common name and a Latin name on their packaging, you should avoid purchasing from them! Most plants may have dozens of different common names that may have different cultural or historic derivations. Each herb, however, will have only one scientific or Latin name. Always be sure you are getting exactly what you want.

Let your food be your medicine and your medicine your food

— Hippocrates

On our farm this quote is prominently displayed on the wall of our farm store. It guides all our herbal advice and all of the products we create. When choosing how to balance the body, we believe that you should **eat** your medicine, not *take* it.

Herbs can be used in a variety of ways: incorporated into home-made baby food; steeped in water for healing, soothing baths, soaks and compresses; made into pills, capsules, boluses and suppositories, depending on the type of need; used in steams; combined with oils to make lotions, creams, salves and balms; applied as liniments or poultices for the pain and symptoms of many health conditions. In fact, the uses are almost endless. And herbs, of course, are also delicious additions to almost any type of recipe, from teas, jams and jellies to soups, stews, bone broths, flavored oils and even spirits.

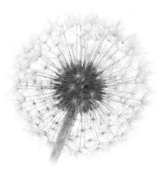

Determining the Quality of Herbs

I ALWAYS TELL MY STUDENTS when they visit the farm, "Herbs are magical, but they aren't magic!" They are magical in the way they can elicit wonder and effect deep, unexpected healing. They are not a sleight of hand or a flash of blue smoke that will bring about instant change. Those of us who are accustomed to Western medicine are used to popping a pill and seeing some relief in fairly short order. Herbs can work like that sometimes, usually when we take a tincture for something minor like a headache. But usually we don't use herbs for the same reasons we use allopathic medicine. Herbs do not merely silence the symptom — they go to the root of the problem and prevent the symptom from appearing again by rebalancing the body. If your car begins to display it's "check engine" light, it is never a good idea to respond by pulling the fuse that is responsible for the power running to your dashboard. The light is merely a symptom that is alerting you to a problem with the engine. Turning off the light may be satisfying in the short term, but the engine trouble is still going on unseen somewhere under the hood. It is sometimes appropriate to use Western medicine to silence a symptom being displayed by our body, but only if we are prepared to follow up with a whole-herb and whole-food protocol to fix the underlying problem. Otherwise you have disconnected the dashboard, but the engine might still seize up and cause a breakdown.

In our society of immediate gratification, not only do we expect our herbs to work quickly, we also expect them to do so when their phytochemical constituents have been almost completely degraded. Herbs aren't magic. There are phytochemical components that lose their usefulness as they are exposed to oxygen, light and heat. Every time a plant part (leaf, berry, bark, etc.) is broken there are more surfaces for oxygen to act upon. Oxygenation is the enemy to these fragile chemical compounds we use for medicine.

Here's a typical scenario of the first-time herbal medicine user. Sarah hears about a wonderful herb that will fix her cholesterol problems. She heads down to the nearest health food store, selects a capsule from the shelf and happily returns home to begin her new healthy life. She makes no changes in her diet. The capsules are made from a powdered herb that was once, long ago, a vibrant plant. Sarah has no idea how the plant was grown, harvested or processed, and can't know how long it sat around after it was harvested, how long ago it was made into capsules or how long it has been a capsule before getting to her. Sarah takes her capsules intermittently for about two weeks and when she

Know Your Herbs

Grow it yourself! When you grow an herb yourself you create a personal relationship with your medicine. You also know how it was grown and processed.

Buy direct from a grower. If you can't grow it yourself, think locally and go to the farm where it's grown. Have a relationship with that grower to know and be comfortable with their practices. Look for a chemical-free, organic or biodynamic farm using non-GMO seeds.

Buy from a reputable retailer. When you don't know the farmer, buy from a business with which you are comfortable based on your research, peer reviews or recommendations. If you don't know the growing practices of a specific herb brand, look for the organic label.

doesn't see any changes in her cholesterol numbers, she throws away the bottle and tells all her friends that herbs are a "bunch of bunk."

Quality matters when it comes to our herbs. So how can you know if you are getting quality? I believe that the closer you can come to the original form of the plant, the better. Here are some keys to consider:

A great start to finding someone you can trust to buy your herbs from is to look for local farms. The benefit of a local herb farm is that you can often ask to visit. A reputable herb farm should be willing and eager to share how they grow, pick and process. Recommendations are often found at the end of your favorite herbals, as they are in this one. They are a great place to start, but don't just take my word on it, read about these farms yourself. If you go to a website because you don't have a local herb farm, you should see good pictures of the herbs, and they should be listed by both their common and their Latin names.

The farm or grower should have some information about how they grow, and it should reveal an understanding and respect for the plants as individuals. Steer clear if their website reads like an infomercial and makes the herbs seem too good to be true. Someone who is growing the herbs solely for a quick buck will most likely produce a plant that is low in healing energy and often low in phytochemical or nutritional value. When you receive a test batch of herbs from the farm of your choice they should pass any test you would put your own herbs through. To obtain the highest quality herbs you will generally want to buy from an organic or biodynamic farm.

Sustainable Suppliers

It is important to be sure you are buying your herbs from a sustainable grower or a supplement maker that is buying from one. As we wake up more and more to the way in which we've lost our health independence to the modern medical machine, we are turning as a very large planet to our plant healers. If we are not careful stewards of these plants, we risk over-harvesting them (or spraying them with weed killer because we don't know what they are) and running out of plant medicine for ourselves and future generations.

There is a very simple solution here! Buy only from people who are growing in a way that ensures native populations are left intact while making the herbs available for us to use. As you read through this herbal, you will note that some of the herbs are marked with a United Plant Savers (UpS) designation. Please be mindful of these herbs — they are the ones we are most at risk of losing forever. When we buy from someone who is selling an endangered herb cheaply or in a suspicious manner, ask questions. If they have stripped a forest community bare of the plant in question, you won't be doing anyone any favors by supporting their questionable harvesting techniques. Our farm, Mockingbird Meadows, and others like it are in a network of UpS Botanical Sanctuaries that are working to repopulate and preserve our native medicinal species. You can read more about UpS in Appendix E.

Herbs retain their viability longer when they are grown, harvested and processed properly. The more "whole" you can get your herbs, the longer they will last. When you get them powdered, or powdered and capsulated, the clock starts ticking pretty fast. Whole herbs should last you several years. Generally, leaves, flowers and dried fruits will last one to two years, and roots, barks and nuts two to three years. If you harvest or buy your own herbs, you should store them in glass away from direct light, heat and moisture. If you begin to wonder if your herbs are still good after some years have passed, here's how to tell:

Ensuring Herbal Quality

Color. The color should still be vibrant

Smell. It doesn't have to smell good. A lot of herbs actually have quite a stinky smell. If it's still good it should have a strong or striking smell.

Taste. Again, it doesn't have to taste good, but it should still taste like it has something going on.

Effect. It should still give you the effect you expect.

Herbs *are* magical. There is so much more to them and what they have to offer us in the way of balance and vitality than can be seen under a microscope. Other systems of traditional medicine, including traditional Chinese medicine and ayurveda, recognize that plants have energetics that can benefit us as much or more than their actual chemical makeup will tell us. Even in our own culture, native peoples practice what is now known as plant spirit medicine. Beyond recognizing the energetics of each plant, this practice recognizes the spirit and essence of the plant as a willful participant in the healing process. These things are difficult to capture in a capsule, but if the plant is grown with respect and honor, and the medicine is created with healing intent, they are most definitely there. These are the things that transcend the mechanics of how you like to take your herbs, or the age and availability of the phytochemicals within. It is something you *feel* when you are using a really well raised and/or made herbal medicine.

Standardized Method versus Simplers Method

In any field of alternative medicine, there is a struggle to gain respect while remaining true to the elements that originally inspired it. Herbal medicine is no different. You can see this in the various ways in which herbs are prepared as well as the cultures in which the preparations are used.

In Europe, herbal therapies have long been accepted as part of the norm. This has brought with it both positives and negatives. Here in the United States we mirror some of this in our standardized medicines. Understandably, there are many in the herbal community who wish to be respected in their healing practices. There is a drive among that portion of the herbal community to be recognized by the medical establishment and respected as equals. Just as in Europe, this brings the practice of herbal medicine even closer to that of modern Western medicine. A standardized tincture is one that has been crafted with complex mathematical formulas to monitor the exact amount of alcohol to water and the exact amount of plant extract to determine the amount of phytochemical constituent in each bottle of medicine.

This means that practitioners who don't make their own tinctures can always be assured of the amount of chemical medicine in the suggested dosage. It is always noted on the label that the formulation is standardized.

In contrast, there is a contingent of herbal practitioners here in the United States who are more folkloric in their approach to the herbs. This group continues to formulate using the simplers method, which is is much more guided by the magical essence of the plant and the intuition of the practitioner. A tincture made by the simplers method goes by proportion and instinct. This is more than likely the method you will use should you decide to make your own tinctures at home. It is no less valid, and no less potent. These are just two different methods. The choice comes down to what you and your health team are more comfortable using.

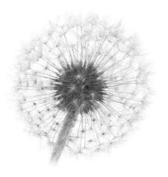

Whole Versus Isolated Constituents:
The Side Effects of Ethnobotany

WHEN THE WORLD OF HERBALISM ventures too close to allopathic medicine it gets very confusing. As a botanist, I became fascinated by the isolated phytochemicals within each plant that we use for medicine. I yearned as a young graduate to travel the world learning from shamans in remote forests. I was driven by the idea that we were losing both of these natural resources, the shaman and the forest, and needed to record the knowledge before it was lost. I was taught that we could harness this knowledge, send samples back from the forest to the lab and isolate chemical constituents that could solve all of humanity's ills. The only thing that kept me from leaping into graduate work in the field was a fear of chemistry. I'm so thankful that I did not follow that path.

Ethnobotany does not have to focus on harvesting chemicals for the pharmaceutical industry. In fact, it just boils down to who you're working for — something I missed in my earlier naïveté. Many of the great ethnobotanists working today are more in line with my changed perspective. I still yearn to walk remote forests and record the shamans' knowledge of the plants before we lose these precious resources. These people are the descendants of those who originally captured the knowledge of how to understand the language of plants.

I had a student once who recalled the biblical story of the Tower of Babel during a plant communication workshop. I knew the story well and had always pictured a large group of scattered humans with no knowledge of how to communicate with one another. This brilliant woman told me she had always envisioned that this story recorded a time in our past when ALL language was scrambled. In her mind, this included our ability to speak and understand the language of the plants and animals. There are many of us today who have learned to converse in this energy-level language. It can be learned from other humans or directly from the plants themselves, but we have to move aside so much cultural indoctrination and suspend belief to such an extent that doing so often requires the help of psychoactive plants. Many of us are called by the plants as children. You are either one of them, or you know one. They are the children who wander happily out into nature on their own as if they are not alone. They freely talk to the fairies and speak about the flowers as individuals with feelings. Our world would be so much better off if we encouraged these children to strengthen their language skills in the plant realm just as we encourage them to learn French or Spanish.

I would no longer wish to be part of an industry that favors the individual components over the whole. Now my interest would be solely in preserving the cultural knowledge and the plant habitat for future generations. It is not so black and white as this, I realize. In a culture obsessed with isolating phytochemicals, many ethnobotanists are straddling the line and sending plants to be evaluated in labs with an eye to the economic benefits of preserving a people and their region. We must move away from the notion that we are cataloging these plants so that we can mine their chemical constituents. Here in the United States we have an enlightened organization called the United Plant Savers that wisely does not call for a moratorium on using endangered plants, but instead for more growers to recognize each plant's individuality. We must preserve habitats where possible and create new ones if necessary, in the soil and not a lab. We must learn to mine the knowledge and the plant intelligence so that we can raise plants sustainably and use them in their whole form.

An obsessive focus on individual constituents within the plants we use for medicine is what gets us into trouble. This focus is so shortsighted and allows us to benefit from only a fraction of what the plants have to offer. It denies their individuality, their "personhood" from a plant perspective. It denies them the ability to use their intention, their energy and their emotion to contribute to a more complete healing process for the human body.

Most of our modern drugs were either based originally on plants or inspired by them. Unfortunately, instead of looking at the whole plant, we isolated what science determined to be the "active" component. We shouted *Eureka*! and blithely pulled out that one special component ... leaving hundreds of other chemicals behind in the plant. Now that we had the one chemical all on its own it could be synthesized so as to have a more direct action, often a much more targeted and harsh action, in the body. Without all the hundreds of other chemicals that this compound once worked with in concert, suddenly there were ... *side effects*.

Let's put it this way. A scientist finds you in the wild and analyzes you based on your parts rather than as a sum total of the whole. He determines that within your circulatory system, it is your heart that is the active component. So he cuts your heart out and puts it under a microscope. Now there's this obnoxious "side effect" involving leaking blood everywhere and the heart only seems to work for a few minutes before it stops beating and requires electrical stimulation.

It is *essential* to use the plants in their whole-plant medicine form. All of the other chemical constituents, some of which we can identify and many more which we can't, have evolved side by side with what science determines to be an "active" ingredient. The plant and its makeup work as a comprehensive system. When we use whole-plant medicine instead of isolated components, either in so-called natural supplements or in allopathic medicine, we don't see the "side effects."[30,31,32,33]

A Word About Supplements

Not all supplements are created equal. I've noticed a disturbing trend as I consult with women. When asked about their diets, many report that they don't really spend very much money or time on whole foods. Instead, they buy cheap food and then spend all their money on dietary supplements. I find this incredibly backward. The myth that "you can't possibly get all your nutrition from food" is just that ... a myth. It's perpetuated by those who will continue to produce subpar food and those who want you to buy supplements.

I do not typically recommend a prenatal vitamin for preconception, pregnancy or nursing. There — I said it. This is not because I don't care about the health of a pregnant mother or her unborn child. In fact, I feel that most of the prenatals on the market do little good and may sometimes cause harm. If you wish to use a prenatal vitamin,

Our Depleted Soils

In one sense, the myth that we cannot get all of our vital nutrients from our food is being propped up by what we know about our soil. Our soils have been overfarmed and underfed to such an extent that the food that is grown on them, by and large, is no longer nutrient-dense. The plants are able to uptake only nutrition that is readily available. Our farming practices have not returned nutrients that were taken many moons ago. We have universally lost the understanding that we must be connected to the soil, the Earth, from which our food originates. Its health is a mirror to our own. As long as our soil is infertile and requires temporary applications of "medicine and nutrition" to prop it up and make it perform... so too will we. Many people are eating chemical-free foods and wondering why they still require supplements. As we have had the opportunity to work our own piece of land and fully devote ourselves through biodynamic farming practices to a vibrant and healthy soil, we have learned this important truth. We must all work on our relationship to the Earth. It must be healed in the same way our bodies need healing, or the human race is heading for real trouble.

don't scrimp. When you look at the ingredients list on any supplement you decide to buy, it should read like a grocery list. The nutrition in the vitamin should come from real food and herbs. If it doesn't, you might as well flush your money down the toilet, because that's where the supplement will go after it runs right through your system. Cheap supplements often get their nutrition from rocks, seashells and the like. Our bodies are not made to absorb this type of nutrition. Some supplements serve up an unbalanced formulation of vitamins; some leave out essential vitamins necessary for the absorption of other vitamins included in the pill. In short, it is much wiser, cheaper and more enjoyable, not to mention easier, to just eat! And by eat, I mean a diet filled with nutrient-dense whole foods.

Homeopathics

Homeopathics work on an energy level. They are based on the theory that like cures like. To protect against poison ivy, for instance, you would take a homeopathic remedy of poison ivy. If you put the homeopathic formulas under a microscope, they have been so diluted as to no longer contain any pharmacologically active compounds. The effect comes from the energy impression created by the original material. This makes homeopathics a mystery to many and makes it difficult to run clinical trials, though multiple clinical trials have proven their effectiveness. For the most part, homeopathic medicines are safe both while you are building a baby and to give directly to your newborn. However, keep in mind that their effectiveness is in tune with the energetics of the ailment and the person who has the imbalance. Not all homeopathics are effective for all people, and not all "safe" homeopathics will be necessarily good for your baby. If you find that your baby is behaving differently while you are using a homeopathic remedy it may be helpful to try something different.

A person could study the therapeutic applications of homeopathics in the body their entire life without knowing the therapeutic use of the herbs themselves — and vice versa. It is very important to understand that we cannot conflate the many different methods of plant medicine. Botanicals and homeopathics are not the same. Becoming aware of these differences helps to better understand why a homeopathic dose of arnica is a remedy for bruising while it could be deadly to ingest arnica, the herb.

Essential Oils

Essential oils have long been used as internal medicines, and are coming back into vogue in the Western world. These powerful medicines are the subject of other wonderful books, but are not my area of expertise. In this book I mainly discuss essential oils that are not safe to ingest while building your baby or for your newborn from an aromatherapy standpoint.

Essential oils are potent medicine and should not be considered safe simply because the plants from which they are made are safe. There is a difference between "lavender oil" and a "lavender essential oil." Lavender oil is created by infusing a small amount of lavender in enough of an oil medium to just cover it for a period of time — somewhere between two and six weeks. This process pulls many different components of the plant into the oil and, when strained, can be used in a gentle way on the skin or in an internal application. It takes large quantities of plant material to make an essential oil, and the process isolates small quantities of extremely concentrated oil. What can start out as a safe and healthy plant can turn into a dangerous or even deadly cocktail in essential oil form.

Although there is definitely a time and place to use essential oils, this form of plant medicine must be approached with respect. I worry that we are building an industry with plasticware-style parties that is creating a culture of using essential oils in place of any other therapy. Too many individuals are now using essential oils as their only form of treatment without any understanding of the immense plant sacrifice it takes to create mere drops.

Be sure to check with your health care team if you are interested in using essential oils internally and are not familiar with their use. These precious drops are not a distillation of everything that makes up the plant, but an isolation of just one component, leaving the rest of the plant to go to waste. It is a double-edged sword that brings alternative therapies into the mainstream but threatens the health and vitality of the plants we depend upon at the same time. I urge readers to use essential oils wisely and with honor for the sacrifice of the plant that gave them up. Using a simple herbal tea that contains all the plant has to offer rather than one isolated compound is a much more balanced approach to building our alternative arsenal. I believe a focus on whole-plant medicine in this way is best for all of us.

Flower Essences

Flower essences are another example of energy medicine. They capture the essence of the plant's soul, vitality or personality and work on emotional wounds, blockages and weaknesses. I don't mention any flower essences in this book as there is no reason to avoid their use while building a baby. Many are recommended by the Flower Essence Society (FES) for administering to infants directly. They are gentle and can be used by anyone of any age in any condition. They tend to help us make a shift from one emotion to another and many mothers have found them helpful in soothing and calming babies. If you are interested in flower essences, pick up a good book on the boch flower essences or from FES, or consult an experienced professional.

General Herbal Components to Watch

As you work through any list of herbs that are contraindicated for women in different phases of their lives, you will see some common chemical constituents. Becoming familiar with these components can help determine the safety of a new herb you don't find in this guide.

Alkaloids

This is a much larger grouping of chemical compounds containing both beneficial and problematic individuals. They are almost all bitter. The important thing here would be to watch which type of alkaloid is occurring in any contraindicated herb. Not all alkaloids should cause concern, but some can be toxic to humans.

Pyrrolizidine Alkaloids (PAs)

PAs are alkaloids that as a whole have exhibited hepatotoxicity, or liver toxicity, in some laboratory studies. You will find different concentrations in different plants and even varying concentrations within those plants depending on the part you work with. PAs are found in plants that have a long historical use in traditional medicine. Usually there is no evidence in literature for toxicity, because the plant is consumed in its entirety rather than in the isolated manner in which PAs are studied. For an in-depth look at one plant that has been placed on a medical blacklist due to its PA content, see Appendix F. As with any herb, you should always examine all the evidence and make your own decision.

Anthraquinones and Cathartics

These are to be avoided in pregnancy and nursing because they are typically harsh and cause evacuation of the bowels, often with painful cramping. As you can imagine, this is not an appropriate action for you or your baby.

Genotoxins

This is a class of chemicals that are known to alter the DNA and potentially contribute to cancer.

Aristolochic Acid

This is an acid group that is carcinogenic, causes mutations and is toxic to the tissues of the kidney. While it also has beneficial effects in humans, the aforementioned problems make it unacceptable while pregnant or nursing.

Beta-asarone

This is one of the lower-risk compounds. It is useful to note because it is a potential liver carcinogen in high and sustained dosages. Usually, the herbs that contain beta-asarone are safe to consume as a food.

Berberine

This alkaloid is the medicinal component of quite a few of our very useful and powerful herbs. There have been no documented issues with the use of berberine-containing herbs in pregnancy. However, there is written historical evidence to show some anti-fertility activity.[34]

Cardiac Glycosides

This group of steroidal glycosides has action on the rhythm and action of the heart muscle. Small, supervised doses can be beneficial, but the risk of adverse effects is high. The negative, cathartic and potentially lethal nature of these herbs makes medical professionals caution against their use in pregnancy and lactation.

Cyanogenic Glycosides

The plants that contain these compounds contain the familiar poison cyanide. In moderate doses, many can cause death due to suffocation at the body's cellular level. Outside of pregnancy and lactation, most plants containing this compound are safe to ingest. In fact, the humble lima bean contains cyanogenic glycosides in a fairly high amount. If limas are properly soaked before eating these levels drop.

Oxalates

This is a class of salts found in the tissues of some of our more common plants. It is the oxalate that makes rhubarb leaves "toxic." In high concentrations they can be toxic, and in any concentration they bind to the calcium in our digestive tract and contribute to mineral deficiencies and bone loss, and can damage our kidneys and contribute to "stones" and "gravel" in our urinary tract. Oxalates appear in herbs as well as in common food plants such as spinach and kale. Eating a regular diet of these vegetables raw can be very dangerous for our health. The good news is that most of the oxalates present in plants can be neutralized by cooking.

Estragole

Like safrole and beta-asarone, the potential for carcinogenic damage to our livers with herbs containing this compound is low. Nonetheless, the safety of this compound is still enough in doubt that herbs containing it are generally not recommended during pregnancy and lactation. As there is no known recorded instance of human toxicity, it is fair to say that this is worth avoiding mainly in very high doses or in its essential oil form taken alone.

Safrole

Like beta-asarone, this is a low threat, but has been found to be mildly carcinogenic and damaging to our livers in high doses. There have been no recorded instances of human toxicity as a result of safrole-rich plant ingestion.[16] It has also not been found to be water-soluble. The safety of this compound is still enough in doubt that herbs containing it are generally not recommended during pregnancy and lactation.

Thujone

You will find this in many herbs that are high in volatile, or essential, oils. Because of the potential for toxicity to the nervous system, generally any herb containing thujone is contraindicated in pregnancy and lactation. It is worth noting that it is not very water-soluble, so it takes a very high dose of these herbs in tea, a moderate (read therapeutic) dose of alcoholic tincture or a straight dose of the essential oil to cause damage.

Cleansing and Detoxing

Many of our customers ask about "detoxing." In our culture, we are taught that we need to detox every once in a while after we have built up a load of toxicity. This is a gut-wrenching experience, literally, that is done with fasting and pills or gritty drinks and results in extended periods of time in the bathroom purging your insides. This model of detox is inappropriate at any time, but especially while trying to build a baby.

So what is appropriate when it comes to detox? If we focus only on the continual need to remove toxicity, we will be caught in a self-perpetuating cycle. Our current supplement market is flooded with products for purging all the chemical buildup out of our bodies. Detox is a buzzword. The underlying message here is, "Continue to immerse your body in chemical body-care solutions, eat all the processed foods you want, we've got this. Just follow our simple three-step system once a month and we'll force your body to purge so you can start again." This logic is so pervasive because we have accepted the notion that our food *has* to be toxic and our Western lifestyle is predetermined.

We need to look at detoxification with different eyes. In a very real sense we are what we eat. I have said this before, but would like to really examine what that means.

When we eat damaged foods our body actually uses their components to make our cells. This means that we are incorporating genetically modified organisms, damaged proteins, improper fat structures and much more. Our food is not just fuel — it is literally the building material that our body uses to keep our house standing. Trans fats are a great example of this, as Sally Fallon Morell tells us in her book *Nourishing Traditions*:

> Partially hydrogenated margarines and shortenings are even worse for you than the highly refined vegetable oils from which they are made because of chemical changes that occur during the hydrogenation process. Under high temperatures, the nickel catalyst causes the hydrogen atoms to change position on the fatty acid chain. Before hydrogenation, pairs of hydrogen atoms occur together on the chian, causing the chain to bend slightly and creating a concentration of electrons at the site of the double bond. This is called the *cis* formation, the configuration most commonly found in nature. With hydrogenation, one hydrogen atom of the pair is moved to the other side so that the molecule straightens. This is

called the *trans* formation, rarely found in nature. Most of these man-made *trans* fats are toxins to the body, but unfortunately your digestive system does not recognize them as such. Instead of eliminating them, your body incorporates *trans* fats into the cell membranes as though they were *cis* fats — your cells actually become partially hydrogenated![4]

The more we eat non-food containing lab-created compounds, the more our tissues are actually built with these same compounds. We become increasingly disconnected from our natural world, not just because we didn't get to the park last weekend, but because we are no longer "of" the natural world. Our cells continue to die off and new ones must be built, so this isn't a life sentence. Those of us who are building our bodies with unnatural substances are like Russian nesting dolls. The layers of disconnected food materials insulate us from the natural world. We are no longer able to "hear" through these layers. When we fully detoxify and replace our cells once again with living material, we begin to taste food again. Moreover, with proper levels of the B vitamins responsible for our ability to taste, we begin to discern the difference between food and chemicals as we are eating. It is an awakening.

You can easily make the argument that one trip through the fast-food drive-through isn't going to make permanent changes. However, with what are you choosing to build the next round of cells? Some of our cells have a longer shelf life than others. What did you eat the day that section of brain cells was laid down?

At any rate, we are continually given the opportunity to reconnect with nature through our food. Traditional societies did not have access to modern processed foods. They were more connected to the rhythm of nature because they recognized that they were part of the cycle. They were connected to what they ate — we are connected to laboratories and food-processing plants. These things are dead at best or were never living, so we have a constant feeling of malaise in our society. We are not comfortable in our own skins and have hormonal imbalances and mental disturbances. The cycles within our bodies that are meant to mirror the natural world (sleep, menstruation, digestion) are out of synch and causing many illnesses.

So what do we do? On some level we seem to grasp that we need to purge the cells that are holding toxins, dyes, harmful fats and more. The focus, sadly, is on tearing out or tearing down. We need to look at detoxification for what it truly is: an opportunity to rebuild. It is very literally a transformation. We should detoxify by balancing and tonifying the digestive system. This can be done with food! Switching to a diet of whole foods that are traditionally prepared is detoxifying. Repopulating our gut with the proper bacteria is also part of detoxification. If we create an environment where this gut flora can flourish, we have detoxified. The catch is that this type of work is ongoing, every day. It is slow, and often triggers a healing crisis that will walk us back through all the dysfunction we have encountered in our body as our toxin-holding cells are replaced with healthy ones. It is important to be prepared for the headaches, rashes, breakouts and even emotional upheaval that may occur during a healing crisis. These are the storm before the calm, the death throes of imbalance and sickness just before they pass out of the body altogether, through organs such as the liver, skin, kidneys or uterus. Many do not see this as an encouraging sign because they do not understand what is happening. Very often this is where someone decides that the "healthy" changes are making them sick and they stop what they are doing. You have to push through a healing crisis if you hope to achieve lasting balance and wellness. That said, detoxification should be slow and gentle. An intense healing crisis is inappropriate as it often signals that we are making too many changes too quickly. Appropriate detoxification is the daily work of our multiple body systems to build this house we live in. It is our daily work to give our home proper building materials. We live in a world where pollution is inevitable. We will always need our plant allies to help when small amounts of pollution are introduced from our environment. We are much better able to deal with such intrusions when our house is built on a strong foundation.

In preconception, it can be helpful to do general detoxification. Whether you do a heavy detox or gentle daily detox is dictated by your specific situation. Were you a heavy drug user or alcoholic? Did you use birth control for thirty years and now want to get pregnant? Are you a fairly healthy eater? In general, a daily detox and a digestive balancer such as triphala would be appropriate. The idea here would be to use bitters, liver supportive herbs and whole foods to remove toxicity from your body in preconception to make fertility possible and to provide the best base for fetal development. After a gentle nudge to "clean clogged filters", I have advised women, who then begin to see improvements with menstrual disorders such as irregularity, cramping and spotting.

While pregnant, any type of internal cleansing is inappropriate unless it is a gentle by-product of everyday whole foods and herbs. We should never be afraid of the tonic herbs and whole foods that aid our body in their natural processes of detox, but fasting is not a good idea. During pregnancy the body already has mechanisms in place, especially during the first trimester, for moving toxicity out of the body. Our urine changes and becomes more efficient at carrying out acidity; we often sweat more; and many experience morning sickness. These are all signs that the body is doing good work! As one of our eliminative pathways is our uterus, we do not want to use any detox products at this time. Good nutrition continues to fuel the body's own detox processes.

While nursing, detoxing is certainly tempting. Your body is shedding a uterine lining, water and much more! It is obvious that our bodies are shedding toxins and waste left over from the pregnancy as we note things like increased body odor. It is not a good idea to do any fasting or harsh detox programs. Your body will go about shedding its extra waste burden on its own without any herbal help. Nursing is not a time to purge or tear down or focus on weight loss. It is a time to allow your body to restock its personal pantry and refuel for the immense job of maintaining health while acting as a food source for your infant.

When I was nursing, I experienced stubborn body odor and changes in my skin texture. This was all indicative of the extra waste my body was trying to shed after the birthing process. There are many good herbs that can gently assist, such as red clover (*Trifolium pratense*), burdock (*Arctium lappa*), triphala and dandelion (*Taraxacum officinale*). My favorite was triphala honey but as a powder it was not a texture or a taste that I was going to do daily over a long period of time. While it is contraindicated during pregnancy, it is safe to use while nursing. Within a week I saw noticeable differences which inspired me to create a triphala honey spread that I routinely offer to nursing mothers.

Prescription, Over-The-Counter (OTC) and Illegal Drugs

It is important at all points in building a baby to think about the chemicals in pharmaceuticals. So different from herbs, many of these chemicals stay resident in our tissues long after we've taken them. The side effects set up chain events that we never intended. Some can inhibit our abilities to get pregnant, causing negative consequences for both men and women. Common high blood pressure medicines, specifically a class called sympathetic nerve inhibitors, contribute to impotence in men.

By inhibiting the body's ability to constrict blood vessels, there is no way for an erection to occur. Ulcer drugs such as Tagamet can also creat impotence in men.

The problem isn't just isolated to prescription drugs, though. OTC antihistamines and decongestants must be used sparingly while you are trying to conceive because they have been known to cause temporary impotence as well. There are so many natural and herbal alternatives to these drugs that it is worth looking into another way of doing things if you would like to rebalance for fertility.

If we understand that what we eat can be passed along to our infant, then we must assume that any chemical we ingest will affect our children. Most any OTC or prescription drug will say that you shouldn't take it without a physician's advice if you are pregnant or nursing. This isn't just legalese — it is there because in most cases, the potential for side effects is just as great, if not greater, for your infant than for you. There may be medications that you cannot avoid taking in order to maintain a health condition. Don't beat yourself up about it; instead inform yourself. What are the listed potential side effects? If you know that your drug carries a warning for stomach pain, you can work to counter that by using herbs that calm and tone the stomach. Looking through the herbs covered in this book you might come across fennel (*Foeniculum vulgare*), which would be a great choice. Using the seed in a tea or tincture would promote a good milk supply while helping to calm an angry stomach and reduce cramping.

Whenever you need to make a choice regarding the use of allopathic drugs for you or your child, consider carefully. Remember that there could be side effects for both of you because these drugs are often based on one chemical constituent (a part rather than the whole) found originally in nature and meant to work in concert with other parts. Ask questions. Most of these drugs will cross the placental or breast milk barrier in some concentration.[60] Ask yourself if you would give this drug directly to your infant or unborn child. If there is a natural alternative, why not use it? If you must use an allopathic remedy, what natural remedies support the body and mediate side effects? In the end, remember that pharmaceuticals are about targeting and killing something off (pain, bacteria, virus, etc.), while botanicals are about balancing and nourishing.

Note: A detailed account of the interaction of specific prescription drugs and over-the-counter medications and breast milk can be found in Thomas Hale's book, *Medications and Mother's Milk 2012: A Manual of Lactational Pharmacology.*

A Final Word

This book is not intended to be an end-all, be-all compendium of any herb you might take and its safety while building a baby. Rather, it is my intention to cover those herbs that are known to cause potential issues for a couple at any point in the process. It is also my intention to bring to light those herbs that might cause issues for a nursing child. Along with the herbs that are contraindicated, you will find some that are often used to treat general health issues. As you read through the list, observe the herbs' active compounds. Should you plan to use an herb not found in this book, do not assume that its absence implies its safety. Rather, compare its active compounds with herbs containing the same to deduce its relative safety or your need for concern.

Always trust your own instinct in regard to the use of herbs. If you read about an herb and it is generally regarded as safe but you still feel in your heart that it may not be right for you — go with that! There are many herbs available to us from all over the planet. While one herb may be specific for addressing a certain type of imbalance, it will rarely be the ONLY herb that can do so. Conversely, if you find an herb that you feel is right for you in the "contraindications" list, work with your health care team and do your research. I have put forth individual reasons each herb is problematic and you may find that the concern does not apply to you. Please use this book as another resource on your health care team, rather than an absolute truth. You are the owner of your own power and the guardian of that of your newborn child. Be sure that you always have the final say in any health care decision.

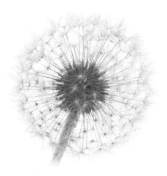

Healthy Baby Herbal Reference Guide

Using the Herbal Guide

HERBS DO NOT HAVE TO BE OVERWHELMING and complicated. For both the everyday person and the practitioner, easily accessible information makes for a better herbal experience.

Plant Name

Depending upon where you live and who you grew up with, an herb may have many different names. These **common names** can provide everyday recognition of a plant, but to be very sure of the herb you intend to use for medicinal purposes, always know the **botanical name**, which will be provided in Latin and italics.

Milk Production

Any herb that can help increase milk production during lactation is denoted as a **galactagogue** at the top of its table.

Part Used

The portion of the plant that is used medicinally is specifically addressed in this herbal. If another part of a plant is commonly used, or it is used in another form that is not listed here, do not assume that the listed analysis applies to the unlisted plant portion.

Main Constituents

This identifies some of the most important phytochemical constituents in the herb. These are not necessarily the "active" constituents and is not intended to be all-inclusive.

Safey Ratings

This is a general guide to the relative safety of each herb. A color-coded, three-category system is provided for easy reference according to the three phases of building a healthy baby (preconception, pregnancy and lactation):

Safety Ratings

No Contraindications (White)

There are no studies or historical writings to indicate there is any problem with the general population using this herb.

Use With Caution (Gray)

There are either reliable medical studies or historical writings that convince me to advise the reader to think carefully before using this herb. It is up to the individual to determine if they are using the herb in the manner that might raise a concern or if their particular constitution warrants concern.

Avoid (Black)

There is sufficient evidence in medical studies or historical writings that convince me to indicate that it is best to find an alternative.

Notes for Caution

For each herb that is listed with contraindications, there is always a reason why. Not every reason to avoid an herb will apply to you and your situation. You may read the reason and feel comfortable discussing the use of this herb with your health care team regardless of the rating.

Alternatives

When a part of a plant, a preparation of it or the *plant* itself is identified as cause for concern, I try to provide alternatives that can be used to effect similar actions in the body.

Male Fertility

Building healthy babies includes both partners. Herbs that can be utilized for the male side of the equation are included with indications as to the effect on the male system.

UpS Designation

Some medicinal herbs are highly endangered or are found in numbers and conditions that warrant concern for their future viability. Herb usage that should take this into consideration is included in two categories: "To Watch" and "At Risk."

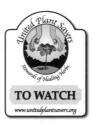

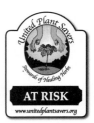

3 PHASES OF BUILDING A HEALTHY BABY
(Grayscale-coded with general safety rating)

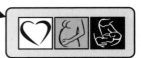

Common name (*botanical / Latin name*)

Galactagogue	[Denotes herbs that support or inhibit milk production]
Part used:	[Part(s) of plant used for herbal preparations]
Main constituents:	[Phytochemical components]
Alternatives:	[Plant(s) that might be substituted for the herb]
Notes for caution:	**During preconception:** (Specific note of concern)
	During pregnancy: (Specific note of concern)
Male fertility:	(Specific notes about male fertility)

MALE HERBS
(Discussion of herb's application to the male system)

NOTES FOR CAUTION
(Grayscale-coded by general safety rating)

REPRODUCTIVE PHASE

 Preconception

 Pregnancy

 Lactation

GENERAL SAFETY RATING

   No Contraindications.
Generally safe to use.

   Use with Caution. There may be
reason for further discussion or
consideration prior to use.

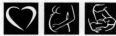 **Generally Avoid.** Regarded as
unsafe due to potential
problems or side effects.

Alfalfa (*Medicago sativa*)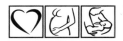

Galactagogue	
Part used:	Aerial portions
Main constituents:	Vitamins A, B$_2$, B$_3$, B$_5$, B$_6$, B$_{12}$, C, E, K; calcium; iron; magnesium; beta-carotene; protein; chromium; cobalt; fiber; fat; phosphorus; potassium; volatile oils; resin; flavonoids (genistein, daidzein, formononetin); coumarin derivatives; saponins; alkaloids (trigonelline, stachydrine, homostachydrine)[35]
Alternatives:	None

Alfalfa is often found in a nutritive blend, perhaps to boost calcium, iron or B-vitamins. It is very balanced in its nutrient load and does not need to be combined with anything else to maximize the absorption of some of its key nutrients; for example, it contains both calcium and the magnesium needed to use calcium properly in the body. Alfalfa is very helpful in all deficiencies related to inflammation, such as inappropriate cholesterol levels. As a homeopathic remedy, alfalfa is known as *Lactuca virosa*, and is used for stimulating milk production.

REPRODUCTIVE PHASE
Preconception   Pregnancy   Lactation

GENERAL SAFETY RATING No Contraindications Use with Caution Generally Avoid

Internal use   External use

           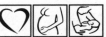

Aloe (*Aloe vera*)

Part used:	Juice from the leaves (fresh or dehydrated)
Main constituents:	Fiber; vitamins B_3, A, C; zinc; sodium; silicon; anthraquinones (aloin, aloe-emodin); anthraglycosides[35]
Alternatives:	Dandelion root (*Taraxacum officinale*) or yellow dock root (*Rumex crispus*)
Notes for caution:	**Internal use during pregnancy:** As a purgative, this herb exerts a downward energy in the pelvic region, which makes it inappropriate during pregnancy. **Internal use during lactation:** It is believed that aloe could have a possible purging effect on the bowels of an infant who is nursing when the mother takes aloe internally.

Internally, aloe is one of the stronger laxatives known as evacuants, which works by chemical stimulation of the brain or bowels and can irritate intestinal lining. This action in a child could cause electrolyte loss, pain or discomfort. Externally, aloe is safe for mother and child so long as it is not used on the nipple while nursing, and can be helpful for minor burns, cuts and rashes — even for diaper rash. Aloe is also a mild and gentle sunscreen, blocking up to 30 percent of the sun's ultraviolet rays.[36]

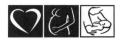

Andrographis (*Andrographis paniculata*)

Galactagogue	
Part used:	Leaves; roots
Main constituents:	Andrographolide
Alternatives:	Shiitake (*Lentinula edodes*)
Notes for caution:	**During preconception:** It is possible that andrographis can reduce sex drive. It is also worth avoiding because of the possibility of abortifacient effects. **During Pregnancy:** There are documented incidents of the use of this herb as an abortifacient.

Andrographis is primarily used in ayurveda and traditional Chinese medicine for its antiviral, anti-inflammatory, immunostimulant and liver-supportive properties.

 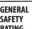

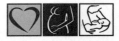

Angelica (*Angelica archangelica*)

Part used:	Aerial portions; seeds; root
Main constituents:	Psoralens; bergapten; beta-sitosterol; coumarins; limonene; umbelliferone
Alternatives:	Appetite stimulant: bitter orange (*Citrus aurantium* spp., *Citrus amara*) Pain Relief: rosemary (*Rosemarinus officinalis*)
Notes for caution:	**During preconception:** This herb is a known emmenagogue.
	During pregnancy: This herb is an emmenagogue and is often used by experienced midwives during labor to facilitate contractions and expel the placenta.[37]
Author's note:	This herb can potentially raise blood sugar. Diabetics should consider its use carefully.

This herb traditionally has been used to reduce the growth of tumors. It is also effective for digestive problems and therefore popular in many bitters formulas. It is effective in reducing the pain associated with coughs, urinary tract infections and the cramping associated with a woman's cycle. Angelica is one of the digestive herbs that have been used successfully to stimulate appetite in the case of eating disorder or debility. Many of the plants in this family have a close affinity with women and are often used as tonics. This particular angelica can encourage the start of a delayed cycle and can be helpful in regulating menstrual irregularities.

REPRODUCTIVE PHASE   Preconception Pregnancy Lactation GENERAL SAFETY RATING No Contraindications Use with Caution   Generally Avoid

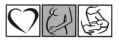

Anise (*Pimpinella anisum*)

Galactagogue	
Part used:	Seeds
Main constituents:	Volatile oil (anethole); fatty oils; choline
Alternatives:	None
Notes for caution:	**During pregnancy:** There should not be an issue with using this herb as a seasoning or tea, but at a therapeutic dose, anise is a recognized emmenagogue.

Anise is used to ease spasms in the digestive tract and to reduce flatulence. It is also often found in natural cough and cold formulas meant to help with the spasms in the respiratory tract that lead to non-productive coughing.

Internal use   **External use**

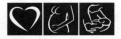

Arborvitae (*Thuja occidentalis*)

Part used:	Leaves
Main constituents:	Thujone; mucilage; tannins
Alternatives:	None
Notes for caution:	**Internal use during preconception:** Arborvitae can act as an abortifacient. Avoid it while trying to get pregnant.
	Internal use during pregnancy: The herb is not appropriate to use either as an essential oil or as an alcoholic extract. It also is not appropriate to take a very high dose of tea or to use tea excessively. If used in any of these ways during pregnancy, it can be act as an emmenagogue or abortifacient.
	Internal use during lactation: The constituent thujone found in arborvitae can have a negative effect through breast milk if the herb is taken improperly while nursing. Do not use the essential oil or an alcoholic extract of arborvitae during this time, and do not take a very high dose of tea or use tea excessively.

This herb has a wide range of traditional uses in Native American groups. Its properties as a diuretic and expectorant made it very useful for issues related to arthritic pain and chest congestion. Due to the presence of thujone, an internal safe dosage is difficult to determine without the assistance of an experienced practitioner. Thujone is not water-soluble. Occasional use of this herb as a small part of a tea formula may not cause a problem.

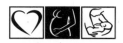

Arisaema (tian nan xing) (*Arisaema triphyllum*)

Part used:	Rhizome
Main constituents:	Calcium oxalate; starch
Alternatives:	Elecampane (*Inula helenium*)
Notes for caution:	**During pregnancy:** Avoid it.[38]

This herb is used in traditional Chinese medicine to relieve deep colds and lung congestion.

Herbal use internal   Homeopathic use

Arnica (*Arnica montana*)

Part used:	Flower (external use only); homeopathic preparations (external use only)
Main constituents:	Essential oil; sesquiterpene lactones; bitter glycosides; alkaloid; polyacetylenes; flavonoids; tannins
Alternatives:	None
Notes for caution:	**Herbal use:** arnica is toxic when taken internally.

When used as an external liniment or cream, arnica is a supreme remedy for bruising or tissue trauma, but it must never be used on broken skin. In addition, it should never be used around the area where a woman nurses or during skin-to-skin contact with her infant. It is very common in homeopathic preparations internally and many new mothers would be wise to take advantage of the herb in this form. It's especially helpful in healing tissues that are bruised and stretched during birth.

REPRODUCTIVE
PHASE
Preconception Pregnancy Lactation

GENERAL
SAFETY
RATING
No Contraindications   Use with Caution   Generally Avoid

Artichoke (*Cynara scolymus*)

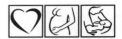

Part used:	Leaf
Main constituents:	Cynarin; beta-sitosterol; luteolin; stigmasterol
Alternatives:	None

Artichoke leaf has been used since ancient times as a digestive aide. It is known to stimulate the gallbladder to provide relief for general gassiness. It also appears to lower total blood cholesterol. Artichoke is a common ingredient in bitters formulas that stimulate the production of bile and aid in proper digestion.

Asefetida (hing) (*Ferula assa-foetida*)

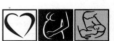

Part used:	Root
Main constituents:	Resin; gum; oil; ferulic acid
Alternatives:	Fennel (*Foeniculum vulgare*); dill (*Anethum graveolens*); anise (*Pimpinella anisum*)
Notes for caution:	**During pregnancy:** asafetida has traditionally been used as an abortifacient and is also an emmenagogue.
	During lactation: Some believe that this herb can cause colic in a nursing infant.

Asafetida is a common seasoning that generally smells and tastes stronger than an onion. Just as the onion has a reputation for causing digestive unrest in a nursing infant, asafetida is believed to do the same.

REPRODUCTIVE PHASE		GENERAL SAFETY RATING			
	Preconception Pregnancy Lactation		No Contraindications	Use with Caution	Generally Avoid

Asarabacca (*Asarum europaeum*)

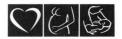

Part used:	Roots; leaves
Main constituents:	Beta-asarone
Alternatives:	Elecampane (*Inula helenium*)
Notes for caution:	Beta-asarone is only mildly toxic, but the purgative effect of this herb is worthy of caution.

At one time, this herb was an ingredient in "snuff," a powder treatment that was snorted to relieve congestion or headache. English botanist, herbalist and physician Nicholas Culpeper used this herb internally for its emetic properties, so it is not appropriate for preconception, pregnancy or nursing.

Ashwaganda (*Withania somnifera*)

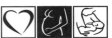

Galactagogue	
Part used:	Root
Main constituents:	Withanolides; glycosides; several different alkaloids
Alternatives:	Ginseng (*Panax ginseng, Panax quinquefolius*); eleuthero (*Eleutherococcus senticosus, Acanthopanax senticosus*)
Notes for caution:	**During pregnancy:** Ashwaganda has a history of use as an abortifacient.
Male fertility:	This herb is excellent for enhancing fertility and sexual performance when they are negatively affected by stress.

Mainly used in ayurvedic medicine, this adaptogenic herb is great for those who are recovering from stress and who are overworked and overwrought. Ashwagandha is much more than a general body tonic. It works on our adrenal glands and can help normalize cortisol and the body's sex hormones. The Latin name, *somnifera*, hints at its power to help with the disturbances in sleep patterns that overstressed adrenal glands can cause.

Astragalus (*Astragalus membranaceous*)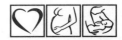

Part used:	Root
Main constituents:	Vitamins B$_1$, B$_2$; zinc; sodium; silicon; selenium; magnesium; iron; fat; fiber; chromium; astragalosides and other immunostimulant polysaccharides; beta-sitosterol; flavonoids (rutin, quercetin)[35]
Alternatives:	None
Male fertility:	Traditionally used to increase the quantity and motility of sperm.

This great adaptogen comes to us from the ayurvedic tradition. It is especially good for recovery from birth, as this herb is used to build resistance to weakness and disease, increase energy and balance the energy of the internal organs. It also stimulates the rebuilding of our bone marrow. After pregnancy and while nursing, many women are low in their nutritional reserves because of the high demands on their bodies, and astragalus is invaluable in rebuilding energy levels.

Bamboo shavings (*Caulis bambusae in taeniis*)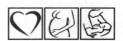

Part used:	Stem
Main constituents:	Cellulose; pentosans; lignin; ash; silica; calcium; phosphorus; iron
Alternatives:	None

Bamboo shavings are used to dissolve phlegm. They are known for treating the tough, yellow, hard-to-get-out phlegm that is part of a respiratory infection. They also can be used for the relief of vomiting, particularly in morning sickness.

REPRODUCTIVE PHASE   GENERAL SAFETY RATING

Preconception Pregnancy Lactation   No Contraindications   Use with Caution   Generally Avoid

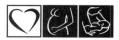

Barberry (*Berberis vulgaris*)

Part used:	Dried berries; roots; bark
Main constituents:	Vitamins B_1, B_2, B_3; tin; sodium; silicon; selenium; manganese; magnesium; iron; fat; fiber; cobalt; calcium; aluminum; alkaloids (berberine, palmatine, jatorrhizine, calumbamine); tannin[35]
Alternatives:	Marsh tea homeopathic (*Ledum palustre*); shiitake (*Lentinula edodes*); elder (*Sambucus nigra*)
Notes for caution:	**During pregnancy:** Berberine is an alkaloid and mild toxin that has a depressant effect on the heart and lungs. There is some evidence that it is also a uterine stimulant in some doses. **During lactation:** Berberine is an alkaloid and a mild toxin that has a depressant effect on the heart and lungs. There is evidence that it is also a uterine stimulant in some doses. This herb could be especially problematic if a baby has been diagnosed with jaundice.

Like goldenseal, this herb is great for an infection. It is antimicrobial and anti-inflammatory. Because goldenseal is a threatened species, barberry is a sustainable substitute, but it must be used carefully. Use barberry *only* for the duration of infection or up to a week at a time.

REPRODUCTIVE PHASE   Preconception   Pregnancy   Lactation   GENERAL SAFETY RATING   No Contraindications   Use with Caution   Generally Avoid

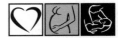

Barley Sprouts (Mai Ya) (*Hordeum vulgare*)

Antigalactagogue	
Part used:	Sprouts
Main constituents:	Potassium; calcium; magnesium; iron; copper; phosphorus; manganese; zinc; beta-carotene; vitamins A, B₁, B₂, B₆, and C; folic acid; pantothenic acid; tin; sodium; silicon; selenium; fat; fiber; cobalt; chromium; aluminum[35]
Alternatives:	Hawthorn berry (*Crataegus* spp.)
Notes for caution:	**During pregnancy:** Barley sprouts exert a strong downward energy in the pelvis that may not be appropriate during pregnancy.
	During lactation: This herb is an antigalactagogue and will decrease milk flow.

Barley sprouts often are used in traditional Chinese medicine for relieving congestion in the digestive system caused by the buildup of too many starches. They are helpful during weaning to dry up a mother's milk supply. For that reason, they should not be used when weaning is not the goal.

 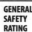

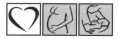
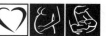

Herb   Essential oil/ Alcoholic tincture

Basil (*Ocimum basilicum*)

Part used:	Aerial portions; essential oil
Main constituents:	Volatile oils such as estragole and safrole
Alternatives:	None
Notes for caution:	**Herb use during pregnancy:** High and prolonged therapeutic doses can have emmenagogue and abortifacient effects. This is not the case, however, when using the herb as a seasoning or as an herbal tea.
	Herb use during lactation: There are possible mutagenic effects for the nursing child due to the accumulation of estragole if the mother is ingesting high quantities of basil.
	Essential oil/alcoholic extract use during pregnancy: Basil contains both estragole and safrole when used as an essential oil or as an alcoholic extract. Although estragole's toxicity is likely small, safrole is a known carcinogen.
	Essential oil/alcoholic extract use during lactation: The essential oil or alcohol extract contains safrole, which is a known carcinogen.

Basil is a common culinary additive put in pizza, pasta, pesto and other foods. There have been no recorded instances of health problems for a baby in pregnancy or while nursing due to a mother's ingestion of basil. However, it contains volatile compounds (estragole and safrole) that could potentially cause problems if taken in certain forms or to excess. Mothers should use in moderation during pregnancy or while nursing.

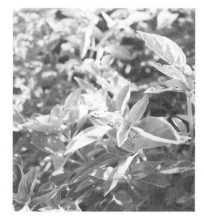

Basil (Ocimum basilicum)

Bearberry (uva ursi) (*Arctostaphylos uva-ursi*)

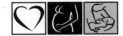

Part used:	Aerial portions
Main constituents:	Vitamin A; iron; silicon; protein; manganese; fat; fiber; chromium; calcium; aluminum; selenium; hydroquinones (arbutin); iridoids; flavonoids; alantoin; resin; volatile oils; tannins (ursolic acid, malic acid, gallic acid)[35]
Alternatives:	Urinary tract toner: dandelion leaf (*Taraxacum officinale*); nettle (*Urtica dioica*)
	Urinary tract infection prevention: cranberry (*Vaccinium vitis-idaea*)
	Kidney and bladder stones: cornsilk (*Zea mays*); goldenrod (*Solidago virgaurea*)
Notes for caution:	**During pregnancy:** This herb can stimulate contractions.
	During lactation: Because of its possible inhibiting effect on B-lymphocyte cell maturation, prolonged use during nursing can affect an infant's liver development.[39]

Bearberry, or uva-ursi, is an important herb that helps the kidneys detoxify the body. It is especially effective for those suffering with a urinary tract infection or kidney or bladder stones. It is a tonic herb and is generally very safe to use. Those who are prone to urinary tract infections (UTIs) should keep a tincture of uva-ursi at home. This herb has an affinity for the genitourinary system and has the ability to kill off *E. coli*. It operates best in an alkaline environment, so refined sugars such as sugary cranberry juice and flours should be eliminated during uva-ursi use. Bearberry is often taken in formula on a regular basis to help strengthen, soothe and tone the urinary tract. Nursing mothers should limit the use of this herb to times when they are contending with an active urinary tract infection. Once the infection is cleared up, use of the herb should be discontinued.

Bee Balm (*Monarda* spp.)

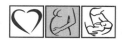

Part used:	Aerial parts
Main constituents:	Thymol; cavacrol; rosmarinic acid
Alternatives:	None
Notes for caution:	During pregnancy: In excessive doses, bee balm can act as an emmenagogue.

This herb has a mild, soothing effect on the nerves and also has antiseptic, antibacterial and stomach-settling actions. It is delicious in salads and an absolute must-have in your kitchen herb garden for its cheeriness and abilities to attract pollinators. It has an interesting patriotic past, being an herb that was used after the Boston Tea Party to replace the lost source of *Camellia sinensis*.

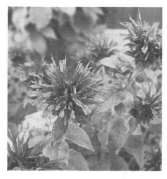

Bee Balm (Monarda *spp.*)

Betel Nut (sopari) (*Areca catechu*)

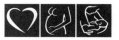

Part used:	Nut
Main constituents:	Alkaloids (arecoline, arecaidine, guvacine, and guvacoline); volatile oils; tannins; gum
Alternatives:	None
Notes for caution:	During preconception, pregnancy and lactation: Although there are no studies to substantiate claims of carcinogenic content, in animal studies betel nut is known to be toxic to a developing fetus.

This herb is a stimulant with a long history of ceremonial use. Today, unless the mother is a member of a traditional society that still chews this nut, she is more likely to come across it in Chinese tooth powders. Avoid it.

Bilberry (*Vaccinium myrtillus*)

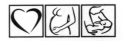

Part used:	Fruit
Main constituents:	Vitamins A. B₁, B₂, B₃, C; zinc; tin; selenium; protein; potassium; phosphorus; manganese; magnesium; iron; fat; fiber; calcium; aluminum; essential oil; resin: anthocyanidins[35]; benzoic acid; caffeic acid; epicatechin; epigallocatechin (EPCG); gallic acid; hydroquinone; isoquercetin; quercetin[41]
Alternatives:	None

Bilberry is often eaten for its positive effects on vision.

Birth Root (*Trillium erectum*)

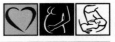

Part used:	Root
Main constituents:	Tannic acid, saponin; gum; resin; starch
Alternatives:	None
Notes for caution:	**During preconception:** Use with caution, as trillium is an emmenagogue.
	During pregnancy: Trillium is a powerful uterine stimulant. Traditionally, it was used only during birth and only by a skilled practitioner.

Trillium is most used in connection with the female reproductive system. It is an emmenagogue and an important tool for midwives during a stalled labor.

 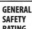

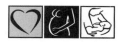

Bitter Melon (*Momordica charantia*)

Galactagogue	
Part used:	Fruits
Main constituents:	Gourmarin
Alternatives:	Jerusalem artichoke (*Helianthus tuberosus*)
Notes for caution:	**During preconception:** Use with caution, as bitter melon is an emmenagogue.
	During pregnancy: The fruit of bitter melon is an emmenagogue and an abortifacient.

This edible melon is currently being used to lower and maintain blood sugar levels in those with diabetes. It is safe and effective, and a delicious vegetable that can be grown right along with other squash in the garden. For those rare people who suffer from favism, it is important to note that bitter melon can bring on typical symptoms such as faintness, anemia, headache, nausea and more. Those with the condition should avoid bitter melon.

   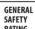

Bitter Orange (*Citrus aurantium* spp.; *Citrus amara*)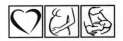

Part used:	Peel
Main constituents:	P-Synephrine; octopamine; hordenine; tyramine; N-methyltyramine
Alternatives:	None

Bitter orange has been under scrutiny in the media because of some inaccurate analysis of its chemical makeup. P-Synephrine, one of the main constituents of bitter orange, is related to ephedrine, although it does not have the same negative effects on blood pressure and heart rate. M-Synephrine has been falsely attributed to the chemical make-up of bitter orange, but it does not appear there naturally and seems to be appearing in products as a result of the addition of a synthetic ingredient.[40] M-synephrine is more like ephedrine in its cardiovascular activity. There are no known adverse effects linked to either animals or humans in response to the use of bitter orange, and the FDA has admitted to misstatements. It can, therefore, be considered safe to ingest.

Bitter orange is found in a number of common foods: fruit juice, teas, liquors such as Triple Sec and marmalade. It is anti-inflammatory, antibacterial and antifungal and is useful for digestive complaints and for loss of appetite, indigestion, diarrhea and constipation.

REPRODUCTIVE PHASE Preconception Pregnancy Lactation GENERAL SAFETY RATING No Contraindications Use with Caution Generally Avoid

Black Cohosh
(*Cimicifuga racemosa; Actaea racemosa*)

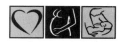

Part used:	Roots
Main constituents:	Vitamins A, B$_3$; silicon; selenium; potassium; phosphorus; magnesium; iron; fat; fiber; cobalt; chromium; calcium; aluminum; resin; bitter glycosides; ranunculin (anemonin when dried); tannins (isoferulic acid, salicylic acid, gallic acid); saponins; volatile oils; cimicifugin[35]
Alternatives:	**As an antispasmodic:** Skullcap (*Scutellaria lateriflora*); chamomile (*Matricaria recutita*) **For pain and relief of inflammation:** Rosemary (*Rosmarinus officinalis*) **For hormone regulation:** Chaste Tree (*Vitex agnus-castus*)
Notes for caution:	**During preconception:** Use with caution because the herb is an emmenagogue. **During pregnancy:** Use only during the last couple weeks of pregnancy to prepare the uterus for effective contractions. Unsafe at any other time during pregnancy. **During Lactation:** There is evidence of an irritant quality for the nursing newborn, as well as a potential toxicity in large doses.

Black cohosh is best known in its role as an aid in menopause. It has many other valuable uses, however, both in the female body and for general use. Black cohosh is a hormonal balancer and regulator. It is estrogenic in nature and can sometimes be given for the healing of tinnitus. It is very valuable for arthritic, neurological and muscular pain. Women who are taking black cohosh on a regular basis for any of these conditions prior to pregnancy and plan to return to use postnatally should wait until they are no longer nursing.

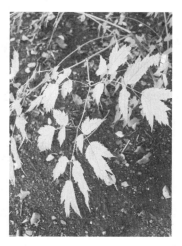

*Black Cohosh (*Cimicifuga racemosa; Actaea racemosa.*)*

Blackberry (*Rubus fruticosus; Rubus villosus*)

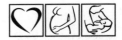

Part used:	Root
Main constituents:	Tannins (gallic acid); villosin; starch; calcium oxalate
Alternatives:	None

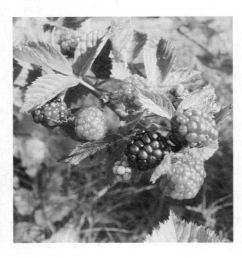

Highly astringent, blackberry root is a very effective remedy for diarrhea or any kind of loose bowel issues.

*Blackberry (*Rubus fruticosus; Rubus villosus*)*

Blackhaw Viburnum (*Viburnum prunifolium*)

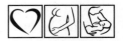

Part used:	Bark from the root, stem or trunk
Main constituents:	Triterpenoids; coumarin; valerianic acid; salicosides; tannin
Alternatives:	None

Black haw often can be used interchangeably with cramp bark. Both are active in relaxing the uterus and relieving cramps. Black haw also is indicated for bringing on a delayed cycle. It has a relaxing effect on blood vessels and is especially useful for reducing blood pressure.

REPRODUCTIVE PHASE Preconception Pregnancy Lactation GENERAL SAFETY RATING  No Contraindications Use with Caution Generally Avoid

Black Walnut Hull (*Juglans nigra*)

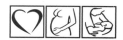

Part used:	Hull of the nut
Main constituents:	Tin; silicon; selenium; potassium; iron; fat; fiber; cobalt; chromium; aluminum; Iodine; resin; flavonoids (quercetin); juglone[35]
Alternatives:	None

Black walnut hull is one of the most popular herbs to use for ridding the body of internal worms. It is also very effective as an external salve for fungi and as a skin wash for yeast infections.

Bladderwrack (*Fucus vesiculosus*)

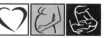

Part used:	Thallus (Leaf)
Main constituents:	Algin; mannitol; carotene; zeaxanthin; iodine; bromine; vitamins B_1, B_2, B_{12}, E; magnesium
Alternatives:	Sea salt
	For hypothyroidism: Eleuthero (*Eleutherococcus senticosus*; *Acanthopanax senticosus*)
	For calcium: Red raspberry (*Rubus ideaus*); oatstraw (*Avena sativa*)
Notes for caution:	**During pregnancy:** Excessive consumption during pregnancy can lead to infantile goiter.[34] It is best to keep the therapeutic dosage of any type of seaweed to no more than 0.25 grams daily.
	During lactation: The high iodine content found in seaweeds can disrupt the iodine used by the thyroid of the nursing infant.

Bladderwrack can be very useful in helping with the symptoms of an underactive thyroid gland and goiter. It is a great source of both iodine and calcium. During lactation, it is best to avoid in more than the small amount naturally occurring in food.

| REPRODUCTIVE PHASE | Preconception | Pregnancy | Lactation | GENERAL SAFETY RATING | No Contraindications | Use with Caution | Generally Avoid |

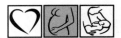

Blessed Thistle (*Cnicus benedictus*)

Galactagogue	
Part used:	Aerial portions; seeds
Main constituents:	Vitamins A, B₁, B₂; tin; sodium; selenium; potassium; phosphorus; magnesium; iron; fiber; cobalt; chromium; calcium; aluminum; sesquiterpene lactone glycoside; cnicin[35]; acetic acid; amentoflavone; arbutin; Esculetin; myristic acid; oleanic acid; salicylic acid; scopoletin; ursolic acid
Alternatives:	Fennel (*Foeniculum vulgare*); bitter orange (*Citrus aurantium* spp., *Citrus amara*)
Notes for caution:	**During pregnancy:** By irritating the digestive tract, this herb can become an emmenagogue. Furthermore, well-known herbalist Susun Weed shares that many thistles have traditionally been used as abortifacients.[42]

Many women come upon blessed thistle for the first time in their milk-producing tea. It is, in fact, a well-known galactogogue. It also contains a bitter component, so it is helpful in digestive issues. This bitter property is responsible for the use of blessed thistle as an appetite stimulant for women with an eating disorder or who have lost interest in eating due to debility.

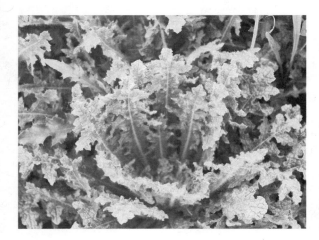

Blessed Thistle
(Cnicus benedictus*)*

Internal use   **External use**

 Bloodroot
(*Sanguinaria canadensis*)

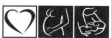   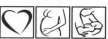

Part used:	Rhizomes
Main constituents:	Sanguinarine; berberine; protopine; chelerythrine; homochelidine; resin; citric acid; malic acid
Alternatives:	Elecampane (*Inula helenium*); mullein (*Verbascum thapsus*)
Notes for caution:	**During pregnancy:** Berberine is an alkaloid and a mild toxin that has a depressant effect on the heart and lungs. There is some evidence that it is also a uterine stimulant in some doses. **During lactation:** Berberine is an alkaloid and a mild toxin that has a depressant effect on the heart and lungs. There is some evidence that it is also a uterine stimulant in some doses. This herb could be especially problematic if your baby has been diagnosed with jaundice.

For internal use, bloodroot is a great herb to have around for bronchitis, asthma or any other respiratory disease that requires either an expectorant or a bronchiole relaxant. Externally, it often is applied to remove skin tags. The use of this herb should be limited as it is currently one of our threatened native plants.

REPRODUCTIVE PHASE   **GENERAL SAFETY RATING**

Preconception Pregnancy Lactation   No Contraindications   Use with Caution   Generally Avoid

Blue Cohosh
(*Caulophyllum thalictroides*)

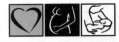

Part used:	Root
Main constituents:	Vitamins A, B_1, B_2, B_3; tin; silicon; selenium; protein; phosphorus; manganese; iron; fat; fiber; cobalt; chromium; aluminum; steroidal saponins (caulosaponin); alkaloids (scaulophylline, anagyrine, baptifoline, and magnoflorine); flavonoids (leontin, hederagenin)[35]
Alternatives:	None
Notes for caution:	**During preconception:** Blue cohosh is an emmenagogue.
	During pregnancy: The herb is a strong uterine stimulant and can be an abortifacient at any other time in a pregnancy other than the last week.

Only an experienced practitioner should administer blue cohosh. It is a strong uterine stimulant that is often used in the last week of a pregnancy to prepare the uterus for contractions. It also can be used in combination with other herbs to move along a stalled labor. The use of blue cohosh should be limited because it is currently one of our threatened native plants.

Blue Vervain (*Verbena hastate*)

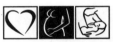

Part used:	Aerial portions
Main constituents:	Mucilage; bitters; iridoid glycosides; caffeic acid
Alternatives:	Goldenrod (*Solidago virgaurea*); cornsilk (*Zea mays*)
Notes for caution:	**During pregnancy:** This herb can cause uterine contractions.

Blue vervain is a diuretic that has been used traditionally for issues with the kidney such as stones and infections. It is also considered to be a "tonic emetic" because it can help expel toxins by way of vomiting. In lower doses, it is often used in the treatment of hot flashes to correct the body's heat pump mechanism if it has gone awry.

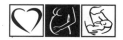

Boneset (*Eupatorium perfoliatum*)

Part used:	Aerial portions
Main constituents:	Vitamin B$_3$; sodium; silicon; selenium; protein; phosphorus; manganese; magnesium; iron; fiber; calcium; sesquiterpene lactones (euperfolin, euperfolitin, eufoliatin); polysaccharides; flavonoids (eupatorin, quercitin. kaempferol, astragalin); saponins; sitosterol; alkaloids; inulin; tannin; resinl chromenes; sesquiterpenes; alpha-amyrin; triterpenes; dendroidinic acid; diterpenes; eupafolin; terpenoids[35, 41]
Alternatives:	Elder (*Sambucus nigra*); echinacea (*Echinacea purpurea*)
Notes for caution:	**During pregnancy:** Boneset's high nitrate content has demonstrated an abortifacient effect in grazing cattle.

This is one of the best herbs available to help with the symptoms of the flu. It can soothe aches and pains, and can also bring down a fever.

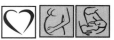

Borage (*Borago officinalis*)

Galactagogue	
Part used:	Aerial portions; flowers
Main constituents:	Saponins; mucilage; tannins; essential oil; vitamin A
Alternatives:	Sunflower (*Helianthus annuus*)
Notes for caution:	**During Pregnancy and lactation:** Borage contains pyrrolizidine alkaloids.

Borage is an important tonic for our adrenal glands and is also often used as a mood lifter. It is a traditional favorite for increasing a mother's milk supply. At a time when many women experience mild baby blues, why not use an herb that will increase their milk production *and* give them a lift? Most of the pyrrolizidine alkaloids in borage are not water-soluble, so if a woman is using borage in a tea, her risk is greatly reduced.

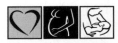

Broom (*Cytisus scoparius*)

Part used:	Tops
Main constituents:	Sparteine; scoparin; volatile oil; tannin; fat; wax; sugar
Alternatives:	Dandelion (*Taraxacum officinale*)
Notes for caution:	**During preconception:** Because this herb can cause contractions, women attempting to conceive should use it with caution.
	During pregnancy: Broom is known to cause contractions.

Broom is a diuretic herb often used when low blood pressure is caused by a weak heart.

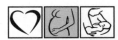

Buchu (*Barosma betulina; Agathosma betulina*)

Part used:	Leaves
Main constituents:	Vitamins A, B$_1$, C[35]; diosphenol; mucilages; diosmin; pugelone[41]
Alternatives:	Dandelion (*Taraxacum officinale*)
Notes for caution:	**During pregnancy:** It is theoretically problematic to treat edema in pregnancy with diuretics because of the potential to reduce plasma volume and thereby decrease placental perfusion. However, studies to date have not shown this to occur.[43]

Buchu has its action in the urinary tract and is often used as an antimicrobial and antiseptic in combination with other urinary tract healing herbs. It can be considered for edema during pregnancy if suggested and overseen by an experienced practitioner.

Buckthorn (*Rhamnus cathartica*)

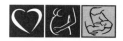

Part used:	Fruit
Main constituents:	Anthraquinones (rhamnocarthrin); vitamin C
Alternatives:	Dandelion Root (*Taraxacum officinale*); yellow dock root (*Rumex crispus*)
Notes for caution:	**During preconception and pregnancy:** High amounts of anthraquinones could potentially be abortifacient.
	During lactation: Because anthraquinones are partially passed through milk, it is believed that this herb can have a laxative effect in infants. There is also the potential to pass along the genotoxins emodin and aloe-emodin.

Buckthorn is one of the stronger laxatives known as evacuants, which works by chemical stimulation of the brain or bowels and can irritate the intestinal lining.

Bugleweed (*Lycopus virginicus; Lycopus europaeus*)

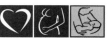

Antigalactagogue	
Part used:	Leaves
Main constituents:	Flavone glycosides; volatile oil; tannins
Alternatives:	Lemon balm (*Melissa officinalis*); motherwort (*Leonardus cardiaca*)
Notes for caution:	**During preconception and pregnancy:** Bugleweed is believed to disrupt hormone production in the pituitary, which can affect fertility.
	During lactation: The herb is believed to reduce milk supply.

Bugleweed is one of the best herbs for an overactive thyroid gland. It also can be very helpful for issues with the heart when there is a build-up of fluid in the body. This herb is not dangerous for mother or baby during the nursing relationship, so if the mother has a condition that requires treatment with it, there is no reason to avoid it. However, she should work with a lactation consultant so that her milk supply can be monitored. Any reduction in milk production can potentially be offset with galactagogues.

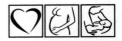

Burdock (niu ban zi) (*Arctium lappa*)

Part used:	Root
Main constituents:	Inulin; polyacetylenes; volatile acids (acetic, proprianic, butyric, isovaleric); non-hydroxyl acids (lauric, myristic, stearic, palmitic); polyphenolic acids; tannins; terpenes; vitamins A, B_1, B_2; calcium; iron; manganese; phosphorus; zinc; tin; sodium; silicon; selenium; protein; potassium; magnesium; fiber; cobalt; chromium; aluminum[35]
Alternatives:	None

Internally, burdock root is especially helpful for super-dry skin conditions such as psoriasis, dry eczema and dandruff. It also can be a liver-cleansing herb and helpful in eliminating acne. Because of its action in the liver, it aids in proper hormonal balance and can be useful in conditions such as endometriosis and uterine fibroids.

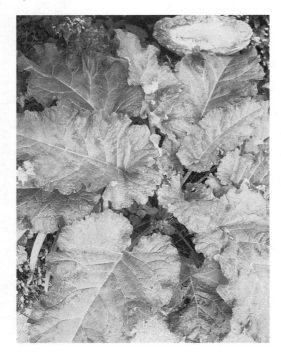

Burdock or Niu Ban Zi

(Arctium lappa)

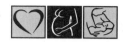

Butterbur (*Petasites hybridus; Petasites officinalis*)

Part used:	Rhizomes
Main constituents:	Essential oil; mucilage; bitter glycosides; tannin
Alternatives:	Elecampane (*Inula helenium*); wild cherry bark (*Prunus serotina*); cramp bark (*Viburnum opulus*)
Notes for caution:	**During preconception:** The herb is an emmenagogue.
	During pregnancy: Butterbur is believed to be an emmenagogue and also to be a fetal toxin due to the presence of pyrrolizidine alkaloids.
	During lactation: It is speculated that pyrrolizidine alkaloids might be toxic to the liver of the nursing infant.

Because of its antispasmodic qualities, butterbur is often used to help control asthma. It is also being used with some success in seasonal allergies. For more information on the safety of pyrrolizidine alkaloids, see Appendix F.

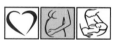

Buttercup (*Ranunculus* spp.)

Part used:	Leaf and root of fresh plants
Main constituents:	Ranunculin
Alternatives:	Topical application of nettles (*Urtica dioica*)
Notes for caution:	**During pregnancy:** Buttercup may possibly stimulate the uterus and cause contractions.

Buttercup is mainly used externally and is extremely irritating. It is known to raise blisters and irritate the tissues over an area, pulling up deep toxicity and inflammation. It is often used to help with the pain of arthritis or gout.

Conceiving Healthy Babies

Calendula (*Calendula officinalis*)

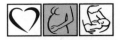

Part used:	Flowers
Main constituents:	Calendulin; beta-carotene; other carotenoids; isoquercitrin; narcissin; rutin; amyrin; lupeol; sterols; volatile oils
Alternatives:	None
Notes for caution:	**During pregnancy:** In early pregnancy, this herb should be used sparingly. In the first trimester, it can have emmenagogue and abortifacient qualities.

Externally, this bright yellow flower has a long history of use for cuts, bruises, burns and minor infections. It has antibacterial, antifungal and anti-inflammatory properties. New mothers can use it combined with comfrey for a sitz bath mixture. Calendula oil or balm are also very useful for cracked or irritated nipples. Many of the creams on the market for this purpose are not safe for an infant to ingest and must be wiped off often, while a preparation of calendula will not only heal the area quickly but also be safe for a nursing infant.

Internally, calendula can be a very helpful regulator of a woman's cycle, and it is this action in the body that demands caution in early pregnancy. It also can be useful for ulcer and gallbladder flare-ups. It is best in formula, as it can be bitter.

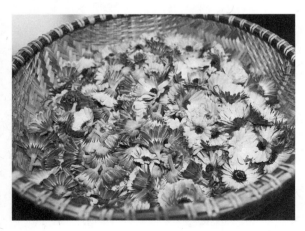

Calendula
(Calendula officinalis)

California Poppy (*Escholtzia californica*)

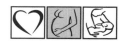

Part used:	Aerial portions
Main constituents:	Alkaloids (cryptopine); flavone glycosides
Alternatives:	Skullcap (*Scutellaria lateriflora*); valerian (*Valeriana officinalis*)
Notes for caution:	**During pregnancy:** This herb may stimulate the uterus due to the presence of the alkaloid cryptopine.

Long used as a safe sedative for young children, this gentle herbal nervine also has applications in colic and sleeplessness.

Camphor Tree (*Cinnamomum camphora*)

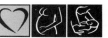

Part used:	Essential oil
Main constituents:	Camphor; linalool; 1,8-cineole; nerolidol; safrole; borneol
Alternatives:	None
Notes for caution:	**During preconception:** The essential oil is an emmenagogue.
	During pregnancy: Camphor oil contains safrole, which is toxic to a developing fetus. Further, it is an emmenagogue and uterine stimulant.
	During lactation: Do not use camphor essential oil on your chest or on the skin of your nursing infant. The inhalation and absorption in small doses of the essential oil can result in central nervous system overstimulation and seizures.[39]

The camphor tree produces three kinds of essential oils: brown, yellow and white. The brown and yellow oils are toxic and carcinogenic because of their high concentrations of safrole; only the white camphor oil is safe to use. It is often used for the effect its vapors have on respiratory ailments and can also be helpful as a topical rub for sore muscles and rheumatic pains.

| REPRODUCTIVE PHASE | Preconception | Pregnancy | Lactation | GENERAL SAFETY RATING | No Contraindications | Use with Caution | Generally Avoid |

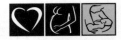

Cascara Segrada (*Rhamnus purshiana*)

Part used:	Aged bark (NOTE: Fresh bark is toxic)
Main constituents:	Vitamin A; selenium; magnesium; iron; fat; fiber; cobalt; calcium; aluminum; anthraquinones; genotoxins (emodin and aloe-emodin); flavonoids; tannins[35]
Alternatives:	Dandelion root (*Taraxacum officinale*); yellow dock root (*Rumex crispus*)
Notes for caution:	**During preconception and pregnancy:** The presence of the genotoxins found in cascara segrada can potentially be mutagenic.
	During lactation: Because anthraquinones are partially passed along in milk, it is believed that this herb could have a laxative effect in infants. There is also the potential to pass along the genotoxins emodin and aloe-emodin.

Cascara segrada is one of a class of stronger laxatives known as evacuants. Evacuants work by chemical stimulation of the brain or bowels and can irritate the intestinal lining. This herb is very important for treating constipation in adults, especially when the condition is chronic. It is, however, not to be taken over the long term as it causes laxative dependency. It is not appropriate for children.

Internal use   External use

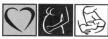   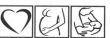

Castor Bean (*Ricinus communis*)

Part used:	Oil of the bean
Main constituents:	Ricin; palmitic acid; fixed oil; ricinoleic acid[41]
Alternatives:	Dandelion root (*Taraxacum officinale*); yellow dock root (*Rumex crispus*)
Notes for caution:	**During preconception:** Castor is an emmenagogue.
	During pregnancy: The oil of the bean is often used to induce labor, but this process involves intense intestinal griping if taken internally and also has mixed results. The oil should never be used internally during pregnancy due to its potential as an emmenagogue and abortifacient.

Castor oil is one of the best external treatments for fatty tumors and cysts — everything from ovarian and uterine cysts to tennis elbow. While castor oil does not affect breast milk production one way or the other, many women use it in conjunction with their breasts. If a woman is prone to fatty lumps in the breast, she may have used castor oil in the past to reduce or dissolve them. While breastfeeding, the recurrence of these lumps could potentially cause milk reduction depending on where they are located, and a mother may be tempted to use the castor oil again. Used internally, however, castor oil is a cathartic laxative and not something an infant should ingest. Keep this oil well away from the nipple and, if possible, wipe it away or place a cloth over the treated area as a barrier between mother and baby.

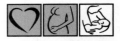

Catnip (*Nepeta cataria*)

Part used:	Aerial portions
Main constituents:	Nepatalactone; sesquiterpene lactones; resin; tannin; essential oil; vitamins A, B_2, and B_6; aluminum; calcium; chromium; cobalt; iron; magnesium; manganese; phosphorus; potassium; selenium; tin[35]
Alternatives:	Rose (*Rosa* spp.); skullcap (*Scutellaria lateriflora*)
Notes for caution:	**During preconception:** Catnip is an emmenagogue.
	During pregnancy: Catnip is a known emmenagogue and abortifacient. Use only in small amounts and/or in tea.

Catnip is an important herb for all nursing mothers. It is not only a relaxant for mother, but is also a mild sedative for the child. It is specific for nursing through to treating a colicky child. A tonic herb, it can be freely drunk by mom and in a pinch can be given directly to baby by dropper, wet and/or frozen washcloth or even a bottle, in baby-sized amounts. Use common sense, and to treat a child for colic, do not give so much that the child is not hungry for the next feeding.

This is also a great tea to drink when you need to break a fever. In combination with such herbs as yarrow, peppermint and elder (when served as a warm tea or a warm bath), it will induce sweating, which will cool the body.

For moms, this herb is specific for unspoken emotions and anxieties that lead to tension. Served warm or cold, it can often be a helpful tonic during this important life transition.

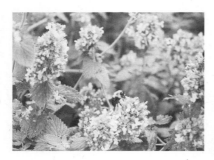

*Catnip (*Nepeta cataria*)*

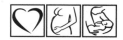

Cayenne (*Capsicum annuum*)

Part used:	Fruit
Main constituents:	Vitamins A, B_1, B_2, B_3, C; zinc; sodium; protein; potassium; phosphorus; magnesium; iron; fat; fiber; cobalt;[35] 1,8-cineole; 2-octanone; alanine; alpha-carotene; alpha-linoleic acid; alpha-phellandrene; arginine; ascorbic acid; beta-carotene; betaine; campesterol; capsaicin; capsanthin; carvone; folacin; glutamic acid; hesperidin; isoleucine; isovaleric acid; kaempferol; myrcene; p-coumaric acid; proline; quercetin; scopoletin; solanine; thujone; tryptophan; valine; zeaxanthin[41]
Alternatives:	None

Cayenne is an important stimulant internally and a rubefacient externally. The capsaicin found in the fruit of this plant is useful for arthritis and sore muscles. It is a warming and activating herb that is often added to digestive formulas to help get the metabolism moving and enable faster absorption. Cayenne is also a vasodilator and has tonic effects in the heart and general circulatory system.

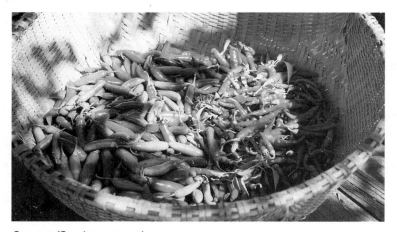

*Cayenne (*Capsium anuum*)*

REPRODUCTIVE PHASE	Preconception	Pregnancy	Lactation	GENERAL SAFETY RATING	No Contraindications	Use with Caution	Generally Avoid

Celandine (*Chelidonium majus*)

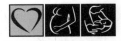

Part used:	Root; aerial portions
Main constituents:	Chelidonine; chelerythrin; homocheledonine; homocheledonine B; protopine; sanguinarine; chelodoxanthin
Alternatives:	Calendula (*Calendula officinalis*); milk thistle (*Silybum marianum, Carduus marianus*); gentian (*Gentiana lutea*)
Notes for caution:	**During preconception:** The alkaloids found in this herb are known to be uterine stimulants.
	During pregnancy: The alkaloids found in this herb are known to be uterine stimulants.
	During lactation: Use this herb sparingly. It is believed that large doses can be toxic to a nursing infant due to the presence of various alkaloids.

Celandine is most often used to treat gallbladder problems by stimulating the production of bile and washing away stones. It is also used in Russian folk medicine to treat cancer.

Celery Seeds (*Apium graveolens*)

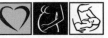

Part used:	Dried seeds
Main constituents:	Volatile oil (apiol); 3-n-butyl-phthalide; alpha-linolenic acid; beta-eudesmol; guaiacol; isoimperatorin; isoquercitrin; p-cymene; umbilliferone
Alternatives:	Dandelion (*Taraxacum officinale*)
Notes for caution:	**During preconception:** Celery seeds are an emmenagogue in therapeutic doses.
	During pregnancy: When used in therapeutic doses (not as a culinary spice) celery seed may act as an emmenagogue and abortifacient.

Celery seed excels at easing rheumatoid arthritis, arthritis and gout. Primarily a diuretic, it is also often used as a seasoning in food. When not taken in therapeutic dose, a woman need not be concerned about ingesting celery seed during preconception, pregnancy or lactation.

Chamomile (*Matricaria recutita*)

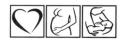

Part used:	Flowers
Main constituents:	Essential oil (bisabolol and chamazulene); flavonoids (apigenin, matricin, rutin, luteolin); coumarins; polysaccharides; vitamins B_2, B_3, and C); calcium; cobalt; iron; magnesium; manganese; tin; sodium; protein; potassium; phosphorus; fat; fiber[35]
Alternatives:	None
Notes for caution:	Watch for any tendency for ragweed allergies. The basis of this concern is in doubt; nonetheless, if either mom or baby develop wheeziness or red or itchy eyes following a cup of tea, find another option.

Chamomile is a favorite for treating the discomfort of teething. A woman may nurse through or give it in a dropper, but by far the best way to administer this tea is in a frozen washcloth to relieve the need to chew and to soothe sore gums. For mom, chamomile is a great anti-inflammatory and painkiller and a fine solution for headaches, anxiety or minor sleeplessness. For those times when mom or baby have eye irritations, chamomile makes a safe, effective eyewash. Finally, if steeped for 15 to 20 minutes, the bitter component becomes available; this is helpful for indigestion, especially if this is associated with a nervous condition.

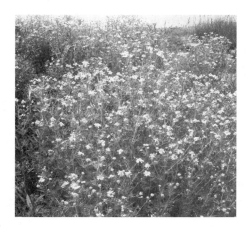

*Chamomile (*Matricaria recutita*)*

Internal use   **External use**

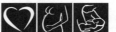   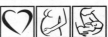

Chaparral (*Larrea tridentata; Larrea divaricate*)

Part used:	Leaves
Main constituents:	Vitamins A, B_1, B_2, C; tin; sodium; silicon; selenium; protein; potassium; manganese; magnesium; iron; fat; fiber; cobalt; chromium; calcium; aluminum; volatile oils; nordihydroguaiaretic acid; terpenes (alpha-pinene; beta pinene, limonene, camphor); cobalt; flavonoids (gossypetin, ternatin); Lignanes; resin; polysaccharides; ketones; vinyl ketones[35]
Alternatives:	**Anti-inflammatory, antifungal:** Calendula (*Calendula officinalis*) **Urinary antiseptic:** Bearberry (*Arctostaphylos uva-ursi*) **Respiratory antiseptic:** Thyme (*Thymus vulgaris*) **Toxin clearing:** Red clover (*Trifolium pratense*); dandelion root (*Taraxacum officinale*)
Notes for caution:	**Internal use during preconception and pregnancy:** This herb is banned in the United States due to concern about hepatotoxicity. **Internal use during lactation:** It is speculated that there is a potential for a greater negative effect for the nursing mother than for her child. The concern is due to the inhibition of RNA, protein and lipid synthesis in the mammary gland following prolactin stimulation.[39]

A highly resinous evergreen shrub of the deserts of Southwest United States, chaparral was traditionally used as a natural antibiotic, anti-inflammatory, antiseptic and antifungal with an affinity for the respiratory and urinary tract. Chaparral contains a powerful antioxidant called nordihydroguaiaretic acid (NDGA) that is believed to be responsible for its anti-tumor effect as well as its many other medicinal applications. It is currently banned for internal use in the United States because of its perceived potential to cause toxic effects on the liver. It is not recommended for internal use during pregnancy or lactation. There is a precedent for using chaparral externally in salves and creams. This is most likely safe if used sparingly and never near the area where your child will be making skin-to-skin contact while nursing.

Chaste Tree (*Vitex agnus-castus*)

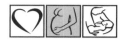

Part used:	Fruit
Main constituents:	Acubin; agnuside; casticin; chrysophanol D; alpha- and beta-pinene; isovitexin; vitexin[44]
Alternatives:	None
Notes for caution:	**During pregnancy:** This herb is a possible emmenagogue unless you have a progesterone deficiency, in which case it is often used to help prevent miscarriage in early pregnancy. If you wish to use chaste tree during pregnancy, seek the advice of a trained clinician.

This is a tonic herb to be taken over a long period of time. It is a hormonal balancer with specific applications for the pituitary gland, luteinizing hormone and progesterone support. In my opinion, this is the best herb for working on the estrogen/progesterone balance and the first herb any woman coming off birth control medication should use to prepare for getting pregnant. It's a great herb for alleviating PMS symptoms and can be very helpful in the first part of pregnancy if there is a risk of low progesterone levels. If taken throughout pregnancy, it can be an aid to milk supply after birth.

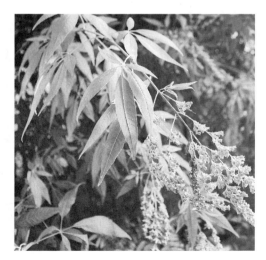

*Chaste Tree (*Vitex agnus-castus*)*

Chervil (*Anthriscus cerefolium*)

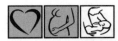

Part used:	Aerial portions
Main constituents:	Flavonoids; volatile oils
Alternatives:	None
Notes for caution:	**During preconception and pregnancy:** This herb is a possible emmenagogue if taken in excessive therapeutic doses rather than as a food or tea additive.

Chervil is a delicious herb that is often added to French cuisine. Its main medicinal properties come from its high volume of volatile oils and its ability to calm the digestive system.

Chickweed (*Stellaria media*)

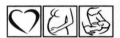

Galactagogue	
Part used:	Aerial portions
Main constituents:	Saponins; vitamins A, B$_1$, B$_3$; calcium; iron; magnesium; manganese; selenium; zinc; sodium; protein; potassium; phosphorus; fat; fiber; cobalt; chromium; aluminum; volatile oil; saturated fatty acids (stearic acid, palmitic); unsaturated fatty acids (linoleic and oleic)
Alternatives:	None

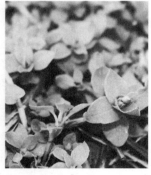

Chickweed (Stellaria media)

This truly delicious little spring weed is available to most, as long as it is not sprayed with chemicals. Chickweed can be eaten fresh in salads, preserved in oil or dried. It is the herbalist's favorite salve herb and can be used topically to gently treat skin problems such as psoriasis, eczema, itchy skin and infections. It is also rumored to be helpful with weight loss because of its diuretic qualities.

Chicory (*Cichorium intybus*)

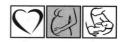

Part used:	Root
Main constituents:	Inulin; vitamin C; calcium; Iron
Alternatives:	None
Notes for caution:	**During pregnancy:** Generally safe in typical food and beverage use. Do not use in excess.

Chicory, a close relative of the dandelion, has long been known as a good coffee substitute. It is usually roasted, which produces a nutty, earthy flavor. While pregnant and nursing, it is important to reduce or eliminate coffee consumption, but you shouldn't have to give up your morning cup experience altogether. The great thing about chicory is that it is healthful. Because it contains vitamin C and inulin, it can help the body absorb calcium and magnesium.

   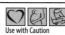

Chinese Motherwort (yi mu cao)
(*Leonurus heterophyllus; Leonurus sibiricus*)

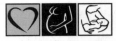

Part used:	Aerial portions
Main constituents:	Alkaloids (stachydrine); volatile oil
Alternatives:	None
Notes for caution:	**During preconception:** The herb is an emmenagogue.
	During pregnancy: The herb is an emmenagogue, and pregnancy is not the time to move pelvic stagnation.

In traditional Chinese medicine, this is the go-to herb for stagnation in the pelvis, irregular menstruation and expulsion of the placenta after birth. It is a uterine tonic, which may mean that it can act as an emmenagogue during pregnancy. Its use to help with the placenta at birth should be monitored only by an experienced midwife. This is a great choice for new moms to get back into their systems; it can help regulate menstrual cycles after weaning a child.

Cinchona (*Cinchona* spp.)

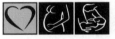

Part used:	Bark
Main constituents:	Alkaloids (quinine, cinchonidin, cinchonine, quinidine, hydrocinchonidine, quinamine, homokinchonidine, hydroquinine); quinic acid; cinchotannic acid
Alternatives:	Catnip (*Cataria nepeta*); yarrow (*Achillea millefolium*); elder (*Sambucus nigra*)
Notes for caution:	**During preconception:** The herb is an emmenagogue.
	During pregnancy: This herb is toxic to a developing fetus.
	During lactation: Excreted through breast milk, cinchona contains the alkaloids quinine and quinidine, making it a toxin.

Cinchona can be used for its fever-reducing abilities, particularly in connection with malaria. It is typically taken in small, occasional doses. Observations about this bark were foundational to the homeopathic idea that "like treats like."

Cinnamon (twak)
(*Cinnamomum zeylanicum;*
Cinnamomum vernum;
Cinnamomum aromaticum)

Bark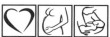

Essential oil/
Alcohol extract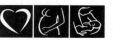

Part used:	Inner bark; essential oil
Main constituents:	Safrole; cinnamaldehyde; eugenol; trans-cinnamic acid; phenolic compounds; tannins; catechins; calcium; iron; mucilage; resin; natural sugars; traces of coumarin
Alternatives:	None
Notes for caution:	There are no contraindications when used as a seasoning.

Essential oil/alcoholic extract during preconception and pregnancy: The essential oil or alcoholic extract will contain safrole, which is a known carcinogen. In these forms, it is an emmenagogue and abortifacient.

Essential oil/alcoholic extract during lactation: The essential oil or alcoholic extract will contain safrole, which is a known carcinogen.

Cinnamon can be found in two forms: "true" cinnamon (*C. Zeylanicum* or *C. verum*) or cassia (*C. bermannii* or *C. aromaticum*). Both will impart a cinnamon flavor and have many of the same health benefits; however, cassia is easier and cheaper to come by and true cinnamon is more expensive but easier for the home cook to use or grate in the kitchen. An email that surfaces frequently contains a list of the things cinnamon is known to cure. It *is* a pretty magical herb, and should not be considered just a flavoring for the holidays. Cinnamon is helpful in controlling blood sugar and is antibacterial, antifungal and anti-inflammatory. It is especially useful in gently calming an upset stomach and allaying nausea. It is completely safe to use cinnamon as a spice in your food or in beverages while you are trying to conceive, are pregnant or are nursing.

REPROCTIVE PHASE				GENERAL SAFETY RATING							
Preconception	Pregnancy	Lactation		No Contraindications			Use with Caution		Generally Avoid		

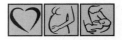

Cocoa (*Theobroma cacao*)

Part used:	Seeds
Main constituents:	Theobromine
Alternatives:	None
Notes for caution:	**During preconception:** Cocoa is not a danger to conception, but should be used sparingly because of its similarities to coffee.
	During pregnancy: Theobromine and caffeine have similar actions in the body although theobromine's effects are much milder. It should be taken into account when monitoring the total amount of caffeine consumed in a day. Caffeine can cause anemia in both mother and fetus. Doses of 200 mg per day (appoximately 10 oz of homemade coffee) or more can lead to miscarriage or birth defect. Caffeine is known to cross the placenta and contribute to low birth weight and preterm delivery.[45]
	During lactation: Theobromine and caffeine have similar actions in the body, although theobromine's effects are much milder. Caffeine has been found to appear in breast milk at half the level in the mother's plasma. It reduces the available iron supply in breast milk.

Cocoa is a stimulant and, sadly, most of us love it. Theobromine has a less marked effect on our central nervous system than caffeine, but it has a greater effect on our muscles, kidneys, heart and immune system.[46]

When pregnant or nursing, a woman should keep in mind the total amount of caffeine and caffeine-like substances she is consuming. If the amount rises above 200 mg per day, there is a risk for low growth rates, birth defects or miscarriage.

Coffee (*Coffea arabica*)

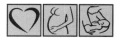

Part used:	Seeds
Main constituents:	Caffeine; tannic acid; caffetannic acid; aromatic oils
Alternatives:	Non-caffeinated beverages
Notes for caution:	**During preconception:** Caffeine is extremely drying to cervical fluids and also places an unnecessary burden on the endocrine system that can lead to hormonal imbalances.
	During pregnancy: Caffeine can cause anemia in both mother and fetus. Doses of 200 mg (approximately 10 oz of homemade coffee) or more per day can lead to miscarriage or birth defect. Caffeine is known to cross the placenta and contribute to low birth weight and preterm delivery.[45]
	During lactation: Caffeine has been found to appear in breast milk at half the level in the mother's plasma. It reduces the available iron supply in breast milk. Coffee specifically can also block the absorption of important nutrients, especially minerals, in very young children.

Coffee is the stimulating beverage of choice for many. It is best to find healthy alternatives to this habit early in your path toward having a baby and to continue the alternative throughout.

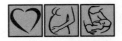

Cola (*Cola nitida; Cola acuminate*)

Part used:	Seeds
Main constituents:	Caffeine; kolanin
Alternatives:	None
Notes for caution:	**During preconception:** Caffeine is extremely drying to cervical fluids and also places an unnecessary burden on the endocrine system that can lead to hormonal imbalances. **During pregnancy:** Cola during pregnancy is believed to cause low birth weight, birth defects and preterm delivery. **During lactation:** Caffeine has been found to appear in breast milk at half the level in the mother's plasma. It reduces the available iron supply in breast milk.

This herb is known as kola nut and used as a condiment and digestive aid in the African countries to which it is native. It is known to have tonic qualities for the nervous system and heart, but is most often used as a stimulant. It is best avoided or used in very limited amounts during preconception, pregnancy and lactation due to its caffeine content.[45]

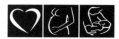

Colocynth (*Citrullus colocynthis*)

Part used:	Dried fruit pulp
Main constituents:	Colocynthin
Alternatives:	Dandelion root (*Taraxacum officinale*); yellow dock root (*Rumex crispus*); triphala
Notes for caution:	**During preconception:** This herb is poisonous if not taken correctly.
	During pregnancy: Colocynth is an abortifacient and poisonous if not taken correctly.
	During lactation: The herb is poisonous if not taken correctly. There is great potential for catharsis in a nursing infant, accompanied with serious cramping and bowel inflammation.

Known as bitter apple or bitter cucumber, colocynth is is by all accounts poisonous unless taken in very exacting small doses. In the wrong dosage it can cause bloody stool, violent cramping and dangerous inflammation of the bowels. Avoid it in favor of the many safer alternatives for relieving constipation.

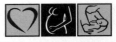

Coltsfoot (*Tussilago farfara*)

Part used:	Leaves; flowers
Main constituents:	Mucilage; flavonoids (rutin and carotene); taraxanthin; arnidiol; faradiol; tannin; essential oil; insulin; sitosterol; zinc
Alternatives:	Mullein (*Verbascum thapsus*)
Notes for caution:	**During preconception:** Coltsfoot is a possible abortifacient.
	During pregnancy: The herb contains pyrrolizidine alkaloids, which are believed to cause liver toxicity, as well as being a possible abortifacient.
	During lactation: It is speculated that due to the presence of potentially toxic glycosides, this plant can pose a threat to a nursing infant's liver. It is best to avoid prolonged use (beyond four to six weeks of steady use in a year). Avoid it altogether in the presence of a known liver issue.

Coltsfoot was once so popular in the United States Pharmacopeia that it was the symbol used on the sign over a physician's door. It is still a very important herb for its ability to help expel mucus from the lungs and calm coughing.

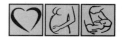

Comfrey (*Symphytum officinale*)

Part used:	Roots; leaves
Main constituents:	Vitamins A, B_1, B_2, B_3, C; silicon; selenium; protein; potassium; phosphorus; manganese; fiber; chromium; aluminum; mucilage; gum; allantoin; tannin; alkaloids; resin; volatile oil; germanium; calcium; saponins; sitosterol; flavonoids[35]
Alternatives:	Marshmallow (*Althaea officinalis*)
Notes for caution:	**During preconception:** Comfrey is not recommended internally due to the presence of pyrrolizidine alkaloids.
	During pregnancy: It is speculated that due to the presence of potentially toxic alkaloids (pyrrolizidine alkaloids or PAs), this plant can pose a threat to the developing fetus's liver. It is best to avoid prolonged use (beyond four to six weeks' steady use in a year) and avoid completely if there is a known liver issue.
NOTE: See Appendix F for more in-depth information on the safety of this herb.	**During lactation:** It is speculated that due to the presence of potentially toxic alkaloids (pyrrolizidine alkaloids or PAs), this plant can pose a threat to the nursing baby's liver. It is best to avoid prolonged use (beyond four to six weeks' steady use in a year) and best avoid completely if there is a known liver issue.

Comfrey is a favorite remedy both internally and externally for wound healing. It is high in mucilage, which makes it very soothing for our mucus membranes, so it is often used for internal ulcers and hemorrhages. It can help to expel mucus in the respiratory system, so it's very useful in a cough formula. Apply it topically to your next bruise and watch the discoloration disappear like magic. It is especially important to women because of its calcium content, for those who find that its internal use is appropriate for them. While *Symphytum officinale* has definitely been shown in lab tests to contain PAs, *Symphytum uplandica*, the cultivated version most often harvested in the United States, does not.[47] The controversy continues over this most valuable herb, so you must decide how you feel.

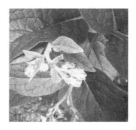

Comfrey (Symphytum officinale)

Cornsilk (*Zea mays*)

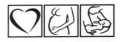

Part used:	Flower tassel
Main constituents:	Vitamins B$_1$, E; zinc; silicon; potassium; phosphorus; magnesium; iron; fat; cobalt; chromium; aluminum;[35] allantoin; saponins
Alternatives:	None

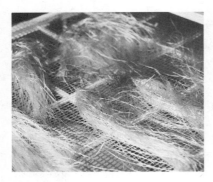

Cornsilk is a very soothing, demulcent herb with an affinity for the urinary tract. It has been used to treat bladder stones, enlargement of the prostate and infection, and even has some application in bedwetting.

*Cornsilk (*Zea mays*)*

Corydalis (yan hu suo) (*Corydalis yanhusuo*)

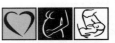

Part used:	Rhizome
Main constituents:	Alkaloids; dehydrocorydaline
Alternatives:	Yarrow (*Achillea millefolium*); ginger (*Zingiber officinale*)
Notes for caution:	**During preconception:** Corydalis is an emmenagogue.
	During pregnancy: Corydalis is an emmenagogue and best avoided during pregnancy.

This is another great herb used in traditional Chinese medicine to move stagnant blood and energy and relieve pain.

REPRODUCTIVE PHASE				GENERAL SAFETY RATING				
	Preconception	Pregnancy	Lactation		No Contraindications	Use with Caution	Generally Avoid	

Cotton Root (*Gossypium herbaceum*)

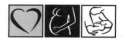

Part used:	Bark of the root
Main constituents:	Resin; tannin; sugar; gum; chlorophyll
Alternatives:	None
Notes for caution:	**During preconception:** Cotton root is an emmenagogue.
	During pregnancy: The herb is a well-known abortifacient.

This herb is used primarily as an abortifacient and should be avoided by any woman trying to have a child.

Cow Parsnip (*Heracleum lanatum*)

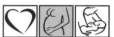

Part used:	Root
Main constituents:	Volatile oil; heraclin
Alternatives:	None
Notes for caution:	**During pregnancy:** It is best not to go overboard eating cow parsnip or using it as a medicine in the first part of pregnancy. Taken in large or frequent amounts, it can act as an emmenagogue.

Cow parsnip is useful as a foraged food supply as well as medicine. It is great for stagnation of the blood or digestion, general sluggishness and depression.

Cramp Bark (*Viburnum opulus*)

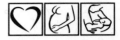

Part used:	Bark
Main constituents:	Calcium; sodium; silicon; phosphorus; manganese; magnesium; iron; cobalt; chromium;[35] coumarins; scopoletin; tannin.
Alternatives:	None

Although cramp bark has an affinity for working with cramps in the uterus, men and women can use it for cramps or spasm in all parts of the body. It may seem like a good solution for the postpartum cramping women may experience during nursing. However, remember that those cramps are doing good work, cleansing the body of remaining blood and shrinking the uterus back to normal size. Don't interfere with this natural cramping action. Take something targeted to relieve pain, such as rosemary or wild lettuce, instead. It is better to encourage these effective contractions by continuing to take raspberry leaf. Save the use of cramp bark for other muscle cramps after a care provider has verified the uterus has returned to its original size.

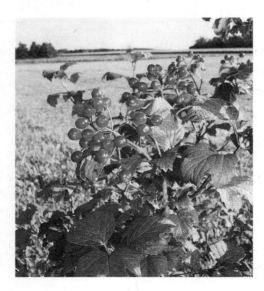

*Cramp Bark (*Viburnum opulus*)*

Cranberry (*Vaccinium vitis-idaea*)

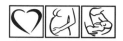

Part used:	Fruit
Main constituents:	Vitamins A, B₁, B₂, B₃, C; sodium; silicon; potassium; phosphorus; manganese; magnesium; fat; fiber; calcium; anthocyanins; flavonals; proanthocyanidins; benzoic and phenolic acids; polyphenols; terpenes; sterols[35]
Alternatives:	None

The cranberry is often used to fight urinary tract infection. Most people use cranberry juice, but it is important to use a pure juice with no sugar added. Bacteria are present during urinary tract infections, because the urine is not acidic enough and there is often also an inappropriate level of sugar. Many natural treatments serve to add acid (vitamin C as an example) to the body's urine output to deal with this. While adding treatments high in natural acids, it is smart to eat an alkaline diet, one free from sugar, to allow the body to rebalance after the bacteria in the kidneys have been destroyed.

Cucumber (*Cucumis sativa*)

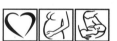

Part used:	Fruit with seeds
Main constituents:	Sodium; potassium; vitamins C and A
Alternatives:	None

Internally, cucumber is a gentle option for expelling worms and parasites. It is also a mild diuretic that can help with any kind of edema or heat.

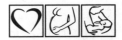

Damiana (*Turnera aphrodisiaca*)

Part used:	Aerial portions
Main constituents:	Vitamins A, B₃, C; zinc, tin, sodium; protein; manganese; magnesium; iron; fat; fiber; cobalt; chromium; calcium; aluminum; chlorophyllins; volatile oil (terpenes); resin; damianin; tannins; flavonoids; beta-sitosterol; glycosides (gonzalitosin, arbutin, tetraphyllin B); polysaccharides[35]
Alternatives:	None
Male fertility:	Damiana is at its best in the male body as an aphrodisiac when a lack of interest is caused by anxiety and depression.

Damiana has a longstanding reputation as an aphrodisiac. It's often associated with men, but its action of increasing blood flow to the abdomen and genitals can benefit women as well. While nursing, it may be difficult to get back into the "mood" from time to time. Damiana is a good option to sip with your significant other when you can get some time alone.

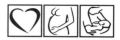

Dandelion (*Taraxacum officinale*)

Galactagogue	
Part used:	All parts
Main constituents:	Vitamins A, C, D, B complex; iron; magnesium; zinc; potassium; manganese; copper; choline; calcium; boron; silicon; bitter taraxacins (eudesmanolides); sitosterol; stigmasterol; alpha- and beta-carotene; carreic acid; mucilage; fatty acids (myristic, palmitic, stearic, lauric); inulin; pectin; flavonoids (lutein); caffeic acid[35]
Alternatives:	None

Women should use this very important herb in as many forms as possible. Dandelion is best known as a liver tonic, and this is definitely a point in our lives when we want to keep our livers healthy. It also an important diuretic, so it helps to keep our kidneys cleansed and healthy as well. For preconception, this herb helps women move toxins out of the body. During pregnancy and nursing, the use of this herb should not diminish. For those who are craving coffee substitutes, dandelion root can be roasted and used along with chicory. Depending on the time of year, enjoy dandelion leaves in salad, casseroles, soups or tea.

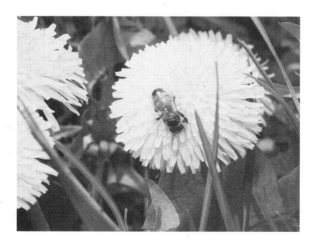

Dandelion
(Taraxacum officinale*)*

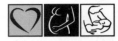

Devil's Claw (*Harpagophytum procumbens*)

Part used:	Tuber
Main constituents:	Vitamin B$_3$; zinc; tin; sodium; silicon; selenium; protein; manganese; magnesium; iron; fat; fiber; cobalt; chromium; calcium; aluminum;[35] iridoid glycosides; quinone; chlorogenic and cinnamic acids; kaempferol; harpogoquinone; sugar
Alternatives:	Chamomile (*Matricaria recutita*); elder (*Sambucus nigra*)
Notes for caution:	**During preconception:** Devil's claw can cause contractions.
	During pregnancy: The herb is known to be oxytocic.

Devil's claw is a strong anti-inflammatory and antirheumatic. It is effective for arthritis, sciatica and nerve pain.

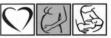

Dill (*Anethum graveolens*)

Galactagogue	
Part used:	Seeds
Main constituents:	Volatile oil; vanadium
Alternatives:	None
Notes for caution:	**During pregnancy:** Dill has been reported to have emmenagogue properties. While it is fine to use this as a condiment or in a tea, it is best to avoid excessive amounts in early pregnancy.

The volatile oils in this seed make it a supreme carminative. Instead of reaching for that popular over-the-counter antacid, just chew a few dill seeds. They will make your breath fresher as a bonus. This can also be a very effective tea for reliving colic, and is in fact one of the traditional ingredients in "gripe water." Dill seeds also can be counted among some of the most popular galactagogues.

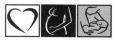

Dong Quai (*Angelica sinensis*)

Part used:	Roots
Main constituents:	Vitamins A, B$_2$, B$_3$, C, E; silicon; protein; potassium; phosphorus; magnesium; fat; fiber; cobalt; chromium; aluminum; butylidene phthalide; ligustilide; n-butylidene-phthalide; volatile oil (sequiterpene lactones, terpenes); carvacrol; dihyrophthalic anhydride; sucrose; beta-sitosterol; iron; saturated fatty acids (stearic, palmitic); unsaturated fatty acids (linoleic, oleic)[35]
Alternatives:	None
Notes for caution:	**During pregnancy:** Dong quai encourages bleeding and is a menstrual and uterine stimulant.
	During lactation: Do not use this herb until after your postpartum bleeding has stopped. Also avoid in each cycle while you are bleeding.

This popular member of the angelica family is often called the "female ginseng." This herb is very gentle and, when used over an extended time, will strengthen and balance the uterus. It doesn't have a specific hormonal action but promotes overall balance, working through the liver and endocrine system. It is specific for irregular or absent cycles.

This is an important herb for returning to hormonal and emotional homeostasis after giving birth. It has been known to increase blood flow if taken during your monthly cycle, so avoid it at this time.

REPRODUCTIVE PHASE
Preconception Pregnancy Lactation
GENERAL SAFETY RATING
No Contraindications   Use with Caution   Generally Avoid

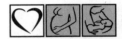

Dulse (*Rhodymenia palmetto*)

Part used:	Thallus (Leaf)
Main constituents:	Alpha-carotene; arsenic;* beta-carotene; calcium; chromium; cobalt; iodine; iron; lead;* lutein; manganese; magnesium; mercury;* phosphorous; potassium; protein; selenium; silicon; sodium; tin; vitamins A, B$_3$, C; zeaxanthin; zinc[35,41]
	Likely contaminates from specimens harvested in contaminated seas.*
Alternatives:	Sea salt
	For hypothyroidism: eleuthero (*Eleutherococcus senticosus, Acanthopanax senticosus*)
	For calcium: Red raspberry (*Rubus ideaus*); oatstraw (*Avena sativa*)
Notes for caution:	**During pregnancy:** Excessive consumption during pregnancy can lead to infantile goiter.[34] It is best to keep therapeutic dosage for any type of seaweed to no more than 0.25 gram daily.
	During lactation: In high doses or in prolonged use, seaweed can overstimulate the thyroid. It is believed that the high iodine content could be a potential toxin to a nursing infant.

All of our available varieties of seaweed are a perfect source of calcium; however, there are conditions that necessitate caution. This food source is best used in moderation while nursing. Be sure to do your research on your choice of seaweed. Many areas from which these superfoods are harvested are now heavily polluted. It can be difficult to find clean suppliers, but these foods should be an important part of our diets, so it is worth the effort.

REPRODUCTIVE PHASE   Preconception Pregnancy Lactation   GENERAL SAFETY RATING  No Contraindications Use with Caution Generally Avoid

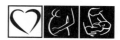

Dyers Broom (*Genista tinctoria*)

Part used:	Aerial portions
Main constituents:	Isofavone genistein; scopnarine; sparteine
Alternatives:	Dandelion root (*Taraxacum officinale*); yellow dock root (*Rumex crispus*)
Notes for caution:	**During pregnancy:** This herb has been known to cause contractions. **During lactation:** As a cathartic, this herb is not appropriate for a nursing infant to receive through breast milk.

Dyers broom has diuretic, cathartic and emetic properties. It is used most often for its perceived abilities to flush toxic elements out of the body.

   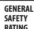

Echinacea (*Echinacea* spp.)

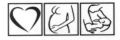

Part used:	All parts
Main constituents:	Vitamins B_1, B_2, B_3, C; zinc; tin; silicon; selenium; manganese; magnesium; iron; fiber; cobalt; chromium; aluminum; complex sugars; polysaccharides (echinacin, gum, inulin); resin (echinaceoside, betaine); essential oil; flavonoids[35]
Alternatives:	None

Many people take echinacea year round as an immune system tonic. While it is safe to do so, I believe it is better to use in isolated instances and to avoid constant stimulation of the immune system. It is better to tone the immune system with diet by focusing on proper gut flora. Echinacea is the best herb to use for a microbial infection, and is effective against both bacteria and viruses. It tones white blood cells and stimulates them to act in the most efficient manner. It is also a great option to use externally for the same sorts of infection. If you plan to take echinacea for longer periods of time, avoid the popular formulation that includes goldenseal, which should be taken for a much shorter time. Better to buy these two tinctures separately.

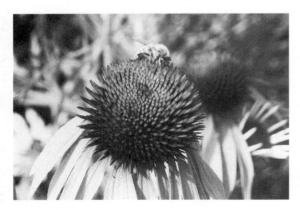

Echinacea
(Echinacea *spp.*)

REPRODUCTIVE PHASE   Preconception   Pregnancy   Lactation   GENERAL SAFETY RATING   No Contraindications   Use with Caution   Generally Avoid

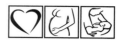

Elder (*Sambucus nigra*)

Part used:	Flowers; berries
Main constituents:	Flavonoids; vitamins A and C; potassium nitrate; sambucin; sambunigrin; sugars
Alternatives:	None

Elder is useful for many things, but it is best known for its beneficial effects during cold and flu season. Both the flowers and the berries can help turn around the symptoms of a cold and are anti-inflammatory. They can also help clear catarrh in the sinuses or upper respiratory tract. Elder has been shown to be effective against eight different strains of influenza and may therefore be an option during flu vaccine season. It can be taken before an infection for prevention or during one to prevent it worsening. Dr. Madeleine Mumcuoglu of Hadassah-Hebrew University in Israel found that elderberry disarms the enzyme that viruses use to penetrate healthy cells in the lining of the nose and throat. In a clinical trial, 20 percent of study subjects reported significant improvement within twenty-four hours, 70 percent by forty-eight hours and 90 percent percent claimed complete cure in three days. In contrast, subjects receiving the placebo needed six days to recover on average.[48, 49]

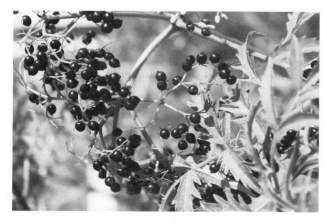

Elder

(Sambucus nigra)

Internal use **External use**

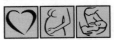

Elecampane (*Inula helenium*)

Part used:	Root
Main constituents:	Vitamins B₁, B₂, B₃; zinc; sodium; protein; potassium; magnesium; fat; fiber; chromium; calcium; essential oil (sesquiterpene lactones, alantolactone); saponins; inulin; helenin
Alternatives:	**External:** Calendula (*Calendula officinalis*); thyme (*Thymus vulgaris*); goldenseal (*Hydrastis canadensis*)
	Internal: None
Notes for caution:	**External use during preconception, pregnancy and lactation:** It has been found that external application of this herb can produce contact dermatitis, which indicates allergic hypersensitivity.

Elecampane is most commonly used for its ability to relieve mucus conditions associated with our lungs. It is typically used in combination with other herbs that are good for colds and congestion. However, there are some indications that it can be very helpful with skin conditions, and for this it is often used both externally and internally. If women use elecampane in this manner, they should be sure that the affected area is not in constant skin-to-skin contact with an infant.

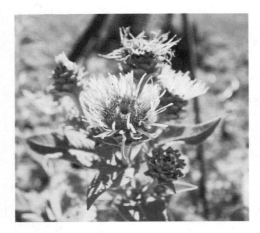

*Elecampane (*Inula helenium*)*

Eleuthero (*Eleutherococcus senticosus; Acanthopanax senticosus*)

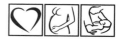

Part used:	Root
Main constituents:	Vitamins A, B₁, B₂, B₃, C; zinc; selenium; protein; potassium; phosphorus; magnesium; fat; iron; fiber; essential oils; eleutherosides B and E; immunostimulant complex polysaccharides
Alternatives:	None

Eleuthero is a member of the ginseng family and has been used in similar fashion for centuries. It has a different energy than red ginseng and can be used for different issues. It is best when used as an adaptogen to increase stamina and energy, especially when under undue stress and demand. It is also an effective herb to support adrenal health and boost the immune system.

Leaf   Essential oil

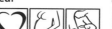

Eucalyptus (*Eucalyptus* spp.)

Part used:	Leaf; essential oil
Main constituents:	Eucalyptol
Alternatives:	**For essential oils:** Rosemary (*Rosemarinus officinalis*); thyme (*Thymus vulgaris*)
Notes for caution:	**Use of essential oil during lactation:** The essential oil is potentially toxic for an infant on the skin, in the air or ingested into the body because of its potential to stress the kidneys or stop the ability to breathe.

As an herb, eucalyptus is important for bacterial infection, especially staphylococci. As an essential oil, it is often used topically as an antiseptic or inhaled as a stimulant and aromatic with decongestant actions. It's also used as a liniment for arthritic pain.

REPRODUCTIVE PHASE   GENERAL SAFETY RATING

Preconception Pregnancy Lactation   No Contraindications Use with Caution Generally Avoid

European Vervain (*Verbena officinalis*)

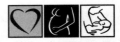

Part used:	Aerial portions
Main constituents:	Mucilage; bitters; iridoid glycosides; caffeic acid
Alternatives:	Goldenrod (*Solidago virgaurea*); cornsilk (*Zea mays*)
Notes for caution:	**During preconception:** European vervain is an emmenagogue.
	During pregnancy: This herb can cause uterine contractions.

European vervain is a diuretic that has been used traditionally for kidney issues such as stones and infections. It is also considered to be a "tonic emetic," which is an herb that helps expel toxins by way of vomiting. In lower doses, it is often used in the treatment of hot flashes.

Eyebright (*Euphrasia officinalis*)

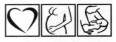

Part used:	Aerial portions
Main constituents:	Vitamins A, B$_1$, B$_2$, B$_3$, C; calcium; iron; magnesium; manganese; zinc; silicon; protein; potassium; phosphorus; fiber; cobalt; aluminum; aucubin; caffeic acid; ferulic acid; tannin; pseudotannin flavonoid[35]
Alternatives:	None

Eyebright is nutritive and when used internally can be helpful for congestion and inflammation caused by cold and flu. It excels as an external eyewash. When an infant has occasional eye irritations or minor infections and inflammations, breast milk applied directly to the eye is often the best medicine. When this simple treatment isn't working, eyebright tea can be applied to solve the problem.

| REPRODUCTIVE PHASE | Preconception | Pregnancy | Lactation | GENERAL SAFETY RATING |  No Contraindications | | Use with Caution | | Generally Avoid |

False Unicorn Root (*Chamaelirium luteum*)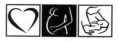

Part used:	Root
Main constituents:	Steroidal saponins
Alternatives:	None
Notes for caution:	**During pregnancy:** This is a powerful uterine tonic that can have a stimulating effect on the uterus that could lead to contractions when not administered by an experienced professional.

False unicorn root has long been used in therapies targeted at balancing hormones in both men and women. It contains precursors to estrogen but is best at balancing hormonal levels overall. It is a threatened plant, and it can be difficult to find a supplier. While it has been used to prevent morning sickness and miscarriage, its use is not to be taken lightly.

Fruit (seed)　　　Essential oil

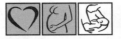

Fennel (*Foeniculum vulgare*)

Part used:	Fruit (seed); bulb (above-ground portion); essential oil
Main constituents:	Volatile oils (anethol, fenchone, D-pinene, phellandrine, anisicacid, anisicaldehyde, limonene); vitamins B$_1$, B$_2$, B$_3$, C; calcium; iron; magnesium; manganese; selenium; tin; sodium; protein; potassium; phosphorus; fat; fiber; unsaturated fatty acids; saponins; flavonoids (quercitin, rutin); coumarin[5]
Alternatives:	Use the fruit (seed) instead of the essential oil.
Notes for caution:	**Use of the fruit (seed) during preconception and pregnancy:** There are no contraindications when used as a seasoning or part of a tea. In therapeutic doses, the fruit can be an emmenagogue.
	Essential oil use during preconception: Fennel essential oil is an emmenagogue.
	Essential oil use during pregnancy: Fennel essential oil is an emmenagogue.
	Essential oil use during lactation: It is believed that the absorption through the skin or inhalation of fennel essential oil may be toxic to the nursing infant.

As an herb, fennel is most often used as a carminative to soothe stomach cramps or gas pains. It's often found in natural cough remedies because it has a calming effect on the respiratory system when there are spasms. Best of all, in relation to nursing, it is a well-known galactagogue. The essential oil can be used internally as a galactagogue, but it is best to use the seed, as it is safer. In aromatherapy, the oil is good for courage and can also be used as an appetite stimulant. The culinary use of the fennel bulb as a vegetable is safe at any time while building a baby.

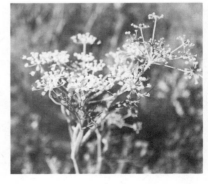

*Fennel (*Foeniculum vulgare*)*

Fenugreek (*Trigonella foenum-graecum*)

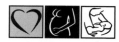

Galactagogue	
Part used:	Seed
Main constituents:	Arginine; beta-carotene; beta-sitosterol; coumarin; diosgenin; gamma-aminobutyric acid (GABA); kaempferol; luteolin; pyridoxine; quercetin; rutin; sulfur; trigonelline; tryptophan; vitexin; vitamins B$_1$, B$_2$, C; tin; sodium; selenium; silicon; protein; potassium; phosphorus; iron; fat; fiber; aluminum[35]
Alternatives:	Bitter orange (*Citrus aurantium* spp., *Citrus amara*); dill (*Anethum graveolens*)
Notes for caution:	**During preconception:** Fenugreek is an emmenagogue.
	During pregnancy: Fenugreek is an emmenagogue, abortifacient and uterine stimulant.

This is another heavy hitter from the Asian culinary spice cabinet. Fenugreek is a strong galactagogue and is believed to help develop breast tissue. It is particularly soothing in cases of indigestion and can be helpful in maintaining blood sugar levels. Externally, it can be used to reduce inflammation.

Feverfew (*Tanacetum parthenium; Chrysanthemum parthenium*)

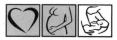

Part used:	Leaves
Main constituents:	Vitamins A, B$_1$, B$_2$, B$_3$, C; tin; silicon; selenium; protein; potassium; phosphorus; magnesium; manganese; fat; fiber; chromium; calcium; parthenolides; terpenes (camphor; L-borneol)[35]
Alternatives:	Skullcap (*Scutellaria lateriflora*); valerian (*Valeriana officinalis*)
Notes for caution:	**During preconception:** Feverfew is an emmenagogue.
	During pregnancy: Because feverfew is an emmenagogue, it is best to avoid therapeutic doses in early pregnancy.

Feverfew is an important nervine. It is one of the best natural remedies for those afflicted with migraine. This is not an acute medicine, however, as it needs to be taken regularly over a period of several weeks to build up a concentration in the blood.

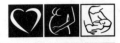

Flax (*Linum usitatissimum*)

Part used:	Ripe seeds
Main constituents:	Mucilage; alpha linoleic acid
Alternatives:	None
Notes for caution:	**During preconception:** Flax is an emmenagogue. **During pregnancy:** Because it can act as an emmenagogue, it is best to avoid using flax during the first trimester.

Because of its high mucilage content, flax can soothe tissues both internally and externally. It is often used as a bulk laxative, but is also good for relieving cough, and is believed to be a galactagogue.

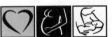

Forsythia (lian qiao) (*Forsythia suspense*)

Part used:	Fruit
Main constituents:	Phenylethanoids; forsythiaside; suspensaside; lignans; phillyrin (+) - pinoresinol; O-p-D-glucoside; phenylethanoids
Alternatives:	Elder (*Sambucus nigra*); shiitake (*Lentinula edodes*)
Notes for caution:	**During preconception:** Forsythia is an emmenagogue. **During pregnancy:** Forsythia is an emmenagogue and believed to be a uterine stimulant.

Forsythia fruit is one of the star players in the honeysuckle and forsythia combination (yin qiao san), a favorite cold and flu remedy in traditional Chinese medicine.

Fo Ti (ho shou wu) (*Polygoniun multiflorum*)

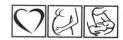

Part used:	Root
Main constituents:	Vitamin B$_3$; zinc; tin; selenium; protein; potassium; magnesium; iron; fat; fiber; cobalt; aluminum;[35] chrysophanic acid; chrysophanol; emodin
Alternatives:	None
Male fertility:	Traditionally used to increase sperm count and quality and improve sperm motility. It has been used in formula for impotence and premature ejaculation.

Fo ti is known for helping us to age well. It might have a lot to offer pregnant and nursing moms because it strengthens the kidneys, liver and blood — all of which are stressed during pregnancy. In traditional Chinese medicine, fo ti is used to maintain muscles, tendons, ligaments and bones.

Frangula (*Rhamnus frangula*)

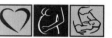

Part used:	Fruit
Main constituents:	Anthraquinones (rhamnocarthrin); vitamin C
Alternatives:	Dandelion root (*Taraxacum officinale*); yellow dock root (*Rumex crispus*)
Notes for caution:	**During preconception:** Anthraquinones can potentially cause birth defects. There is concern that this herb also may be an abortifacient.
	During pregnancy: Anthraquinones can potentially cause birth defects. There is concern that this herb also may be an aborifacient.
	During lactation: Because anthraquinones are partially excreted in milk, it is believed that the herb has a laxative effect in infants. There is also the potential to pass along the genotoxins emodin and aloe-emodin.

Frangula is one of the buckthorn species and a strong laxative known as an evacuant. It works by chemical stimulation of the brain or bowels and can irritate the intestinal lining.

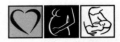

Fritillary (chuan bei mu) (*Fritillaria* spp.)

Part used:	Processed bulb
Main constituents:	Alkaloids; fritimine
Alternatives:	Bamboo shavings (*Caulis bambusae in taeniis*)
Notes for caution:	**During preconception:** This herb has been known to cause uterine contractions.
	During pregnancy: The herb has been known to cause uterine contractions.

In traditional Chinese medicine, this herb is used as the energetic counterpart to the herb arisaema. Fritillary is for chronic, unproductive cough caused by heat and phlegm in the chest.

Garlic (*Allium sativum*)

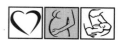

Galactagogue	
Part used:	Bulb
Main constituents:	Vitamin B_1; sodium; selenium; protein; potassium; phosphorus; cobalt; chromium; allicin; citral; geraniol; linalool; phellandrene; S-methyl-1-cysteine sulfoxide[35]
Alternatives:	None
Notes for caution:	**During pregnancy:** Excessive use is not a good idea because of potential emmenagogue and uterine-stimulating effects. It is believed that standardized preparations of garlic do not have these effects.
Male fertility:	Traditionally believed to be an aphrodisiac, garlic can be used in place of prescription male enhancement products due to its ability to sustain erection.

I wouldn't go into cold and flu season without garlic. Its antimicrobial action includes bacteria, viruses, fungus and some internal parasites. It is also being used successfully to reduce blood pressure and cholesterol levels. Garlic and onions are an important dietary choice for any mother fighting thrush. They are in the same plant family and are often grouped in a cautionary note during breastfeeding. While it is worth seeing if a child reacts negatively after the mother has eaten a lot of either one, there is no negative health impact on the child. If a child does become colicky or refuses the breast, it is best to avoid garlic or use it only in the case of illness.

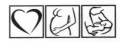

Gentian (*Gentiana lutea*)

Part used:	Root
Main constituents:	Vitamins A, B$_1$, B$_2$, B$_3$; zinc; tin; selenium; protein; phosphorus; magnesium; iron; fiber; chromium; calcium; aluminum; amarogentin; gentiopicroside; gentiobiose; volatile oils; alkaloids (gentianine, gentialutine); flavonoids (gentisein, gentisin) [35]
Alternatives:	None

Gentian is the classic "bitters" herb. It is used to stimulate and tone the liver and gallbladder to begin producing bile in anticipation of the proper digestion of your food. It is safe to continue using bitters with gentian while you are building a baby.

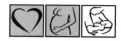

Ginger (*Zingiber officinale*)

Galactagogue	(when fresh)
Part used:	Rhizome
Main constituents:	Vitamins B$_2$, B$_3$, C; tin; sodium; silicon; selenium; potassium; phosphorus; manganese; magnesium; iron; fiber; cobalt; aluminum; 1,8-cineole; 6-gingerol; 6-shogaol; 8-shogaol; acetic acid; alpha-linolenic acid; alpha-phellandrene; alpha-pinene; alpha-terpinene; alpha-terpineol; arginine; ascorbic acid; beta-bisolene; beta-carotene; beta-pinene; beta-sitosterol; boron; caffeic acid; camphor; capsaicin; chlorogenic acid; curcumene; gingerols; sesquiphellandrene; zingiberene; resins; starches; fats[35]
Alternatives:	None
Notes for caution:	**During preconception and pregnancy:** Ginger is not a problem when used as a spice or as part of herbal teas. Excessive use is not a good idea because of potential emmenagogue and abortifacient effects.

This is another herb that I would not go into cold and flu season without. Ginger is a heat producer that has been used traditionally in poultice form to bring heat and blood flow to the pelvis for treatment of various female complaints. It is also used as a diaphoretic in breaking a fever. It is antiviral and helpful with allergies and asthma as well as cholesterol. It's also effective against internal worms, which is the reason it accompanies the raw fish in sushi. In traditional Chinese medicine, oil of ginger is often used to help turn a baby in the womb. It is massaged into the lower back and has a fairly high success rate. Definitely something to look into if you are dealing with a baby who won't turn in the final weeks of pregnancy, along with finding a chiropractor who is familiar with the Webster Technique.

REPRODUCTIVE PHASE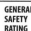
Preconception Pregnancy Lactation GENERAL SAFETY RATING No Contraindications Use with Caution Generally Avoid

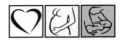

Ginkgo (bai guo) (*Ginkgo biloba*)

Part used:	Leaf
Main constituents:	Vitamins A, B_1, B_3; zinc; sodium; selenium; potassium; phosphorus; iron; fat; fiber; chromium; calcium; terpenes; tannins; flavonoids (ginkgo heterosides, ginkgolic acid, pro-anthocyanidines)[35]
Alternatives:	None
Notes for caution:	Wait to use ginkgo until postpartum bleeding has passed. The herb can act as a blood thinner that might promote blood flow.
Male fertility:	Ginkgo has applications for impotence because it enhances blood flow to the penile artery, sustaining erection without any negative effects for blood pressure.

Ginkgo is best known for its ability to cross the blood-brain barrier and increase blood flow. Aging issues such as memory loss often occur as we lose more and more blood flow to all parts of our brain. Washing our brain in blood keeps our mind sharp. Ginkgo is often combined with gotu kola for this purpose. It's also great to promote better circulation to the extremities.

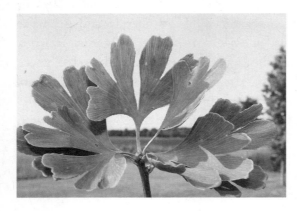

Ginko aka: Bai guo
(Ginkgo biloba)

REPRODUCTIVE PHASE	Preconception	Pregnancy	Lactation	GENERAL SAFETY RATING	No Contraindications	Use with Caution	Generally Avoid

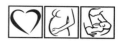

Ginseng (*Panax ginseng; Panax quinquefolius*)

Part used:	Root
Main constituents:	Acetic acid; adenine; adenosine; alanine; ascorbic acid; benzoic acid; beta-sitosterol; caryophyllene; cysteine; ferulic acid; at least 11 different ginsenosides; essential oil (panacene); 6 different panaxosides; glycine; guanidine; histidine; isoleucine; kaempferol; magnesium; salicyclic acid; tannins (malic acid); tyrosine; vanadium; zinc; vitamins B_2, B_3; germanium; manganese; selenium; fat; fiber; chromium[35]
Alternatives:	None
Male fertility:	Traditionally believed to be an aphrodisiac, ginseng may be used in place of prescription male enhancement products due to its ability to sustain erection.

Ginseng invigorates and increases vitality. It can have a positive effect on depression, low energy and general weakness. It is an adaptogen that tends to help the body in times of stress and overwork. There are two different types of ginseng: *Panax ginseng,* which comes from Asia, and *Panax quinquefolius,* which comes from America. They have different energies and often address different types of problems. *Panax quinquefolius* is more often used for women's issues as it provides a "cool" or "moist" yin energy more appropriate for adding balance when women get too "hot" and "dry." *Panax ginseng* tends to be more "hot" or yang in energy and can be used when that type of heat is needed for balance.

   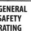

Goat's Rue (*Galega officinalis*)

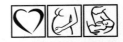

Galactagogue	
Part used:	Aerial portions
Main constituents:	Galegine; tannins; chromium
Alternatives:	None

Goat's rue is an important galactagogue used not only to promote milk supply but also to grow glandular tissue in the breast. It is applicable in cases of tubular hypoplastic breasts, for women who are hoping to nurse an adopted child or to increase general milk supply for all others. It is also one of the herbs used in natural diabetic therapies to reduce blood sugar levels.

Gokshura (*Tribulus terrestris*)

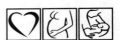

Part used:	Fruit
Main constituents:	3,7,11,15-tetramethyl-2-hexadecen-1-o1; N-hexadecadienoic acid; hexadecadienoic acid; ethyl ester; phytol; 9, 12-octadecadienoic acid; 9,12,15-octadecatrienoic acid; octadecanoic acid; 1,2-benzenedicarboxylic acid; disooctyl ester; α-Amyrin
Alternatives:	None
Male fertility:	This is a tonic herb that has traditionally been used to improve libido and treat impotence. It has been shown to increase sperm survival time. Research has also shown that it increases the endogenous production of luteinizing hormone, possibly stimulating endogenous testosterone and increasing potency in both men and women.[51]

Gokshura is an ayurvedic treatment that excels in the genitourinary tract and as a circulatory tonic. This herb is worth looking at if you are having erratic or missed ovulations and suspect that you are not producing an appropriate level of luteinizing hormone.

Goldenrod (*Solidago virgaurea*)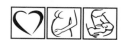

Galactagogue	
Part used:	Aerial portions
Main constituents:	Flavonoids (kaempferol, rhamnetin, quercetin, quercitrin, astragalin afzetin); saponins; gemacrene; essential oil (pinene, limonene); hydoxycinnamic acid; tannins (caffeic acid)
Alternatives:	None

Goldenrod has traditionally been used to treat stones in the urinary tract. It is useful for any kind of inflammation in the kidneys or bladder and is used to tone the muscles of the bladder. It would be a nice addition to body work and nutrition for regaining tone in the pelvic floor when dealing with urinary incontinence.

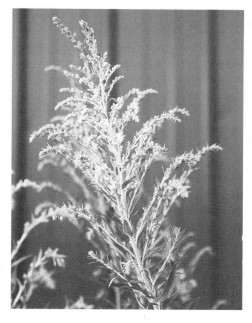

*Goldenrod (*Solidago virgaurea*)*

REPRODUCTIVE PHASE			GENERAL SAFETY RATING		
Preconception	Pregnancy	Lactation		No Contraindications	Use with Caution	Generally Avoid

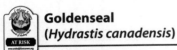

Internal use   **External use**

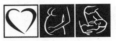   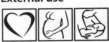

Part used:	Root
Main constituents:	Vitamins B_1, B_2, B_3, C; zinc; tin; silicon; selenium; protein; manganese; magnesium; iron; fat; fiber; cobalt; chromium; aluminum;[35] hydrastine; berberine; berberastine; canadine; candaline; hydrastinine; fatty acids; resin; polyphenolic acids; meconin; chlorogenic acid; phytosterins; volatile oil
Alternatives:	Marsh tea homeopathic (*Ledum palustre*); shiitake (*Lentinula edodes*); elder (*Sambucus nigra*)
Notes for caution:	**Internal use during pregnancy:** Berberine, an alkaloid, is a mild toxin that has a depressant effect on the heart and lungs. There is some evidence that it is also a uterine stimulant in some doses.
	Internal use during lactation: Berberine, an alkaloid, is a mild toxin that has a depressant effect on the heart and lungs. There is some evidence that it is also a uterine stimulant in some doses. This herb could be especially problematic if your baby has been diagnosed with jaundice.
Author's note:	Because of the number of volatile oils in this root, use the infusion, rather than the decoction, method when making a tea.

A natural antibiotic, goldenseal has a strong affinity for the mucus membranes and is most effective in these areas of our bodies and with the illnesses that attack them. It is just as effective externally as internally when there is infection. Do be careful, though, as it is a Native American dye plant and will quickly stain things yellow. While goldenseal should not be used with impunity, it would still be my first choice over an allopathic antibiotic and its possible side effects, for either me or my nursing child. During pregnancy or lactation, it is best to consult with an experienced herbal practitioner if you wish to use goldenseal. Having a good relationship with your physician is also important, and if for some reason the infection does not immediately respond to goldenseal, you can always use a prescription antibiotic.

Goldthread (*Coptis groenlandica*)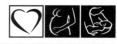

Part used:	Dried rhizome; roots; stems; leaves
Main constituents:	Berberine; coptine; albumen; sugar
Alternatives:	Hops (*Humulus lupulus*); artichoke (*Cynara scolymus*)
Notes for caution:	**During pregnancy:** Berberine, an alkaloid, is a mild toxin that has a depressant effect on the heart and lungs. There is some evidence that it is also a uterine stimulant in some doses.
	During lactation: Berberine, an alkaloid, is a mild toxin that has a depressant effect on the heart and lungs. There is some evidence that it is also a uterine stimulant in some doses. This herb could be especially problematic if your baby has been diagnosed with jaundice.

This herb is a classic bitter and has actions in the digestive system as well as in the liver. As it contains berberine, it has been routinely substituted for goldenseal.

Gotu Kola (*Centella asiastica*)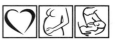

Part used:	Aerial portions
Main constituents:	Triterpenoid saponins; sapogenins; vitamins A, B_1, B_2, B_3, C; zinc; tin; sodium; selenium; protein; phosphorus; manganese; magnesium; fat; iron; fiber; cobalt; chromium; calcium; aluminum; pectins; terpenes[35]
Alternatives:	None

Gotu kola is best known for increasing cognitive functioning and is often paired with ginkgo. It might be of special interest to women recovering from a C-section as the topical application has been found to decrease the time a wound takes to heal after surgery. It is a delicious salad herb that can be grown in a pot if you don't live in a tropical location, and it is easy to obtain in dried form for tea.

Guarana (*Paullinia cupana*)

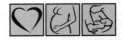

Part used:	Seeds
Main constituents:	Guaranine; tannic acid; catechutannic acid
Alternatives:	None
Notes for caution:	**During preconception:** Guaranine is identical to caffeine, which is extremely drying to cervical fluids and also places an unnecessary burden on the endocrine system, which can result in hormonal imbalances.
	During pregnancy: Guaranine is identical to caffeine, which has been found to cross the placenta and contribute to low birth weight, preterm birth and birth defects.
	During lactation: Guaranine is identical to caffeine, which has been found to appear in breast milk at half the level in the mother's plasma. It reduces the available iron supply in breast milk.

Guarana is a stimulant and primarily acts on the nervous system. It is often used for headache, and some drink it on a regular basis as a health tonic. Currently it is found in many natural energy drinks and bars. The chemical constituent, guaranine, is chemically identical to caffeine and therefore warrants the same cautions.[45]

Gymnema (*Gymnema sylvestre*)

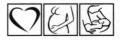

Galactagogue	
Part used:	Leaf
Main constituents:	Vitamins A, C; sodium; selenium; protein; potassium; phosphorus; iron; fat; chromium; gymnemic acid; parabin; tannin[35]
Alternatives:	None

Gymnema is an important galactagogue, but is also known as "destroyer of sugar." It is being used successfully in natural therapies for maintaining blood sugar levels.

Hawthorn (*Crataegus* spp.)

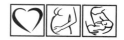

Part used:	Berry; leaf; flower
Main constituents:	Flavonoids and oligomeric procyanidins; tin; potassium; fat; fiber; chromium; calcium; selenium; volatile oil; saturated fatty acids (lauric, palmitic); unsaturated fatty acids (linoleic, linolenic); catechin; alkaloids (tyramine); coumarins. The berries contain more hyperoside than the leaves and flowers, and the leaves and flowers contain more vitexin rhamnoside than the berries[35, 44]
Alternatives:	None
Male fertility:	Hawthorn is an important circulatory tonic for the support of fertility.

Hawthorne berries are specific to the health of the heart. They have an amphoteric effect on the heart, either stimulating or depressing as needed, and can help with returning proper blood pressure levels after carrying a child. Hawthorne berries are also helpful with palpitations, but be sure to check with a chiropractor to ensure proper spinal alignment. A chiropractor may explain that heart palpitations are common when either the upper cervical or lower thoracic spine is out of place. This type of misalignment is common not only due to the posture required for nursing but also as a result of changes in posture during pregnancy. Hawthorne berries are also specific for orthostatic hypotension, a condition causing dizzy spells and loss of blood pressure when standing up, which can sometimes be a complication after a particularly difficult birth.

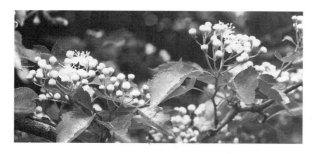

Hawthorn

(Crataegus *spp.*)

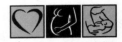

Hemp Agrimony (*Eupatorium cannabinum*)

Part used:	Aerial portion
Main constituents:	Volatile oil; tannins; alkaloids (pyrrolizidine alkaloids)
Alternatives:	**For fever:** Peppermint (*Mentha piperita*); catnip (*Cataria nepeta*); elder (*Sambucus nigra*)
	As a laxative: Dandelion root (Taraxacum officinale); yellow dock root (Rumex crispus)
Notes for caution:	**During preconception:** Hemp agrimony is an emmenagogue.
	During pregnancy: An emmenagogue, hemp agrimony also has abortifacient effects coupled with possible hepatotoxicity from pyrrolizidine alkaloids.
	During lactation: It is speculated that hemp agrimony is toxic to the nursing infant's liver. The herb may also have a negative laxative effect.

Hemp agrimony is not used very often today. It was known in its time as a valuable cathartic and fever reducer.

REPRODUCTIVE PHASE	Preconception	Pregnancy	Lactation	**GENERAL SAFETY RATING**	No Contraindications	Use with Caution	Generally Avoid

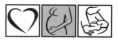

Hibiscus (*Hibiscus sabdariffa*)

Galactagogue	
Part used:	Flower
Main constituents:	Vitamins A, C; tin; sodium; silicon; selenium; manganese; cobalt; chromium; aluminum; citric acid; malic acid; tartaric acid; anthocyanins (delphinidins and cyanidins); ibiscic acid; saponins; mucilage; pectins[35]
Alternatives:	None
Notes for caution:	**During pregnancy:** Excessive use in early pregnancy should be avoided as it can act as an emmenagogue and abortifacient.

Often used for its vitamin C content, hibiscus is also slightly astringent. The combination makes it helpful in the case of mild colds and flus. Currently popular for its use as a circulatory and heart tonic, the herb has successfully reduced blood pressure in clinical trials.[50] There is evidence that it might prove useful in lowering cholesterol levels as well.

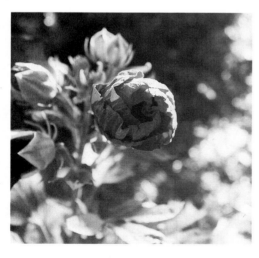

*Hibiscus (*Hibiscus sabdariffa*)*

| REPRODUCTIVE PHASE | Preconception | Pregnancy | Lactation | GENERAL SAFETY RATING | No Contraindications | Use with Caution | Generally Avoid |

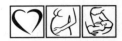

Holy Basil (tulsi) (*Ocimum sanctum*)

Galactagogue	
Part used:	Leaf
Main constituents:	Eugenol app.; beta-caryophyllene; sesquiterpenes; monoterpenes; ascorbic acid; carotene; calcium; iron; selenium; zinc; manganese; sodium[41]
Alternatives:	None

Holy Basil is a very important adaptogen in ayurveda. It is used to help the body restore balance after some type of stress, and is often suggested for use after birth. It is highly regarded for a host of physical ailments and is generally taken routinely over a long period of time as a tonic.

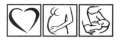

Hops (*Humulus lupulus*)

Galactagogue	
Part used:	Dried flower
Main constituents:	Terpenes; bitter resin; choline; tannins; flavonoid antioxidants; lupulone; humulene; vitamins B_1, B_2, B_3, B_{12}, C; calcium; magnesium; manganese; potassium; selenium; zinc; tin; silicon; protein; phosphorus; fat; fiber[35]
Alternatives:	None

Hops is the first herb anyone should try for sleeplessness. It is also a very important nervous system tonic. Women can use hops in tea form if they don't mind the taste, but most people use a tincture. Hops are an important and long-storied galactagogue. In many cultures, a daily small beer was given to women to increase their milk supply. For many years in this country that practice was frowned upon, but recent research has shown that minimal alcohol use while nursing will not do an infant any harm.[51] If you decide to use beer to increase your supply, be sure to pick one that has been brewed to feature a heavy amount of hops. Your beer should reek of hops and taste extremely bitter. Don't bother with the generic brewers who use hops as an afterthought. You will just be wasting calories and introducing alcohol to your system for no good purpose. Whatever hops brew you drink should be offset by (and not considered a part of) an appropriate amount of water, because alcohol is an antidiuretic that can be drying in the body.

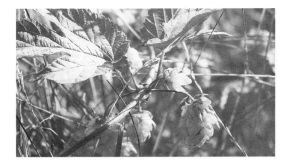

*Hops (*Humulus lupulus*)*

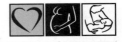

Horehound (*Marrubium vulgare*)

Part used:	Leaf
Main constituents:	Marrubium; volatile oil; tannin; fat; sugar
Alternatives:	Elecampane (*Inula helenium*); mullein (*Verbascum thapsus*)
Notes for caution:	**During preconception:** Horehound is an emmenagogue.
	During pregnancy: Horehound is a known emmenagogue and abortifacient due to uterine stimulation.

Horehound has a long history of use with tenacious phlegmy coughs. It is best when it is fresh, but can be used dry. For children, horehound made into candies, syrups or teas; given in small, frequent doses it can aid with croup and also be a tonic for the stomach. This is currently a popular ingredient in natural cold and cough remedies.

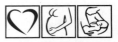

Horny Goat Weed (*Epimedium sagittatum, E. grandiflora*)

Part used:	Aerial portion
Main constituents:	Icariin
Alternatives:	None
Male fertility:	Traditionally used to increase sperm count and help with impotence and premature ejaculation. It is one of the herbs that can be used in place of prescription male enhancement drugs to sustain an erection without negative side effects.

This herb is helpful in the genitourinary tract, but also has applications for rheumatic pain in joints and for irregular menstruation that comes as a result of liver weakness

Horsetail (*Equisetum* spp.)

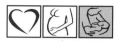

Part used:	Aerial portions
Main constituents:	Silica; vitamins A, B_2, B_3, C, and D; calcium; chromium; iron; magnesium; manganese; potassium; selenium; sulfur; tin; sodium; protein; phosphorus; fat; fiber; cobalt; aluminum; tannin; saponins; flavonoids; alkaloids[35]
Alternatives:	**Calcium supplement:** Oatstraw (*Avena sativa*) **Diuretic:** Dandelion (*Taraxacum officinale*)
Notes for caution:	**During lactation:** Because of its high inorganic silica content, it is best to keep the use of this herb to a minimum to prevent a negative reaction in a nursing mother.

Horsetail contains thiaminase, which breaks down vitamin B_1 (thiamine) and can cause a deficiency if taken for too long. A deficiency of thiamine can lead to beriberi or eating disorders. It can also lead to reduced levels of hydrochloric acid and thereby contribute to digestive issues.[4] Horsetail is most often used for its ability to help the kidneys rid the body of toxins through increased urine output. It is also highly nutritional (especially if silica is needed) and found in many herbal vitamin blends.

Hyssop (*Hyssopus officinalis*)

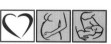

Part used:	Aerial portions
Main constituents:	Alpha-glucosidase inhibitors; essential oil
Alternatives:	Elecampane (*Inula helenium*); mullein (*Verbascum thapsus*)
Notes for caution:	**During preconception:** Hyssop is an emmenegogue. **During pregnancy:** Hyssop is an emmenagogue and abortifacient.

Hyssop is another great herb for both the lungs and the digestion. It is most often used for expelling mucus from the lungs, especially when there is a fever, and is frequently found in combination with horehound. It is generally taken warm, which encourages its diaphoretic action.

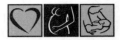

Ipecac (*Cephalelis ipecacuanha*)

Part used:	Roots; rhizome
Main constituents:	Elemitine; cephaeline; psychotrine; ipecacuanhic acid; choline; resin; pectin; starch; sugar; calcium oxalate; volatile oil
Alternatives:	None
Notes for caution:	**During preconception:** The alkaloid emetine is a uterine stimulant.
	During pregnancy: The alkaloid emetine is a uterine stimulant.
	During lactation: The herb is known to be toxic in large doses (emetic dose). It is best to use only standardized preparations and to work with a trained herbal practitioner if you choose to use this herb. *Proper dosage levels are important.*

Ipecac was used mainly as an emetic. Taken in smaller doses, it has also been used for dysentery and respiratory disorders. Ipecac was most commonly obtained over the counter as syrup of ipecac. It is no longer available in your local drugstore or grocery and is not recommended by poison control centers as a typical remedy for poisoning. It became clear that not every case of poisoning called for an emetic because vomiting often caused more harm than good. It is now recommended that you call your local poison control line first in the event of suspected poisoning.

Jaborandi (*Pilocarpus* spp.)

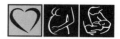

Part used:	Leaf
Main constituents:	Volatile oil; dipentene; tannic acid; potassium chloride; alkaloids (pilocarpine, isopilocarpine, pilocarpidine, jaborine)
Alternatives:	**Diuretic:** Dandelion (*Taraxacum officinale*)
	Diaphoretic: Yarrow (*Achillea millefolium*); elder (*Sambucus nigra*)
Notes for caution:	**During preconception:** The alkaloid pilocarpine can cause uterine contractions when taken internally.
	During pregnancy: The alkaloid pilocarpine can cause uterine contractions when taken internally.
	During lactation: The alkaloid pilocarpine acts on the autonomous nervous system and can have negative effects on the functioning of the heart and lungs of a nursing infant.

This herb has a number of alkaloids that are helpful in the treatment of glaucoma. Internally, it is a diuretic and diaphoretic. By stimulating the autonomous nervous system, it has a wide range of effects such as stimulating salivation and perspiration.

 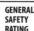

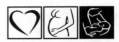

Jamaica Dogwood (*Piscidia erythrina*)

Part used:	Bark
Main constituents:	Resin; fat; piscidin; piscidic acid
Alternatives:	**Toothache:** Clove essential oil
	Asthma: Elecampane (*Inula helenium*); wild cherry bark (*Prunus serotina*); cramp bark (*Viburnum opulus*)
Notes for caution:	**During lactation:** In large doses, this herb is toxic, and in small doses is believed to cause nervous system irritation and/or act as a neuromuscular depressant in nursing infants.

While some people find this herb useful for toothache or spasmodic lung issues such as whooping cough and asthma, an equal number who've tried it have had negative effects. It is best avoided while you are nursing. While there are no contraindications attached to this herb for preconception or pregnancy, I advise women to seek out a qualified herbal practitioner if they want to take this herb at any point while building a baby.

   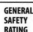

Flowers   Berries

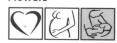

Jasmine (*Jasminum officinale*)

Antigalactagogue	
Part used:	Flowers
Main constituents:	Alpha-terpineol; benzaldehyde; benzoic acid; benzyl acetate; benzyl alcohol; eugenol; farnesol; geraniol; jasmone; linalyl acetate; nerolidol, salicyclic acid; vanillin[41]
Alternatives:	None
Notes for caution:	**Flower use during lactation:** The flowers of jasmine are believed to interfere with a mother's milk supply.
	Berries during preconception, pregnancy and lactation: A reported case of childhood toxicity is listed in the 1861 *Dispensatory of the United States of America*.[52]

Several different types of jasmine are used commercially, all for different purposes. While jasmine is not toxic unless you eat the berries, it is best to be aware of your intake of jasmine tea while nursing and monitor any changes in your milk supply.

Jatamansi (*Nardostachys jatamansi*)

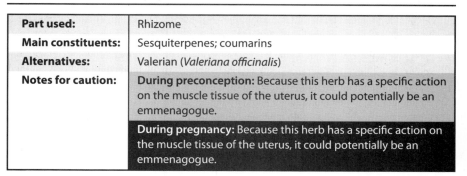

Part used:	Rhizome
Main constituents:	Sesquiterpenes; coumarins
Alternatives:	Valerian (*Valeriana officinalis*)
Notes for caution:	**During preconception:** Because this herb has a specific action on the muscle tissue of the uterus, it could potentially be an emmenagogue.
	During pregnancy: Because this herb has a specific action on the muscle tissue of the uterus, it could potentially be an emmenagogue.

Jetamansi is an ayurvedic sedative and antispasmodic that is used in similar fashion to valerian. It is believed to have a specific action on the pelvic region and therefore has been used in the past to treat a lack of menstruation. It is also used in ayurveda for relief of mental and psychological distress.

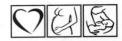

Jerusalem Artichoke (*Helianthus tuberosus*)

Part used:	Tuber
Main constituents:	Inulin; vitamins A, B_1, B_2, B_3, B_6, B_9, C; calcium; potassium; phosphorus magnesium; iron; zinc
Alternatives:	None

This bright yellow, sunflower-like flowering plant is native to my area of the country. We dig its tubers and use them much like very flavorful potatoes. They are important in the maintenance of health for diabetics as they have the ability to control blood sugar.

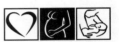

Job's Tears (*Coix lacryma-jobi*)

Part used:	Seed
Main constituents:	Starch; sugar; protein; amino acids; coixol; coixenolide; coixans
Alternatives:	Dandelion (*Taraxacum officinale*)
Notes for caution:	**During pregnancy:** Avoid it.[38]

It's a shame that this herb isn't appropriate for pregnancy, as it is great for draining inflammation, swelling and edema. Job's tears is anti-inflammatory and diuretic in nature. This herb is excellent for rheumatism and arthritis.

Joe Pye Weed (*Eupatorium purpureum*)

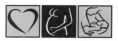

Part used:	Root
Main constituents:	Euparin; eupurpurin; pyrrolizidine alkaloids
Alternatives:	Goldenrod (*Solidago virgaurea*)
Notes for caution:	**During preconception:** In large doses, joe pye weed can be an abortifacient.
	During pregnancy: The herb has been shown to be abortifacient in grazing cattle.
	During lactation: Because this herb is known to contain a certain amount of pyrrolizidine alkaloids, it is speculated that it may be toxic to the nursing infant's liver.

Also commonly known as queen of the meadow, joe pye weed is a common herb to use for kidney and bladder stones.

Jujube Seeds (da zao) (*Ziziphus spinosa*)

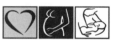

Part used:	Fruit
Main constituents:	Vitamins A, B_1, B_2, B_3, B_6, and C; calcium; iron; magnesium; phosphorus; potassium;[53] triterpenes; betulic acid; oleanic acid; jujubosides
Alternatives:	Skullcap (*Scutellaria lateriflora*)
Notes for caution:	**During preconception:** Jujube seeds are known to be an emmenagogue and some sources list them as an anti-fertility herb.
	During pregnancy: Jujube seeds are known to be an emmenagogue.

Jujube date is found in traditional Chinese and Middle Eastern medicine. It has quite a laundry list of uses, but is most often eaten for its nutritional content, its ability as a nervous system sedative for insomnia and its use in building overall body system vitality.

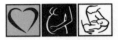

Juniper (*Juniperus communis*)

Part used:	Leaf; essential oil
Main constituents:	Essential oil (monoterpenes, sesquiterpenes); sugar; flavone; glycosides; resin; tannin[44]
Alternatives:	Goldenrod (*Solidago virgaurea*)
Notes for caution:	**During preconception:** Because it is a urinary tract irritant, juniper can have a secondary effect as a uterine stimulant.
	During pregnancy: Because it is a urinary tract irritant, juniper can have a secondary effect as a uterine stimulant

Juniper leaf is an antiseptic diuretic. It has application for arthritis or kidney diseases, and has a calming effect on disorders of the digestive system.

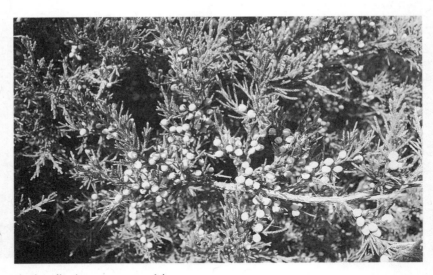

*Juniper (*Juniperus communis*)*

REPRODUCTIVE PHASE   Preconception   Pregnancy   Lactation   GENERAL SAFETY RATING   No Contraindications   Use with Caution   Generally Avoid

Kava Kava (*Piper methysticum*)

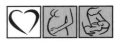

Part used:	Root
Main constituents:	Kavalactones (kavain, dihydrokavain, methysticin, dihydromethysticin, yangonin, desmethoxyyangonin); pyrones
Alternatives:	Lemon balm (*Melissa officinalis*); rose (*Rosa* spp.); lavender (*Lavendula angustifolia*)
Notes of caution:	**During pregnancy:** The chemical constituent of pyrone can potentially cause loss of uterine tone.
	During lactation: Kava is contraindicated in cases of depression. There have been 31 documented cases of liver toxicity in conjunction with the use of this herb. Ten cases were reversed; four needed a liver transplant; and one died. There were extenuating circumstances in all cases involving excess dosage, alcoholism and concurrent prescription drug use. Nonetheless, it has not been determined conclusively that kava is safe. All formulations (water, alcohol and acetone) have been implicated in the case studies.[54] There is also the possibility of the passage of pyrones in breast milk.

Kava is one of the best herbal therapies for anxiety. There is currently quite a bit of concern about its use and many studies are being conducted. The root contains no pipermethystine, an alkaloid that is being looked at as a source of possible problems. If your supply of kava has been adulterated with any other part of the plant, this chemical compound will be present. If you choose to use this herb, it is important to verify that you are getting an authentic product. It must always be used exactly as instructed. Kava is a powerful nervine sedative that has been used for thousands of years in traditional societies. It is a ceremonial beverage that was used in treaty making, marriage bargains and other uncomfortable situations. It has the ability to loosen the tongue, lighten the mood and ease tension. If you are experiencing serious postpartum anxiety, this is an herb to explore carefully with your health care team.

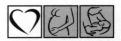

Kelp (*Nereocystis luetkeana*)

Part used:	Thallus (Leaf)
Main constituents:	Vitamins A, B$_3$, C, K; calcium; iron; zinc; tin; sodium; silicon; selenium; potassium; phosphorus, manganese; magnesium; fat; fiber; aluminum; saturated fatty acids (palmitic, stearic, myristic, squalane); unsaturated fatty acids (oleic, arachidonic); saponins (cholesterol, fucosterol, beta sitosterol); algin; iodine[35]
Alternatives:	Sea salt **For hypothyroidism:** Eleuthero (*Eleutherococcus senticosus, Acanthopanax senticosus*) **For calcium:** Red raspberry (*Rubus ideaus*); oatstraw (*Avena sativa*)
Notes for caution:	**During pregnancy:** Excessive consumption during pregnancy can lead to infantile goiter.[34] It is best to keep any therapeutic dosage of any type of seaweed to no more than 0.25 gram daily. **During lactation:** With high doses or prolonged use, seaweed can overstimulate the thyroid. It is believed that the high iodine content could be a potential toxin to the nursing infant.

Kelp and other seaweeds like it are often used as good sources of calcium. Kelp is one of the best natural solutions for mild underactive thyroid dysfunction due to its iodine content. Women who use kelp to help the thyroid should be under the supervision of a medical professional who can monitor their progress with blood testing. They should go slowly and start with very low doses until they see if it is improving their numbers.

Khella (*Ammi visnaga*)

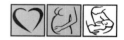

Part used:	Fruit; seeds
Main constituents:	thymol; isothymol; A-pinene; P-cymene; Y-terpinene; limonene; coumarin; furocoumarin (khellin, visnagin); volatile oil[55]
Alternatives:	Elecampane (*Inula helenium*); wild cherry bark (*Prunus serotina*); cramp bark (*Viburnum opulus*)
Notes for caution:	**During preconception:** Khella can act as an emmenegogue. **During pregnancy:** Khella has been known to be a uterine stimulant and an emmenegogue.

The use of khella originated in Egypt. It is antibacterial and anti-spasmodic and a bronchial dilator. All of these properties combine to make this herb very useful in respiratory and related cardiac ailments, as well as in asthma. The high volatile oil component makes it great in the digestive system and for indigestion or flatulence.

Knot Grass (*Polygonum aviculare*)

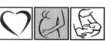

Part used:	Aerial portions
Main constituents:	Volatile oils; quercitol; salicyclic acid; tannins; silica; kaempferol
Alternatives:	Plantain (*Plantago lanceolata, Plantago major*)
Notes for caution:	**During pregnancy:** Excessive use is believed to make this herb an abortifacient.

This unassuming weed is diuretic and astringent. It can be used to stop bleeding in a pinch, or can help with internal hemorrhages and varicosities. This is also a great little plant to know about if you're camping and wind up with diarrhea.

Lady's Mantle (*Alchemilla vulgaris*)

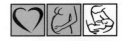

Part used:	Aerial portions
Main constituents:	Tannins; flavonoids (quercitin); salicyclic acid
Alternatives:	Blackberry root (*Rubus fruticosus, Rubus villosus*)
Notes for caution:	**During preconception and pregnancy:** In some sources, the tonic nature of the herb is viewed as a possible uterine stimulant.

This wonderful herb is not used as much as it should be in the Americas. It is easy to grow and very beautiful. It is astringent and therefore helps in any disorder that could use a little tightening, such as diarrhea, irregular menstruation, etc. It is a perfect restorative to add to your teas after labor.

Lavender (*Lavendula angustifolia*)

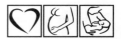

Galactagogue	
Part used:	Flower
Main constituents:	Volatile oil; linalyl acetate; linalol; geraniol; cineole; limonene; sesquiterpenes
Alternatives:	None

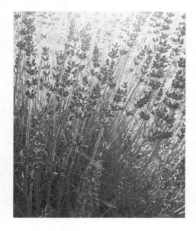

Lavender is used to best effect for depression, and can be helpful during the postpartum time of hormonal shifts. It is also helpful for tension headaches and to promote the soothing and calming needed to get a good sleep. When harvested at peak medicinal potency, it contains bitter components that soothe the digestion.

*Lavender (*Lavendula angustifolia*)*

Lemon Balm (*Melissa officinalis*)

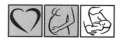

Galactagogue	
Part used:	Aerial portion
Main constituents:	Essential oils (citral, citronella, geraniol, linalol); bitter flavones; flavones; resin
Alternatives:	**For depression/anxiety:** Rose (*Rosa* spp.)
Notes for caution:	**During preconception:** The herb is an emmenagogue in therapeutic doses.
	During pregnancy: Lemon balm has some recorded instances of use as an emmenagogue. It also tends to inhibit thyroid and gonadotropic hormones. It is best to use in a nontherapeutic dose as a flavor in herbal teas or in food, not as an active herbal therapy during pregnancy.
Author's note:	Women with hypothyroidism should avoid lemon balm at all phases.

Lemon balm is extremely gentle while being exceedingly powerful. It is highly effective as a general soother for our nervous system, subsequently aiding in anxiety and depression. It has been tested over the years and found to be very helpful for those who suffer from seasonal affective disorder. It has also been found to help with the attention deficit spectrum of disorders. Because it is tasty, lemon balm is easy to eat in salads, drink in tea or make into glycerite. It is also an important herb for both internal and external treatment of things that "sleep" at the nerve endings, such as viruses including shingles, chicken pox and herpes, some of which often crop up periodically in times of stress or low body resistance.

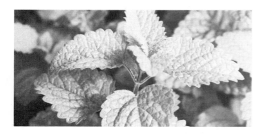

Lemon Balm (Melissa officinalis)

Lemongrass (*Cymbopogon citratus*)

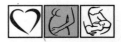

Part used:	Aerial portions
Main constituents:	Essential oil (citral, myrcene, nerol, limonene, linalool); beta-caryophyllene; fat; cobalt; chromium; aluminum; iron; magnesium; manganese; selenium; sodium; silicon; potassium; phosphorus[41,35]
Alternatives:	Cramp bark (*Viburnum opulus*); eucalyptus (*Eucalyptus* spp.)
Notes for caution:	**During pregnancy:** In therapeutic doses, lemongrass is reported to be an emmenagogue. Use this only as a flavoring ingredient in your food and beverage during pregnancy.

Lemongrass is used mainly as a flavoring in traditional Thai and Indonesian cuisine, and in many herbal tea blends. It does have some medicinal actions, mainly in cooling the body, helping with digestion and relieving headaches and menstrual cramping. It has also been shown to contain some antimicrobial action against *E. coli* and *Stapylococcus aureus*. In our culture, it is not used heavily in healing and should never be taken to excess. However, it is safe to use in your food or in a favorite blend you drink during lactation.

Dried rhizome   Fresh root

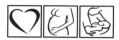

Leptandra (*Veronica virginica*)

Part used:	Dried rhizome; fresh root
Main constituents:	Volatile oil; tannins; gum; resin; sugar
Alternatives:	Gentian (*Gentiana lutea*); dandelion root (*Taraxacum officinale*); yellow dock (*Rumex crispus*)
Notes for caution:	**Fresh root during preconception, pregnancy and lactation:** The fresh root is violently cathartic and emetic and has been shown to be an abortifacient.

Even in small doses, the dried rhizome of this herb is powerful. It is often employed to aid the body in cleansing the liver or gallbladder. This relatively strong herb should not be used without the guidance of an experienced practitioner.

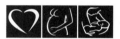

Levant Wormseed (*Artemesia cina*)

Part used:	Aerial portions
Main constituents:	Santonin; artemisin; cineol
Alternatives:	Pumpkin seeds (*Curcurbita* spp.); garlic (*Allium sativum*); black walnut hull (*Juglans nigra*)
Notes for caution:	**During preconception, pregnancy and lactation:** Santonin has resulted in several recorded cases of fatal poisoning.

Levant wormseed has been used in the United States to remove intestinal worms in children. Even in small doses, it has been known to have negative side effects. It is best to avoid this herb in favor of others if you or your child suffers from a worm infestation.

REPRODUCTIVE PHASE   GENERAL SAFETY RATING

Preconception   Pregnancy   Lactation   No Contraindications   Use with Caution   Generally Avoid

Licorice (*Glycyrrhiza glabra*)

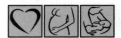

Galactagogue	
Part used:	Root
Main constituents:	Glycyrrhizin; glycyrrhizic acid; glycyrrhetic acid; sugar; starch; gum; protein; fat; tannin; asparagine; resin; volatile oils; vitamins B$_1$, B$_3$, C; chromium; iron; magnesium; tin; sodium; silicon; potassium; manganese; fiber; cobalt; calcium; aluminum; terpenes (acetol, thujone, fenchone); saturated fatty acids (caprylic, hexanoic, palmitic); unsaturated fatty acids (linoleic, linolenic); salicyclic acid; flavonoids (quercitin, apigenin); coumarins; alkaloids (tryptamine, pryrazine, pyrrolidine); pectin[35]
Alternatives:	Borage (*Borago officinalis*)
Notes for caution:	**During preconception and pregnancy:** Licorice can be used as an emmenagogue. **During lactation:** The concentration of glycyrrhetinic acid in the herb might cause an unsafe retention of sodium and potassium in the nursing mother or child. This is especially dangerous for those already suffering from high blood pressure.
Male fertility:	Licorice can be very important for men due to its ability to support the adrenals. A common cause of sexual dysfunction is stress that leads to weakened adrenals. This herb is important to return full vitality to the male reproductive system.

Known as the great harmonizer, licorice is found in many herbal formulas as a balancer and sweetener. Its main component, glycyrrhizin, is structurally similar to adrenal cortical hormones. This makes it an important herb for helping with balance in the female body and in supporting our adrenal glands. The main reason for the fear surrounding its use is due to its history as a cough suppressant. When a Dutch pharamacist began using it heavily in his new cough medicine, it was discovered that the high concentration of glycyrrhetinic acid caused sodium and potassium retention. This can contribute to problems with high blood pressure. The presence of asparagine in licorice is believed to counteract this negative reaction if you are using it in its natural plant form rather than as a synthetic compilation. It still may warrant caution during your pregnancy or nursing relationship, especially if you are suffering from high blood pressure.

Life Root (*Senecio aureus*)

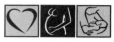

Part used:	Aerial portions
Main constituents:	Senecin; senecionine; florosenine; otosenine; floridanine
Alternatives:	**For respiratory applications:** Thyme (*Thymus vulgaris*) **For reproductive applications:** Pennyroyal (*Mentha pulegium*)
Notes for caution:	**During preconception:** Life root can be used as an emmenegogue.
	During pregnancy: The toxic alkaloid senecionine can cross the placenta and cause a potential danger to the developing fetus' liver.
	During lactation: Because it contains pyrrolizidine alkaloids (senecionine), life root is speculated to be a potential toxin to the liver of the nursing infant.

Life root, also known as groundsel, is astringent in nature. This astringency is often employed in the respiratory system for wasting diseases associated with phlegm in the lungs. It has also been used for bringing on delayed menstruation and aiding in pain relief and labor facilitation.

Liverwort (*Hepatica nobilis*)

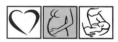

Part used:	Leaves; flowers
Main constituents:	Tannins; flavonoids; saponins; sugar; mucilage
Alternatives:	Gentian (*Gentiana lutea*); dandelion root (*Taraxacum officinale*); yellow dock (*Rumex crispus*)
Notes for caution:	**During pregnancy:** High doses may irritate the urinary tract, resulting in uterine stimulation.

As its name suggests, this is an herb that can be very helpful in treating the liver and its diseases. It is mostly astringent and works to tighten and tone the liver, gallbladder and lungs.

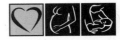

Lobelia (*Lobelia inflate*)

Part used:	Aerial portions; seeds
Main constituents:	Vitamins A, B$_1$, B$_3$, C; potassium; phosphorus; manganese; magnesium; iron; fat; fiber; calcium; aluminum; alkaloid (lobeline)[35]
Alternatives:	Elecampane (*Inula helenium*); wild cherry bark (*Prunus serotina*); cramp bark (*Viburnum opulus*)
Notes for caution:	**During preconception:** Lobelia can potentially interfere with uterine tone and can threaten fetal viability with the toxicity of the alkaloid lobeline.
	During pregnancy: Lobelia can potentially interfere with uterine tone and can threaten fetal viability with the toxicity of the alkaloid lobeline.
	During lactation: In large doses, lobelia is a potential toxin for the nursing infant. In smaller doses it carries the risk of emesis. Lobeline is similar in chemical makeup to nicotine and may carry the same risk of transmission to an infant, leading to immediate changes in respiration and oxygen saturation. It may also alter a child's intelligence and behavioral development.

Lobelia is one of those special herbs that have different qualities in different doses. In small doses, it is an important herb to help with controlling asthma. In larger doses, it's an emetic. It is not a good risk in either dose while building a healthy baby. Avoid it.

Lovage (*Levisticum officinale*)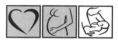

Galactagogue	
Part used:	Aerial portion; root
Main constituents:	Quercetin; the root also contains 1,8-cineole; camphor; coumarin; eugenol; limonene; menthol[41]
Alternatives:	**For respiratory issues:** Elecampane (*Inula helenium*); wild cherry bark (*Prunus serotina*); cramp bark (*Viburnum opulus*)
Notes for caution:	**During preconception and pregnancy:** In high therapeutic doses, this herb can be an emmenagogue. Use in food or beverage is acceptable.

Lovage is a perennial herb that can be swapped for celery in the kitchen. Like most kitchen herbs, it is carminative, but lovage has much more for us. It is antispasmodic, diuretic, diaphoretic and expectorant. It is helpful in the digestive tract, but also in the respiratory tract for issues such as bronchitis, asthma, allergies and even the common cold. Eating more than a serving of it a day or eating large portions at a time can bring on menstruation.[41]

 Lomatium (*Lomatium dissectum*)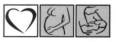

Galactagogue	
Part used:	Root
Main constituents:	Tetron acid; luteolin
Alternatives:	Elderberry (*Sambucus nigra*)
Notes for caution:	**During pregnancy:** High doses can induce nausea. There are no known studies on safety during pregnancy.
	During lactation: High doses can induce nausea.

Lomatium root is one of nature's antibiotics. It is both antibacterial and antiviral, and is now extremely rare in the wild.

Homeopathic   **Root**

Long Birthroot
(*Aristolochia clematis*)

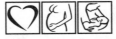 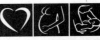

Part used:	Homeopathic; root
Main constituents:	Aristolochic acid
Alternatives:	None
Notes for caution:	**Root during preconception:** Long birthroot is an emmenegogue. **Root during pregnancy and lactation:** Aristolochic acid is strongly carcinogenic and nephrotoxic. It is best avoided during pregnancy and while nursing.

Long birthroot is used in homeopathy for depression that is expressed as loneliness and fear for the future. The homeopathic preparation of this herb does not have any contraindications. Due to the presence of aristolochic acid, this herb is not used internally anymore. It is highly damaging to the kidneys and is a known carcinogen

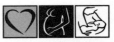

Lycium (*L. barbarum; L. chinensis*)

Galactagogue		
Part used:	Berry	
Main constituents:	Beta-sitolsterol; betaine; beta-carotene; niacin; pyridoxine; ascorbic acid[41]	
Alternatives:	**For vision:** Bilberries (*Vaccinium myrtillus*)	
Notes for caution:	**During preconception:** Betaine is a known emmenagogue and abortifacient.	
	During pregnancy: Betaine is a known emmenagogue and abortifacient.	

Lycium is commonly known as wolf berry or goji berry. This berry has an affinity for the liver, kidney and lung and is used to build and tonify the body. It is very commonly used for blurry vision or problems with night vision.

Maca (*Lepidium meyenii, L. peruvianum*)

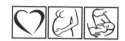

Part used:	Root
Main constituents:	Calcium; magnesium; phosphorus; potassium; iron; zinc; sterols; essential fatty acids; lipids; amino acids
Alternatives:	None
Male fertility:	Maca is a nutritive tonic for male fertility.

Maca is a nutritive tonic for female fertility. In Peru it is taken for infertility and belived to positively affect ovarian function. It has been shown to stimulate follicle development. This plant is highly endangered, so use it responsibly.

Madagascar Periwinkle (*Vinca rosea*)

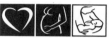

Part used:	Whole plant
Main constituents:	Alkaloids (vinblastine, vincristine, alstonine, ajmalicine, leurocristine, reserpine)
Alternatives:	**For diabetes:** Jerusalem artichoke (*Helianthus tuberosus*)
Notes for caution:	**During preconception and pregnancy:** This herb is teratogenic and is capable of causing birth defects.

Vinca is used in folk remedies to treat diabetes and malaria. Its strong anti-tumor properties have attracted attention from those researching cancer treatments. It is the chemicals that deliver those same properties that give us a reason to be careful with the use of vinca during pregnancy.

| REPRODUCTIVE PHASE | Preconception | Pregnancy | Lactation | GENERAL SAFETY RATING | No Contraindications | | Use with Caution | Generally Avoid |

Madder (*Rubia tinctorum*)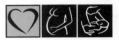

Part used:	Root
Main constituents:	Rubin; rubiadin; ruberythric acid; purpurin; tannin; sugar; alzarin; pseudopurpurin; xanthopurpurin
Alternatives:	None
Notes for caution:	**During preconception:** Madder is an emmenagogue.
	During pregnancy: Madder is an emmenagogue that is genotoxic for the fetus.
	During lactation: Madder is believed to be a genotoxin for infants.

Madder is little used today. At the height of its popularity, the herb was used as an internal dye that helped doctors study the bones, urine and milk of animals. Avoid it.

Magnolia (hou po) (*Magnolia officinalis*)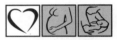

Part used:	Bark
Main constituents:	Honokiol; magnolol; eudesmol; benzylisoquinoline alkaloids (magnoflorine, magnocurarine, salicifoline with traces of oxoushinsunine, anonaine, michelabine)[56]
Alternatives:	None
Notes for caution:	**During pregnancy and lactation:** Recent reports have indicated that the levels of magnocurarine in products made with magnolia are a danger to fetus, infant and child due to the potential for respiratory paralysis or renal failure. It has come to light that magnolia itself is safe and it is the common adulterants that should be considered with caution. If you are sure of your supply of magnolia bark, there should be no contraindication against its use during pregnancy or lactation.[56]

Magnolia is used in traditional Chinese medicine to regulate digestion and ensure proper assimilation of food. It is also believed to aid in abdominal bloating and menstrual cramping and help with allergies, nervous system imbalances and memory loss.

Ma Huang (*Ephedra sinica; Ephedra vulgaris*)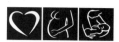

Antigalactagogue	
Part used:	Aerial portions
Main constituents:	Vitamins A, B₁, B₂, B₃, C; zinc; tin; sodium; silicon; selenium; protein; potassium; phosphorus; manganese; magnesium; fiber; fat; iron; cobalt; tannins; alkaloid ephedrine and pseudoephedrine[35]
Alternatives:	Elecampane (*Inula helenium*); wild cherry bark (*Prunus serotina*); cramp bark (*Viburnum opulus*)
Notes for caution:	**During preconception and pregnancy:** Ephedrine is an alkaloid that can stimulate the uterus.
	During lactation: It is believed that in a nursing infant, ephedra can stimulate the sympathetic nervous system. This stimulation can cause increased heart rate, lowered digestive activity and contraction of the peripheral blood vessels.

The chemical ephedrine found within ephedra acts on the sympathetic nervous system in a fashion similar to that of adrenaline. It is an activator with antispasmodic properties, used often for opening air passages in the case of respiratory disease or asthma. Ephedra is sometimes found in natural cough and cold preparations or formulas.

Male Fern (*Dryopteris felx-mas*)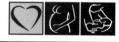

Part used:	Rhizome
Main constituents:	Filmaron; filic acid; tannin; resin; dye; sugar
Alternatives:	Pumpkin seeds (*Curcurbita* spp.); garlic (*Allium sativum*); black walnut hull (*Juglans nigra*); cucumber (*Cucumis sativa*)
Notes for caution:	**During preconception:** Male fern is an abortifacient.
	During pregnancy: Male fern is an abortifacient.
	During lactation: It is believed that male fern poses a threat as a toxin to the nursing infant.

The extracted oil is the most often used preparation of the male fern. It is known for its ability to rid the body of worms.

Marijuana (*Cannibis sativa*)

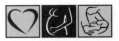

Part used:	Flowering tops of the female plant
Main constituents:	Cannabinoids (cannabidiol, cannabichromene); volatile oil; steroidal compounds; THC
Alternatives:	For its historical use as an anti-inflammatory and pain reliever, especially in regard to menstrual and pelvic disorders, there is some evidence that hemp seed oil can be taken internally.
Notes for caution:	**During preconception:** Marijuana is an emmenagogue.
	During pregnancy: The herb causes uterine contractions and can be abortifacient.
	During lactation: There are no specific warnings for the nursing relationship. It is important to keep in mind that if you are using the herb recreationally, any effects might be amplified in a newborn. Potential side effects of paranoia, disorientation and disruption of motor skills, among others, are not things you want a developing child to experience. Further, THC is known to be excreted in breast milk.
Male fertility:	Use of this herb can reduce the ability for or interest in erection.

Marijuana acts on the higher nerve centers. It produces a feeling of euphoria and often hallucinations and is used for its calming action on the nervous system. It can help with sleep, convulsions, nausea, loss of appetite and nerve pain. Most of the anti-inflammatory action harnessed in the traditional use of this drug came from a fairly low dose. It is most often used as a recreational drug. There are no reliable studies demonstrating a danger to the health and development of either a growing fetus or a nursing child. If you are afflicted with a disease that makes this herb a viable treatment option, please discuss any ramifications with your health care team before beginning use. If this is an herb that you choose merely for recreational purposes, it is best to avoid it until after you have weaned your baby.

REPRODUCTIVE PHASE			GENERAL SAFETY RATING		
Preconception	Pregnancy	Lactation		No Contraindications	Use with Caution	Generally Avoid

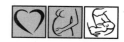

Marjoram (*Origanum marjorana*)

Galactagogue	
Part used:	Aerial portions
Main constituents:	Essential oils (thymol, carvacrol); tannins; bitters
Alternatives:	None
Notes for caution:	**During preconception and pregnancy:** Excessive doses can make marjoram an emmenagogue.

Marjoram is often used in cooking, but don't forget its medicinal qualities. It is an antiseptic, antispasmodic, diaphoretic and expectorant. It is helpful for a headache, for colds and flu, and some references even hint at its ability as a drawing agent. For the purposes of building a baby, don't eat more marjoram than you would typically add to your food or beverage, as it becomes an emmenagogue at larger doses.

REPRODUCTIVE PHASE   Preconception Pregnancy Lactation GENERAL SAFETY RATING No Contraindications Use with Caution   Generally Avoid

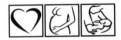

Marshmallow (*Althea officinalis*)

Galactagogue	
Part used:	Leaf; root
Main constituents:	Vitamins B$_3$, C; tin; sodium; silicon; selenium; protein; potassium; phosphorus; manganese; magnesium; iron; fiber; chromium; calcium; aluminum; mucilage; volatile oils; tannins; saponins[35]
Alternatives:	None

Marshmallow is one of our best mucilaginous herbs, whether the root or the leaf is used. It is a supreme soother. The leaf tends to have its best showing in relation to our lungs and our urinary tract, and the root in relation to digestion and our skin. It is helpful anywhere there is inflammation, either internally or externally. It is typically used in combination with other herbs that are having a direct action on the body; marshmallow goes along as a partner to soothe that action. It can be used in cough formulas and could also be a great addition to a salve for cracked nipples during lactation.

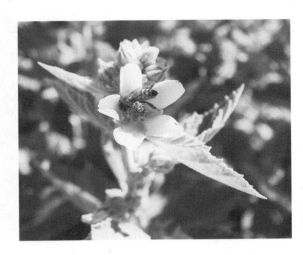

Marshmallow
(Althea officinalis*)*

REPRODUCTIVE PHASE   Preconception   Pregnancy   Lactation   **GENERAL SAFETY RATING**   No Contraindications   Use with Caution   Generally Avoid

Homeopathic   Herb

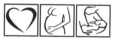 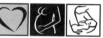

Marsh Tea (*Ledum paulstre*)

Part used:	Homeopathic; aerial portions
Main constituents:	Ledum camphor; valeric acid; ericinol; tannin[57]
Alternatives:	For essential oils: Rosemary (*Rosemarinus officinalis*); thyme (*Thymus vulgaris*)
Notes for caution:	Herb use during preconception: As a strong diuretic, this herb has the tendency to irritate the urinary tract and lead to uterine stimulation, which could result in miscarriage.
	Herb use during pregnancy: As a strong diuretic, this herb has the tendency to irritate the urinary tract and lead to uterine stimulation, which could result in miscarriage.

Marsh tea homeopathic is used for inflammation or infection and is safe to use. The herb as a tea, syrup or tincture is often used as a diuretic and therefore has much to offer in cases of rheumatism, gout and arthritis.

 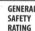

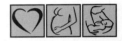

Mate (*Ilex paraguayensis*)

Part used:	Leaves
Main constituents:	Caffeine; tannin
Alternatives:	None
Notes for caution:	**During preconception:** Caffeine is extremely drying to cervical fluids and places an unnecessary burden on the endocrine system. It can lead to hormonal imbalance. **During pregnancy:** Caffeine has been found to cross the placenta and contribute to low birth weight, preterm delivery and birth defects.[44] **During lactation:** Caffeine has been found to appear in breast milk at half that of the level in the mother's plasma. It reduces the available iron supply in breast milk.

Mate is a daily drink for many in South America. It is named for the special bulbous cup and straw typically used. It is a tonifying stimulant unlike many other stimulating drinks. Medicinally it is used to aid the kidneys or cool the body during a fever. In large doses, it can cause vomiting.

Mayapple (*Podophyllum peltatum, Podophyllum hexandrum*)

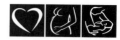

Part used:	Root
Main constituents:	Podophyllotoxin; peltatin; quercitin; sugar; starch; fat
Alternatives:	Gentian (*Gentiana lutea*); dandelion root (*Taraxacum officinale*); yellow dock (*Rumex crispus*)
Notes for caution:	**During preconception and pregnancy:** Podophyllotoxin and peltatin are teratogenic and can lead to the death of a fetus. **During lactation:** Mayapple is a deadly poison unless administered by an experienced practitioner.

Mayapple is a powerful herb that has amazing benefits for our body, but it is not an herb to be used by a layperson. Do not try to use it without an experienced practitioner. It is best for obstructions of the liver, gallbladder and digestion. Mayapple can also be used topically, but even then only with great care.

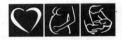

Meadow Saffron (*Colchicum autumnale*)

Part used:	Corm; seed
Main constituents:	Cholchicine
Alternatives:	**Laxative:** Dandelion root (*Taraxacum officinale*); yellow dock (*Rumex crispus*)
	For arthritis: Turmeric (*Curcuma longa, Curcuma domestica, Curcuma aromatica*); ginger (*Zingiber officinale*); ashwaganda (*Withania somnifera*)
Notes for caution:	**During preconception:** If a woman has colchicine in her system while trying to get pregnant, it can interfere with cell division before she is aware she has conceived.
	During pregnancy: Colchicine is believed to interfere with cell division, leading to birth defects.
	During lactation: Colchicine is considered a poison that can cause deep depression, catharsis and/or vomiting.

Known more commonly as "naked ladies" or "surprise lilies," these beauties are considered by some as a known poison and by others as a valuable medicine. Taken in small, appropriate doses, they can help with rheumatic pain, relieve severe constipation and serve as a useful emetic. Without the help of an experienced herbalist, however, it is best to look to other, gentler ways to help with these problems, especially while pregnant or nursing.

REPRODUCTIVE   GENERAL
PHASE   SAFETY
       Preconception Pregnancy Lactation RATING No Contraindications Use with Caution Generally Avoid

Meadowsweet (*Filipendula ulmaria*)

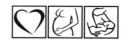

Part used:	Aerial portions
Main constituents:	Salicylic acid; spiraeine; gaultherin; tannins; ascorbic acid; mucilage; volatile oil; flavonoids
Alternatives:	None

Meadowsweet is best used for its abilities to calm the stomach and reduce acid, especially in times of nausea or heartburn. It has diuretic properties and can be used as a mild urinary astringent in cases of urinary tract distress. It is also a great anti-inflammatory and can be used anytime you would normally reach for an aspirin.

Milk Thistle (*Silybum marianum, Carduus marianus*)

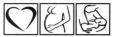

Galactagogue	
Part used:	Seeds
Main constituents:	Vitamins A, B$_1$, B$_2$; flavones (silybin, silydianin, silychristin); essential oil; bitter principle; mucilage; iron; selenium; zinc; tin; protein; phosphorus; manganese; magnesium; fat; fiber; cobalt; chromium; calcium; aluminum; resin[35]
Alternatives:	None

Milk thistle is one of the known galactagogues. It can be used interchangeably with blessed thistle; it also has some great action on the liver. This herb is used to counteract heavy liver toxins or to rebuild liver tissue that has been damaged due to cirrhosis. It can also be used to heal the liver in cases of jaundice. It would, therefore, be a great choice to nurse through for a baby with true jaundice (not just typical slight yellowing that can occur in a newborn in the first few days). Common newborn jaundice can be remedied simply by nursing on demand. Milk thistle is also known to safely help increase the bile secretion from both the liver and the gallbladder, giving implications to its application for digestive, blood sugar and gallbladder stone issues.

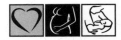

Mistletoe (*Viscum album*)

Part used:	Whole plant
Main constituents:	Aluminum; calcium; chromium; cobalt; fat; iron; magnesium; manganese; phosphorus; potassium; protein; selenium; tin; zinc; amines (acetylcholine, choline, histamine, GABA, tyramine); antioxidant flavonoids (quercitin, chalcone, flavone derivatives); terpenoids (beta-amyrin, betulinic acid, oleanic acid, beta-sitosterol, stigmasterol, ursolic acid, lupeol); tannins (caffeic acid myristic acid); mucilage[41]
Alternatives:	Chaga (*Inonotus obliquus*)
Notes for caution:	**During preconception:** Mistletoe is an emmenagogue due to the presence of quercitin, which stimulates uterine contractions.[42]
	During pregnancy: Lectins cross the placenta and are toxic to red blood cells and the heart.[34] There is also a concern due to quercitin, which stimulates uterine contractions, making the herb an abortifacient.
Additional note:	This herb should be used only sporadically. Used as part of an intensive, daily treatment protocol, it is advisable *only* if used under the guidance of an experience practitioner.

Mistletoe is included in this listing mainly because many people who use natural medicine are now turning to it for its anti-tumor or tumor-reducing abilities. For a new mother who has been diagnosed with cancer and is researching her options while hoping to continue breastfeeding, this is definitely an herb to discuss with your health care team. Mistletoe reduces both heart rate and blood pressure, and is good for symptoms that accompany those health issues in a nursing mother. The mother must monitor the effects on her infant. If she notices a depressant effect in her child while using mistletoe, it is best to switch to another herb for symptom remediation.

| REPRODUCTIVE PHASE | Preconception | Pregnancy | Lactation | GENERAL SAFETY RATING | No Contraindications | Use with Caution | Generally Avoid | |

Motherwort (*Leonurus cardiaca*)

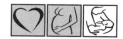

Part used:	Aerial portions
Main constituents:	Bitter glycosides (leonurin, leonuridine); alkaloids (leonuinine, stachydrene); volatile oil; tannin
Alternatives:	**For erratic heart:** Valerian (*Valeriana officinalis*)
Notes for caution:	**During preconception:** Motherwort is an emmenagogue.
	During pregnancy: Excessive use should be avoided in early pregnancy to prevent miscarriage.

As the Latin name suggests, this herb is a great support to heart health. It can be specific for fast or erratic heart beat when the cause is anxiety, stress or tension. It is also a general tonic to anyone with heart conditions that are brought on or exacerbated by a "stressed-out" or anxious emotional state. Motherwort is also a great support for the female reproductive system as it can help bring on a delayed cycle.

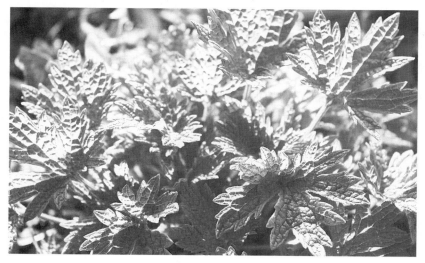

Motherwort (Leonurus cardiac)

REPRODUCTIVE PHASE			GENERAL SAFETY RATING		
Preconception	Pregnancy	Lactation	No Contraindications	Use with Caution	Generally Avoid

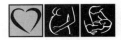

Mugwort (*Artemesia vulgare*)

Part used:	Leaves; root
Main constituents:	Essential oils (cineole, linalool, camphor, thujone); bitter principle; tannin; resin
Alternatives:	Gentian (*Gentiana lutea*); dandelion root (*Taraxacum officinale*); artichoke (*Cynara scolymus*)
Notes for caution:	**During preconception:** Mugwort is an emmenagogue.
	During pregnancy: Mugwort is a uterine stimulant. **During lactation:** The constituent thujone can have a negative effect through breast milk if the herb is taken improperly while breastfeeding. It is not appropriate to use either the essential oil or an alcoholic extract of mugwort during this time. Use this herb sparingly. Do not take a very high dose or use excessively as a tea. It is so bitter that the bitter qualities are known to transmit through the milk and have historically been used to help with weaning a baby. Don't drink too much, and reduce usage if you notice your baby beginning to pull away.

The bitter principle of this herb gives it its great abilities in perking up lazy digestion and stimulating the production of digestive secretions. It is also one of the best herbs to use to encourage regularity and balance of the menstrual cycles. It is often used for girls entering puberty, and can again be very helpful to women when they reach the point in their lactation when cycles begin to reappear. A tea of mugwort at this time can help your body return to balance if you no longer wish to nurse or have already weaned. As mentioned in the cautionary note, keep a close watch on your baby if you use mugwort in this way while you are still nursing.

 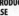

Muira Puama (*Ptychopetalum olacoides*)

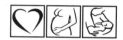

Part used:	Roots; bark; wood
Main constituents:	Alkaloids; sterols; long chain fatty acids; coumarin; chromium; essential oils
Alternatives:	None
Male fertility:	This herb has traditionally been used to alleviate performance anxiety and to treat impotence.

Muira puama has been known to markedly boost libido in women. It is safe to take for long periods of time because it is tonic in nature. It is a nervous system tonic, aiding in the ability to deal with stess. It is believed that it raises testosterone levels.

Mullein (*Verbascum thapsus*)

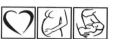

Part used:	Leaves; flowers
Main constituents:	Mucilage; saponins; tannin; vitamins A, B_3, C; calcium; iron; magnesium; manganese; tin; sodium; silicon; protein; potassium; phosphorus; fiber; cobalt; chromium; aluminum[35]
Alternatives:	None

Mullein is well known for both its external and internal applications. Internally, it is great for breaking up congestion while soothing the mucus membranes in the chest during a cold. It is most often used in conditions in which there is a painful, non-productive cough. Externally, it is best known for mullein flower ear oil. Dropped into the ear canal, it is specific for relieving pain and inflammation involved in an ear infection. A mullein/garlic ear oil is even better. The addition of the garlic will help heal the infection.

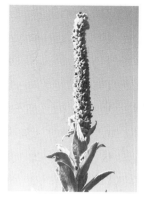

Mullein
(Verbascum thapsus)

Mushroom
Turkey Tail (*Trametes versicolor*)
Shiitake (*Lentinula edodes*)
Reishi (*Ganoderma lucidum*)
Maitake (*Grifola fondosa*)
Chaga (*Inonotus obliquus*)
Cordyceps (*Cordyceps sinensis*)

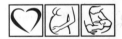

Part used:	Fruiting body
Main constituents:	Various
Alternatives:	None

Mushrooms are safe and recommended for use from preconception through nursing. Most of them are highly useful in fighting infection and for both stimulating and toning the immune system. A few of the more medicinal mushrooms are also highly indicated in the natural treatment of cancer and are part of the conversation you should have with your health care team if you are a new mother researching this diagnosis.

Mustard (*Brassica nigra, Brassica alba*)

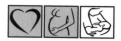

Part used:	Seed
Main constituents:	Fixed oil; mucilage; volatile oil; sinigrin[44]
Alternatives:	None
Notes for caution:	**During preconception and pregnancy:** In excessive amounts, mustard can be an emmenagogue and abortifacient.

Mustard seed can be used internally as a diuretic, stimulant or alterative. It is most often used as a seasoning in food and in this application, there are no contraindications. It is only when used in a repeated therapeutic dose that mustard becomes an issue.

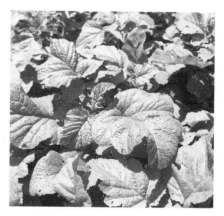

*Mustard (*Brassica nigra, Brassica alba*)*

Myrrh (mo yao) (*Commiphora myrrha*)

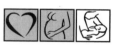

Part used:	Bark resin
Main constituents:	Gums; resins; sterols; volatile oils
Alternatives:	None
Notes for caution:	**During preconception:** Myrrh can cause contractions.
	During pregnancy: Myrrh can be a uterine stimulant that can cause contractions. Confine the use of this herb to the occasional tooth product additive while you're pregnant.

You'll most often find this little gem in toothpaste, mouthwash or in topical products meant to disinfect cuts. It is great for topical antibacterial use.

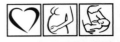

Nettle (*Urtica dioica*)

Galactagogue	
Part used:	Aerial portions
Main constituents:	Vitamins A, B$_1$, B$_2$, B$_3$, B$_5$, C, D, E, and K; calcium; chromium; cobalt; fat; fiber; iron; manganese; magnesium; phosphorus; potassium; protein; silicon; selenium; tin; zinc; histamine; formic acid; chlorophyll; minerals; amino acids; serotonin; carotenoids; tannins; sterols; flavonoids; glucosamine[35]
Alternatives:	None

In my opinion, *everyone* should be using nettle often. It is an awesome general tonic for women, excellent for girls entering their moon cycles and for women in menopause. It helps reduce water retention, is excellent for PMS symptoms and is specific for excessive menstruation. It is especially good for strengthening the kidneys and adrenals. Nettle is highly nutritious and has applications toward supporting our veinous integrity. For women who bruise easily or are prone to varicose veins or hemorrhoids, nettle can be a big help. If used throughout a pregnancy, it can be an aid in the prevention of hemorrhage at birth. This is a great herb to use for nursing through to help an infant to build up his or her vitamin K reserves if the mother wishes to avoid the vitamin K shot at birth.

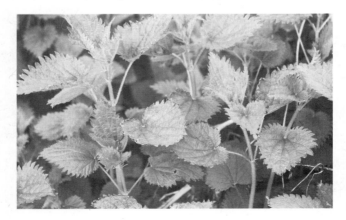

Nettle
(Urtica dioica)

Nettle is important for those who are working naturally to allevi-ate allergy symptoms. While I normally recommend using the herb in its most natural state, this is an exception. The freeze-dried prepa-ration of nettle in capsules provides the best allergy relief, but teas, tinctures and capsules are still helpful. Nettle is the herb I most rec-ommend to mothers recovering from heavy blood loss during birth as its high chlorophyll content aids the body's ability to oxygenate the red blood cells. Because of this action, preparations of nettle can relieve the feeling of extreme exhaustion that occurs while a woman's body is working to rebuild her blood supply.

	Seed/aril (mace)	Essential oil/ Alcoholic extract
		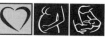

Nutmeg (*Myristica fragrans*)

Part used:	Seed; aril (mace); essential oil
Main constituents:	Essential oil (camphene, P-cymene, phellandrene, terpinene, limonene, myrcene, linalool, geraniol, terpineol, myristicin, elemicin, safrol, eugenol and eugenol)[41]
Alternatives:	None
Notes for caution:	**Use of essential oil/alcoholic extract during preconception:** The essential oil or an alcoholic extract will contain safrole, which is an emmenagogue, abortifacient and known carcinogen.
	Use of essential oil/alcoholic extract during pregnancy and lactation: The essential oil or an alcoholic extract will contain safrole, which is an emmenagogue, abortifacient and known carcinogen.

It is safe to use both nutmeg and mace as a spice in your food or drinks, even while building a baby. However, avoid using the essential oil on your skin during pregnancy and anywhere near your nipple or where skin-to-skin contact will be made with your infant while nursing.

Oats (*Avena sativa*) aka milky oats or oat tops
Oatstraw (*Avena fatva, Avena sativa*)

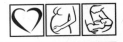

Galactagogue	
Part used:	**Oats:** Milky, unripened stage of the oat **Oatstraw:** Aerial portions
Main constituents:	Starch; alkaloids (trigonelline, avenine); sterols; saponins; flavones; vitamins A, B_1, B_2, B_3, B_6, C, E, and K; calcium; chromium; iron; magnesium; selenium; sodium; silicon; phosphorus; fiber[35]
Alternatives:	None
Male fertility:	Milky oats are especially useful when male impotence is associated with stress.

All parts of the oat plant are nutritious and soothing especially for the nervous system, including our morning oatmeal. Oats are specific for stress, exhaustion and nervous debility associated with depression. They are also soothing externally for irritated skin.

Ocotillo (*Fouquieria splendens*)

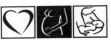

Part used:	Bark
Main constituents:	Adoxoside; fouquierol; isofouquierol; ocotillol; asperocotillin; asperuloside; caffeic acid; kaempferol; leucocyanidin; p-coumaric acid; ellagic acid; quercetin; scopoletin[58]
Alternatives:	**For the liver and gallbladder:** Gentian (*Gentiana lutea*); dandelion root (*Taraxacum officinale*); yellow dock (*Rumex crispus*)
Notes for caution:	**During pregnancy:** This herb's action focuses on creating movement and removing obstruction in the pelvic region, so it is not appropriate for use during pregnancy.

This desert plant is used to help improve circulation in the pelvis. It helps in all types of pelvic congestion in both men and women, positively affecting the prostate and the hormonal levels around menstruation. It also has an effect on digestion and the liver, helping with fat metabolism.

Oregon Grape Root
(Mahonia aquifolium, Berberis aquifolium)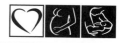

Part used:	Root
Main constituents:	Berberine; calumbamine; hydrastine; jatrorrhizine; oxyacanthine; tetrahydroberberine; tannin
Alternatives:	Marsh tea homeopathic (*Ledum palustre*); shiitake (*Lentinus edodes*); elder (*Sambucus nigra*)
Notes for caution:	**During pregnancy:** Berberine, an alkaloid, is a mild toxin that has a depressant effect on the heart and lungs. There is some evidence that it is also a uterine stimulant in some doses. **During lactation:** Berberine, an alkaloid, is a mild toxin that has a depressant effect on the heart and lungs. There is some evidence that it is also a uterine stimulant in some doses. This herb could be especially problematic if your baby has been diagnosed with jaundice.

Antibacterial, antiviral, antifungal and vermifuge, this herb used to be a sustainable alternative to goldenseal. However, these days in much of our country Oregon grape is now also in danger of being overharvested. As with goldenseal, seek out a sustainably grown supply. Oregon grape also has a love for the mucus membranes and takes special care with them. It is also being used to treat psoriasis somewhat successfully.

 Osha *(Ligusticum porter)*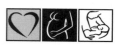

Part used:	Root
Main constituents:	Furanocoumarins; mucilage[41]
Alternatives:	None
Notes for caution:	**During preconception:** Osha is an emmenagogue.
	During pregnancy: Osha is an emmenagogue.

An expectorant and anti-inflammatory herb steeped in Native American history, this herb is the last line of defense for stubborn respiratory infections that nothing else can touch. It also has great applications in the digestive tract.

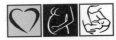

Pareira (*Chondrodendron tomentosum*)

Part used:	Dried root; bark; leaves
Main constituents:	Resin; fecula; tubocurarine; D-tubocurarine; L-curarine; calcium; malate; salt; potassium nitrate
Alternatives:	**Laxative:** Yellow dock (*Rumex crispus*) **Diuretic:** Dandelion (*Taraxacum officinale*)
Notes for caution:	**During preconception:** Pariera is an emmenagogue.
	During pregnancy: Pariera is an emmenagogue.

This diuretic and laxative herb is the source of the paralyzing poison curare. This herb can be taken safely *only* if it does *not* touch a cut or sore between your fingers and your stomach.

Aerial Portions   Root

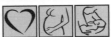

Parsley (*Petroselinum crispum*)

Antigalactagogue	
Part used:	Aerial portions; root
Main constituents:	Vitamins A, B_2, B_3, C, D; calcium; cobalt; fat; fiber; iron; magnesium; manganese; phosphorus; potassium; protein; selenium; silicon; sodium; tin; volatile oils; resins; flavonoids; coumarins[35]
Alternatives:	None
Notes for caution:	**Aerial portion during preconception and pregnancy:** Use sparingly as a culinary herb. In therapeutic doses, it can act as an emmenagogue.
	Aerial portion during lactation: The herb will potentially reduce milk volume, but it will take significant intake to create an effect. Therefore, it is not a problem if women use in their food unless they are overly sensitive. Monitor milk flow if using the herb and avoid foods in which parsley is a primary ingredient.
	Root during pregnancy: Parsley root is an emmenagogue, an abortifacient and a uterine stimulant.

This delicious culinary herb is high in vitamin C and is helpful in relieving flatulence and colic pains.

Partridgeberry (*Mitchella repens*)

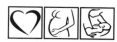

Part used:	Leaves; berries
Main constituents:	Tannin; bitter principle; saponins; mucilage; unspecified alkaloids; glycosides; resin
Alternatives:	None

Many doctors warn against the use of partridgeberry. It is, however, one of the best herbs for toning and nourishing the uterus. It is an herb whose use was passed to us from the Native peoples of the United States. In my research, I did not come across any specific contraindications that were backed by science. Partridgeberry has been included often in formulas to prevent miscarriage. It is also highly useful for infertility caused by a hormonal imbalance.

If a woman has been given a list that includes this herb as something to avoid but is still interested in using it, she should talk with an experienced practitioner. I believe it winds up on these lists because of its traditional use in labor formulas. Indeed, it is useful during labor, not because of its stimulant action on the uterus but because of the balance it provides in the body for blood pressure. It will also stop hemorrhage and provide nourishment and support to the uterus, enabling an efficient and successful labor. In short, it seems that the misconception about raspberry leaf (*Rubus ideaus*) being oxytocic falls on partridgeberry as well.

REPRODUCTIVE PHASE   **GENERAL SAFETY RATING**

Preconception   Pregnancy   Lactation   No Contraindications   Use with Caution   Generally Avoid

Passionflower (*Passiflora incarnata*)

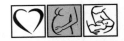

Part used:	Leaves
Main constituents:	Vitamins A, B₃; tannin; alkaloids (harmine, harman, harmaline, harmol, passiflorine); chrysin; sterols; flavonoids[35]
Alternatives:	Chamomile (*Matricaria recutita*); skullcap (*Scutellaria lateriflora*)
Notes for caution:	**During pregnancy:** This herb is a possible uterine stimulant due to the presence of the alkaloids harman and harmaline.

Passionflower is a nice little nervine for all ages. It is calming, pain relieving and antispasmodic in its action and helps with issues such as insomnia, headaches, asthma and nervous tremors.

Pau D'arco (*Tabebuia impetiginosa*)

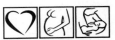

Part used:	Inner bark
Main constituents:	Zinc; silicon; fiber; cobalt; chromium; calcium; tannins; lapachol; lapachone; isolapachone; saponins; volatile oils; resins; pseudo tannins[35]
Alternatives:	None

Pau d'arco is often found in cold, flu and sore throat preparations, and is also used to treat yeast infections.

Bark/leaf   Seed

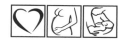

Peach (tao ren) (*Prunus persica*)

Part used:	Bark; leaf; seed
Main constituents:	Cyanogenic glycoside; amygdalin; fats; oils
Alternatives:	None
Notes for caution:	**Seed use during preconception:** Peach pits can act as an emmenagogue.
	Seed use during pregnancy: A high concentration of cyanogenic glycosides makes this particular part of the plant potentially deadly, not to mention an emmenagogue and abortifacient. Pregnancy is not the time to move pelvic stagnation.
	Seed use during lactation: A high concentration of cyanogenic glycosides make this particular part of the plant potentially deadly.

Peach pit, or seed, is a traditional Chinese remedy for diseases caused by stagnant blood. These include menstrual irregularities and blunt force trauma. Peach leaf is called for most often as a tincture or fresh. It is used for nausea or inflammation and irritation of skin and joints. Peach bark is believed to have some of the same effects as leaf, but is primarily a diuretic and used to help remove toxicity from the body by way of the genitourinary tract.

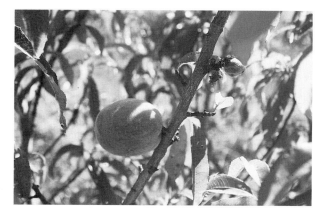

Peach aka: Tao Ren

(Prunus persica)

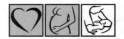

Pennyroyal (*Hedeoma pulegoides, Mentha puleguim*)

Part used:	Aerial portions
Main constituents:	Aluminum; calcium; chromium; fiber; fat; iron; magnesium; manganese; phosphorus; potassium; protein; selenium; silicon; sodium; zinc;[35] volatile oil; tannins; bitters; flavone glycosides
Alternatives:	**For colds:** Elder (*Sambucus nigra*)
	For digestion: Dill (*Anethum graveolens*)
Notes for caution:	**During preconception and pregnancy:** Pennyroyal is a well-known emmenagogue and abortifacient.

Pennyroyal is a delicious herb that acts on the female reproductive system; it also helps with digestion. It can help bring on a delayed menstruation while its volatile oils also help with flatulence and colic. It brings blood flow to the pelvis and stimulates uterine contractions. For this reason, it is great for menstrual cramps, congestion and irregular cycles. During labor, a glass of pennyroyal tea can strengthen contractions and move a stalled labor along. In the U.S. Pharmacopeia it is listed as an aid for colds. It is only the essential oil of pennyroyal that is dangerous; it would be nearly impossible to drink enough tea to have the same effects. *Ingestion of any amount of pennyroyal essential oil can be extremely dangerous and even deadly.*

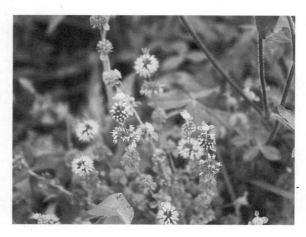

Pennyroyal
(Hedoma pulegoides,
Mentha puleguim)

Peony (bai shao) (*Paeonia officinalis*)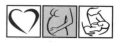

Part used:	Root
Main constituents:	Paeonine; volatile oil; tannin; resin[26, 59]
Alternatives:	**For pain:** Rosemary (*Rosemarinus officinalis*)
	For swelling: Poultice of yarrow (*Achillea millefolium*)
Notes for caution:	**During pregnancy:** Excessive use should be avoided in early pregnancy, as it acts as an emmenagogue.

Peony is used in traditional Chinese medicine to alleviate pain and swelling. Both the red and white varieties are used in different ways and are not harmful so long as excessive doses are avoided.

Leaf   Essential oil

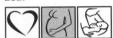 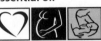

Peppermint (*Mentha piperita*)

Part used:	Leaves; essential oil
Main constituents:	Terpenes (menthol, menthone, cineol); azulene; resin; tannin; flavonoids; vitamins A, B$_1$, B$_2$, B$_3$, C; calcium; cobalt; fat; fiber; iron; magnesium; manganese; phosphorus; potassium; protein; selenium; sodium[35]
Alternatives:	None
Notes for caution:	**Using leaves during pregnancy:** Excessive use should be avoided in early pregnancy. Volatile oils can cross the placenta, and can act as an emmenagogue.
	Using essential oil during pregnancy: Peppermint essential oil is believed to be an emmenagogue.
	Using essential oil during lactation: Inhalation of essential oil by infants can cause adverse nervous system reactions.

Peppermint is a favorite additive to teas and is perfectly safe for both mother and nursing infant. It is the essential oil of peppermint that has been known to cause adverse effects in a nursing infant and to potentially encourage menstruation in women. Women who are trying to get pregnant or are already pregnant should use peppermint essential oil in moderation. It is often used as an inhalant to calm the nausea of morning sickness, but it is best to try it internally as a tea instead. In respect to a newborn, it is advisable to avoid this essential oil in humidifiers, home air infusers and any products a woman applies near the breasts or anywhere there will be skin-to-skin contact with her baby.

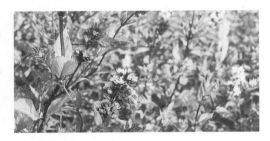

*Peppermint (*Mentha piperita*)*

Phellodendron (huang bai)
(*Phellodendron amurense, P. chinense*)

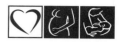

Part used:	Bark
Main constituents:	Berberine; jatorrhizine; phellodendrine; palmatine
Alternatives:	Shiitake (*Lentinula edodes*)
Notes for caution:	**During pregnancy:** Berberine, an alkaloid, is a mild toxin that has a depressant effect on the heart and lungs. There is some evidence that it is also a uterine stimulant in some doses.
	During lactation: Berberine, an alkaloid, is a mild toxin that has a depressant effect on the heart and lungs. There is some evidence that it is also a uterine stimulant in some doses. This herb could be especially problematic if your baby has been diagnosed with jaundice.

This herb is used mainly in traditional Chinese medicine for its anti-inflammatory and antibacterial properties in conjunction with the kidneys, bladder and intestine.

Conceiving Healthy Babies

Pine (*Pinus* spp.)

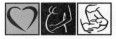

Part used:	Needles; bark; buds
Main constituents:	Tannin; terpenes; resin; essential oil; pinipricin;[44] flavonols; proanthocyanidins; bitters; volatile oil[60]
Alternatives:	Elecampane (*Inula helenium*); mullein (*Verbascum thapsus*)
Notes for caution:	**During preconception:** Pine has abortifacient qualities.
	During pregnancy: Pine has abortifacient qualities.

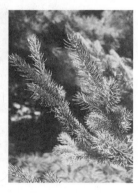

Pine is often used as a stimulant to help with respiratory issues. The resin is the most medicinal component and can be used internally for the lungs, digestion and heart. Externally it's a great skin healer with drawing properties. It is relatively safe to use externally while building a baby, but it's not advisable to soak in a bath tea made from pine.

Pine (Pinus spp.)

Pinellia (ban xia) (*Pinellia ternate*)

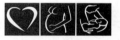

Part used:	Prepared rhizome
Main constituents:	Pinellic acid
Alternatives:	Elecampane (*Inula helenium*)
Notes for caution:	**During preconception:** In the United States, pinellia is currently considered to be toxic.
	During Pregnancy: Because of its action in moving qi downward, as well as warnings against possible bleeding issues, pinellia should be avoided.
	During lactation: In the United States, pinellia is currently considered to be toxic.

Used in traditional Chinese medicine, pinellia is good at moving cold, stagnant phlegm in situations of congestion.

Plantain (*Plantago* spp.)

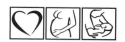

Galactagogue	
Part used:	Leaf
Main constituents:	Vitamins A, C; calcium; iron; potassium; mucilage; glycosides; chlorogenic; ursolic acid; silicic acid
Alternatives:	None

This is an important herb to know. In my opinion, it is the premier drawing herb and when used as a poultice, can remove everything from splinters to infection. It is also highly nutritive and can be added fresh or dried to everyday foods. Plantain excels in the treatment of poison ivy. Powdered plantain poultices mixed with green clay are a wonderful way to pull the oils out of the skin. For even more relief, mix the paste with peppermint essential oil (so long as the rash is well away from the breasts). Be sure to wash the dried paste from the skin with cool water regularly. Ice packs can be helpful to numb the nerve endings, but above all, *never* take hot baths or showers. Hot water lifts the oil to the skin's surface, leaving it free to run and spread elsewhere. As this is one of the most common plant families in the world, it can be found growing almost everywhere. If gathered for first aid or edible use, be sure to get it from an area that is not polluted or chemically contaminated.

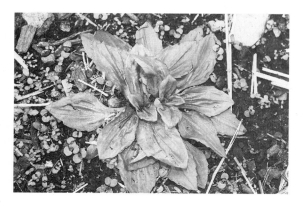

Plantain (Plantago spp.)

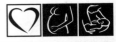

Pleurisy Root (*Asclepias tuberosa*)

Part used:	Root
Main constituents:	Essential oil; cardiac glycosides
Alternatives:	Elecampane (*Inula helenium*); mullein (*Verbascum thapsus*)
Notes for caution:	**During pregnancy and lactation:** The side effects of cardiac glycosides can have uterine stimulant and estrogenic activity.

This beautiful landscaping ornamental is native to Ohio and is full of powerful remedy for the respiratory system. In the case of lung infection involving inflammation, such as bronchitis, pnuemonia, pleurisy and even flu, pleurisy root is a superstar in formula with other respiratory herbs.

Poke Root (*Phytolacca americana*)

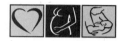

Part used:	Root; spring shoots (*Note: berries are toxic*)
Main constituents:	Sugar; jagilonic acid; oleanolic acid; bitter tannin; histamine; betalain alkaloids; triterpene saponins; GABA; spinasterol; sterols; starch; potassium salts; lectins[41]
Alternatives:	**To dissolve lumps in breast tissue while breastfeeding:** Poultice of turmeric (*Curcuma longa; Curcuma domestica; Curcuma aromatica*)
Notes for caution:	**During preconception:** The lectins in all parts of poke are toxic and can lead to the clumping of red blood cells and rapid and uncontrolled cell growth.[34]
	During pregnancy: The lectins in all parts of poke are toxic and can lead to the clumping of red blood cells and rapid and uncontrolled cell growth.
	During lactation: Poke root is mentioned here because it is a popular ingredient in breast balm and is used often in breast self-exams and routine massage. It is suspected that poke root may have an undesired laxative effect in a nursing infant.

Poke root is often used internally for inflammation, immune system stimulation and cancer, but can be done safely only under the guidance of an experienced herbalist. *The seed should be considered toxic under all conditions.* I have heard some say that they routinely eat pokeberry pie. It is the seed that is the most toxic component here, but it is best to avoid in any case as the idea of a pie with these berries is either an incorrect plant identification or the result of much luck or skill. It is wise during the nursing relationship to avoid any breast massage balm containing poke root (and to discontinue any internal use), as it is a known cathartic and may cause very strong reactions in an infant's body. Applying it externally anywhere but on the breasts while nursing is a relatively safe way to treat with poke. Homeopathic poke is safe to use for rheumatism and arthritis when trying to build a healthy baby.

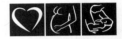

Pomegranate (*Punica granatum*)

Part used:	Root bark
Main constituents:	Punicotannic acid; gallic acid; mannite; pelletierine; methyl-pelletierine; pseudo-pelletierine; isopelletierine[52]
Alternatives:	Pumpkin seeds (*Cucurbita* spp.); garlic (*Allium sativum*); black walnut hull (*Juglans nigra*)
Notes for caution:	**During preconception, pregnancy and lactation:** Pomegranate bark is harsh, purgative and can be an emmenagogue and uterine stimulant.

All parts of the pomegranate are used in herbal treatments, but it is the bark that is problematic during preconception, pregnancy and lactation. The bark is used to rid the body of tapeworms, but it is a harsh and purgative treatment that is not appropriate for this time in a woman's life.

Prickly Ash (*Zanthoxylum americanum; Xanthoxylum americanum*)

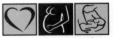

Part used:	Bark
Main constituents:	Volatile oil; fat; sugar; gum; acrid resin; alkaloid berberine; xanthoxylin
Alternatives:	Cayenne (*Capsicum annuum*)
Notes for caution:	**During preconception:** Prickly ash is an emmenagogue.
	During pregnancy: Prickly ash is an emmenagogue.
	During lactation: The herb is believed to be a possible stomach irritant to a nursing infant. The presence of berberine may be a danger to an infant who has been diagnosed with jaundice.

This herb is a stimulant and when swallowed actually produces a heating effect in the stomach and oftentimes in the extremities. For that reason, it is helpful in poor blood flow that results in cold hands and feet. It is also used routinely for fever and for toning the digestive system.

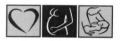

Pulsatilla (*Anemone pulsatilla; Pulsatilla vulgaris*)

Part used:	Aerial portions
Main constituents:	Anemonin; anemonic acid
Alternatives:	Elecampane (*Inula helenium*); wild cherry bark (*Prunus serotina*); cramp bark (*Viburnum opulus*)
Notes for caution:	**During preconception:** Pulsatilla is an emmenagogue.
	During pregnancy: Pulsatilla is an emmenagogue.
	During lactation: The herb is believed to cause a gastrointestinal irritation in nursing infants. There is also some concern about the depressant effect on the nervous system caused by the active ingredient anemonin, which leads to decreased respiration and circulation. This depressant effect is likely more pronounced in doses above a few drops of tincture in a spoonful of water.[39]

Also known as pasque flower, this herb is a potentially important heroic medicine due to its antispasmodic actions for bronchitis, asthma or whooping cough. For all other non-emergency times, it is best to avoid the use of pulsatilla, as it should be taken only in the appropriate small dose.

REPRODUCTIVE
PHASE
Preconception Pregnancy Lactation

GENERAL
SAFETY
RATING   No Contraindications   Use with Caution   Generally Avoid

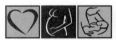

Purslane (ma chi xian) (*Portulaca oleracea*)

Part used:	Aerial portions
Main constituents:	Oxalates; vitamins A, C; calcium; iron; magnesium; phosphorus; salt; potassium; manganese; selenium
Alternatives:	Dandelion greens (*Taraxacum officinale*)
Notes for caution:	**During preconception:** Eat this only when it is cooked. High levels of oxalic acid bind to the body's supply of calcium and create deficiencies.
	During pregnancy: When raw, purslane contains high amounts of oxalic acid that can potentially be damaging to developing kidneys.
	During lactation: Eat this only when it is cooked. High levels of oxalic acid bind to the body's supply of calcium and create deficiencies.

Purslane is a nutritive herb that has applications as well for its "cooling" effect on inflammations of the body. Steaming purslane inactivates the oxalates and makes it a safe potherb for anyone. Traditional Chinese medicine makes use of its mild diuretic qualities to treat the genito-urinary tract.

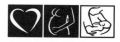

Quassia (*Quassia amara*)

Part used:	Wood; bark; leaves
Main constituents:	Quassin; phytochemicals; quassimarin; simalikalactone D.[41]
Alternatives:	Fennel (*Foeniculum vulgare*); bitter orange (*Citrus aurantium* spp., *Citrus amara*); artichoke (*Cynara scolymus*)
Notes for caution:	**During preconception and pregnancy:** In vitro studies suggest that quassia has anti-fertility effects due to the presence of quassin.[61]

Quassia is a common ingredient in bitters formulas. It helps with sluggish digestion by stimulating gastric juices and can also help when there is a lack of appetite and an out-of-control sweet tooth. Its bitter components are also useful in treating a sluggish liver or gallbladder problems. Externally as well as internally, it is a vermifuge and also can be used as a topical lice treatment. It would be wise to use caution even when using this herb externally.

Seed   **Aerial portions**

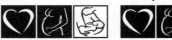

Queen Anne's Lace
(*Daucus carota*)

Part used:	Seed; aerial portions
Main constituents:	Acetone; acetylcholine; alpha-linolenic acid; alpha-pinene; alpha-tocopherol; aapigenin; arachidonic acid; arginine; asarone; ascorbic acid; bergapten; beta-carotene; beta-sitosterol; caffeic acid; camphor; chlorogenic acid; chlorophyll; chrysin; citral; citric acid; coumarin; elemicin; esculetin; ethanol; eugenol; falcarinol; ferulic acid; folacin; formic acid; fructose; gamma linolenic acid; geraniol; glutamine; glycine; HCN; histidine; kaempferol; lecithin; limonene; linoleic acid; lithium; lupeol; lutein; luteolin; lycopene; magnesium; manganese; methionine; mufa; myrcene; myricetin; myristicin; niacin; oleic acid; pantothenic acid; pectin; phenylalanine; potassium; psoralen; quercetin; scopoletin; stigmasterol; sucrose; terpinen-4-ol; thiamin; tryptophan-3; tyrosine; umbelliferone; xanthotoxin[62]
Alternatives:	**For urinary stones:** Cornsilk (*Zea mays*); goldenrod (*Solidago virgaurea*)
	For digestive tract: Dill (*Anethum graveolens*)
Notes for caution:	**Seed use during preconception and pregnancy:** The seeds of Queen Anne's lace are abortifacient.
	Aerial use during preconception and pregnancy: The herb is a uterine stimulant and should be avoided.
Additional caution:	Queen Anne's lace looks very similar to poisonous hemlock and should only be harvested in the wild by a professional.

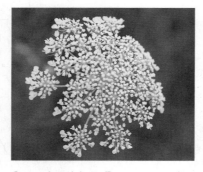

*Queen Anne's Lace (*Daucus carota*)*

The herb and root of wild carrot have a mild diuretic quality that can be used for gout or stones in the urinary tract. The seeds are carminative and can alleviate pains and gas in the digestive system. They are also strongly emmenagogue and abortifacient. As the long list of constituents may suggest, this herb is receiving a lot of attention and is being studied for its potential to help with a number of our worst diseases. *Queen Anne's lace looks very similar to the poisonous hemlock and should only be harvested in the wild by a knowledgable professional.*

Red Clover (*Trifolium pratense*)

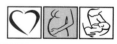

Galactagogue	
Part used:	Flower
Main constituents:	Vitamins A, B$_1$, B$_2$, B$_3$, C; calcium; chromium; magnesium; manganese; molybdenum; potassium; isoflavones: tin; protein; phosphorus; fat; fiber; aluminum; essential oil; resin; salicyclic acid; coumaric acid; coumestrol; saponins; flavonoids; polysaccharides[35]
Alternatives:	Dandelion root (*Taraxacum officinale*); burdock (*Arctium lappa*)
Notes for caution:	**During pregnancy:** Red clover contains natural coumarins, which are a class of blood thinner. It seems as though this action is actually very mild and has not been seen to cause a problem in either animals or humans. To date, the concern with the anticoagulant nature of this herb is only suspected. That being said, it is important for women to be mindful if they choose to use this herb during pregnancy, as this is a time when blood volume is changing often.
	You also should be aware that red clover is suspected to amplify the effects of allopathic blood thinners.

Red clover was traditionally used in the spring as a blood cleanser, as it helps the liver properly remove toxins from the blood. It is a favorite for women in all phases of life, especially for those working to improve their fertility. It is highly recommended (internally and externally) in the case of childhood skin problems, especially eczema, but may be used for people of all ages. It is also helpful both externally and internally for psoriasis.

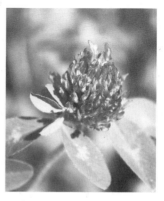

Red Clover *(Trifolium pratense)*

Red Raspberry (*Rubus idaeus*)

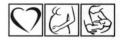

Galactagogue	
Part used:	Leaf
Main constituents:	Vitamins A, B₁, B₂, B₃, C, E; calcium; iron; magnesium; manganese; selenium; fragarine; protein; potassium; phosphorus; chromium; aluminum; citric acid; malic acid; volatile oil; resin; tannin; flavonoids; pectin[35]
Alternatives:	None
Male fertility:	There are many indications that red raspberry is an important tonic for the male reproductive system just as it is for the female.

The herb par excellence for women's health! Red raspberry is good for us at any stage of our lives. It is a uterine tonic, helping that muscle perform its job to the best of its ability. Contrary to current popular belief, it does not act to cause contractions. Instead, it enables the body to contract effectively by toning the muscle beforehand. During labor, it can be very helpful to ensure complete delivery of the placenta. Highly nutritive, this herb delivers much of what we need to keep our reproductive system healthy and also supports the nervous system and many other parts of the body.

Rhubarb (*Rheum palmatum; Rheum officinale*)

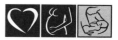

Part used:	Root
Main constituents:	Rheopurgarin; chrysophanic acid; rheochrysidin; emodin; aloe-emodin; rhein; phaoretin; calcium oxalate; iodine; phosphorus
Alternatives:	Dandelion root (*Taraxacum officinale*); yellow dock root (*Rumex crispus*)
Notes for caution:	**During preconception:** Rhubarb is a uterine stimulant with potential mutagens that are not good to be resident in pre-pregnancy tissues.
	During pregnancy: The herb is a uterine stimulant with a strong downward energy, as well as a potential mutagen due to the presence of anthraquinones. Rubarb also carries a risk of kidney damage due to its high oxalate content.
	During lactation: Because anthraquinones are partially excreted in milk, it is believed that this herb can have a laxative effect in infants. There is also the potential to pass along the genotoxins emodin and aloe-emodin.

Turkey rhubarb, or rhubarb root as it is commonly known, is an important laxative that can potentially cause griping. It is best taken with seeds containing volatile oils (dill, anise, fennel) to soothe the digestion and prevent these cramps.

   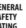

Roman Chamomile (*Chamaemelum nobile*)

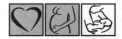

Part used:	Flower
Main constituents:	Volatile oil; tannic acid; anthemic acid
Alternatives:	German chamomile (*Matricaria recutita*)
Notes for caution:	**During preconception and pregnancy:** Extremely high doses can be an emmenagogue and abortifacient.

While Roman chamomile has some of the same effects in the body as German chamomile, it carries some extra warnings. Both chamomiles have sedative effects in the nervous system and can be used as carminatives. Roman chamomile has a slightly more bitter taste. Its use is often suggested in very large therapeutic doses, and it is only in such doses that Roman chamomile could potentially pose a threat to a pregnancy.

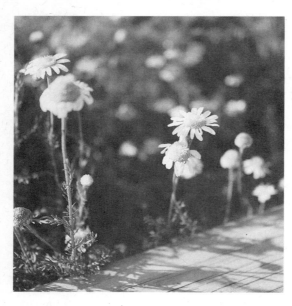

Roman Chamomile
(Chamaemelum nobile*)*

REPRODUCTIVE PHASE   Preconception   Pregnancy   Lactation

GENERAL SAFETY RATING   No Contraindications   Use with Caution   Generally Avoid

Rose (*Rosa* spp.)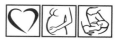

Part used:	Petals; hips (fruit)
Main constituents:	Vitamins A, B$_1$, B$_2$, B$_3$, C, E; calcium; iron; manganese; selenium; zinc (in hips)
Alternatives:	None

In Eastern ayurvedic medicine, rose is used to open the heart chakra. In Western herbalism, we use it often as an emotional medicine as well. Preparations of the petals can help with loss, grief, depression and anxiety. It is also astringent and can be used internally as well as externally to tighten pores. The hip, or fruit, of the rose is high in vitamins and minerals and provides support to the immune and nervous systems.

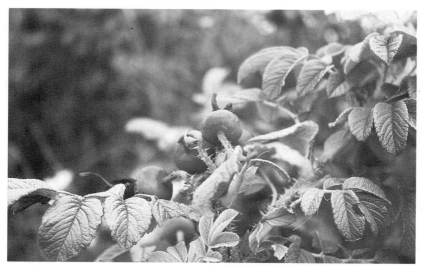

Rose (Rosa spp.)

REPRODUCTIVE PHASE   Preconception Pregnancy Lactation   GENERAL SAFETY RATING   No Contraindications   Use with Caution   Generally Avoid

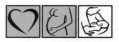

Rosemary (*Rosmarinus officinalis*)

Part used:	Leaves
Main constituents:	Rosmarinic acid; volatile oils; borneol; linalol; camphene; cinceole; camphor; resin
Alternatives:	None
Notes for caution:	**During preconception:** Rosemary is an emmenagogue in therapeutic doses.
	During pregnancy: Taking rosemary in therapeutic doses during pregnancy is not appropriate because of its potential emmenagogue and abortifacient effects. This is not the case if you are using it in the occasional herbal tea or as a seasoning.

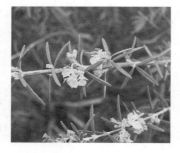

Rosemary is the herb of remembrance and has a long history of traditional and ceremonial use. It is an anti-inflammatory and a pain reliever that can help with just about any kind of pain, whether muscular, nerve or digestive.

*Rosemary (*Rosmarinus officinalis*)*

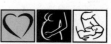

Rue (*Ruta graveolens*)

Part used:	Aerial parts
Main constituents:	Caprinic; pagonic; caprylic acid; oenanthylic acid; rutin[41]
Alternatives:	None
Notes for caution:	**During preconception:** Rue is an emmenagogue.
	During pregnancy: Rue is an emmenagogue that causes contractions.

Rue is an herb that should be taken only internally in small, supervised doses. *It can be very dangerous otherwise.* In small doses it can be used as an emmenagogue, but it would not be the best and safest choice. It is most often used externally for sprains and strains.

Safflower (*Carthamus tinctorius*)

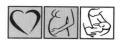

Part used:	Flowers (stamens only)
Main constituents:	Vitamins A, B₂; sodium; silicon; selenium; protein; potassium; phosphorus; magnesium; iron; fat; fiber; chromium; aluminum; essential fatty acids (linoleic, linolenic); carotenes; tannin; flavonoids;[35] carthamin; carthamadin[41]
Alternatives:	**For a laxative:** Yellow dock (*Rumex crispus*)
	As a febrifuge: Elder (*Sambucus canadensis*); catnip (*Nepeta cataria*)
Notes for caution:	**During preconception and pregnancy:** Safflower is an emmenagogue and can cause problems with cell division and growth in a developing fetus when taken in a therapeutic dose.

Safflower is often used as a laxative and febrifuge, though it is more commonly known as an oil for cooking. If you want to continue to use safflower oil in your food preparation from preconception on, it is best to use it in small amounts and only occasionally. Do not combine the use of safflower oil in your food with herbal therapeutic doses, even if they are low doses. Coconut oil is a much better alternative.

Saffron (*Crocus sativus*)

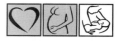

Part used:	Flowers (stigmas only)
Main constituents:	Zeaxanthin; lycopene; beta-carotene vitamin B₂; crocin[41]
Alternatives:	**For fever:** Elder (*Sambucus nigra*); yarrow (*Achillea millefolium*)
Notes for caution:	**During preconception and pregnancy:** Saffron is an emmenagogue when taken in therapeutic or excessive doses. There is no reason for caution when used as a seasoning or in a tea when consuming under 1.5 grams per day.[34]

Saffron is a seasoning known to many for its exorbitant price. It is an important dye and has traditionally been used in digestive system disorders, to reduce fevers and to bring on menstruation. It has special application when there is old blood in the cycle that needs to be moved out of the body.

	Leaf	Essential oil/ Alcoholic extract

Sage (*Salvia officinalis*)

Antigalactagogue	
Part used:	Leaf
Main constituents:	Volatile oil (thujone, cineole, borneol); resin; tannins; phenolic acids (salvin, rosmarinic); flavonoids; picrosalvin; carnosol; vitamins A, B_1, B_2, B_3, C; magnesium; potassium; zinc; sodium; silicon; protein; iron; fat; fiber; calcium; aluminum[35]
Alternatives:	**For sore throat:** Pau d'arco (*Tabebuia impetiginosa*); thyme (*Thymus vulgaris*)
Notes for caution:	**Leaf during pregnancy:** Due to thujone content, it is not recommended to take a very high dose of tea or to use the herb excessively. If used in this way, it can be an emmenagogue or an abortifacient. **Leaf during lactation:** Sage is a known anti-galactagogue and will reduce milk supply.
	Essential oil/alcoholic extract during preconception and pregnancy: When taken internally can be an emmenagogue and abortifacient. **Essential oil/alcoholic extract during lactation:** Due to the presence of thujone, when taken interally can have a negative effect on the breastfeeding baby.

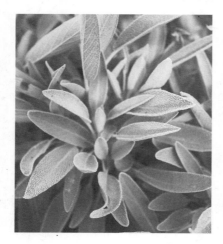

Sage may be the herb commonly used for sore throats, but its use should be limited during nursing. As it is also a common culinary herb, be aware of what's in that breakfast sausage or Thanksgiving stuffing. If, however, a mother is experiencing an infection, mastitis or engorgement in her breast

*Sage (*Salvia officinalis*)*

while nursing and needs to reduce her milk for a short period of time while healing, sage tea is specifically indicated.

 Sandalwood (chandana) (*Santalum album*)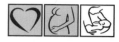

Part used:	Wood; essential oil
Main constituents:	Essential oil (alpha- and beta-sanitol)
Alternatives:	Chamomile (*Matricaria recutita*)
Notes for caution:	**During preconception and pregnancy:** Sandalwood is an abortifacient in excessive doses.

Sandalwood is a popular incense, but in ayurveda it is a common herbal treatment as well. It is a cooling herb that has application in the body for all types of inflammation.

Root bark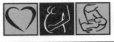

Essential oil/
Alcoholic extract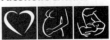

Sassafrass (*Sassafrass albidum; Sassafrass officinale*)

Part used:	Root bark; essential oil; extract in alcohol
Main constituents:	Volatile oil; safrole; sassafrid; tannic acid; gum; albume; starch; lignan; salts
Alternatives:	Red clover (*Trifolium pretense*); burdock (*Arctium lappa*)
Notes for caution:	**Root bark use during preconception:** Sassafrass is a possible uterine stimulant. Don't use for prolonged periods of time (daily for more than 3 months).
	Root bark use during pregnancy: Sassafrass is a possible uterine stimulant. It is most problematic during early pregnancy. Don't use for prolonged periods of time (daily for more than 3 months). The constituent safrole is known to have toxic and hepatocarcinogenic effects in animals.
	Root bark use during lactation: Don't use for prolonged periods of time (daily for more than 3 months). Safrole is known to have toxic and hepatocarcinogenic effects in animals.
	Essential oil/alcoholic extract during preconception and pregnancy: The essential oil or alcoholic extract will contain safrole, which is an emmenagogue and abortifacient.
	Essential oil/alcoholic extract during lactation: The essential oil or alcoholic extract will contain safrole, which is a known carcinogen.

Sassafrass is a Southern herb that was traditionally used in spring tonics meant to cleanse the blood after winter. In this capacity it is specifically used for skin conditions such as psoriasis and eczema. It is also specific for conditions such as gout, in which the blood needs cleansing of uric acid. It is used mainly as a tea. The toxic ingredient, safrole, is insoluable in water and therefore is not available in this type of preparation. As an essential oil or alcoholic extract, safrole is made available because it is soluble in alcohol. Sassafrass essential oil is highly regulated and is not readily available. This herb was a familiar flavoring agent found in many teas (think root beer) before the FDA banned its use.

Savin (*Juniperus sabina*)

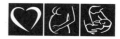

Part used:	New buds (dried)
Main constituents:	Volatile oil; resin; gallic acid; chlorophyl extractive; lignin; calcareous salts; fixed oil; gum; salts of potassium[52]
Alternatives:	None
Notes for caution:	**During preconception, pregnancy and lactation:** Savin is toxic when taken internally.

Savin is a strong emmenagogue and abortifacient that is an internal irritant and toxin.

Seaweed (*Laminaria* spp.)

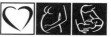

Part used:	Thallus (leaf)
Main constituents:	Iodine; calcium
Alternatives:	Sea salt
	For hypothyroidism: Eleuthero (*Eleutherococcus senticosus; Acanthopanax senticosus*)
	For calcium: Red raspberry (*Rubus ideaus*); oatstraw (*Avena sativa*)
Notes for caution:	**During pregnancy:** Excessive consumption during pregnancy can lead to infantile goiter. It is best to keep the therapeutic dosage of any type of seaweed to no more than 0.25 grams daily
	During lactation: In high doses or with prolonged use, seaweed can overstimulate the thyroid. The high iodine content could be a potential toxin to a nursing infant.

Seaweeds are often eaten as a good source of calcium. They are also often used to aid in mild thyroid dysfunction due to their iodine content.

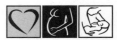

Senega (*Polygala senega*)

Part used:	Root
Main constituents:	Methyl salicylate; triterpenoid saponins (senegin); polygalitol; plant sterols
Alternatives:	Elecampane (*Inula helenium*); wild cherry bark (*Prunus serotina*); cramp bark (*Viburnum opulus*)
Notes for caution:	**During preconception:** Senega is an emmenagogue.
	During pregnancy: Senega is an emmenagogue.

Senega is a purgative herb that causes vomiting, sweating or coughing. It is used most often for inflammation of the respiratory tract such as in emphysema, bronchitis and asthma.

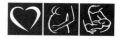

Senna (*Cassia* spp.; *Senna* spp.)

Part used:	Leaves; pods
Main constituents:	Anthraquinones; glucosides (cathartic acid, chyrsophanic acid, sennacrol sennapicrin); rhein; aloe-emodin; kaempferol; isormamnetin; myricyl alcohol
Alternatives:	Dandelion root (*Taraxacum officinale*); yellow dock root (*Rumex crispus*)
Notes for caution:	**During preconception:** Possibilities exist for uterine stimulation. Of more concern is the possibility for genotoxins to be resident in the body's tissues at the time of conception. **During pregnancy:** Possibilities exist for uterine stimulation. Of more concern is the potential for genotoxins to cross the placenta. There have been animal cases that have found a therapeutic dose to be safe for pregnancy, but controversy continues between the world's herbal safety governing bodies, and a determination has not yet been made. **During lactation:** Senna is a strong laxative in adults. While there have not been any studies that have demonstrated enough secretion of the laxative component through breast milk to have a laxative effect in a nursing infant,[39] a purgative effect is found in historical references. There have been reported cases of occasional diarrhea in an infant receiving senna directly by mouth. It is also a potential genotoxin.

Senna is a strong herb capable of assisting with purging the body of waste material. Unfortunately, on its own, it causes significant gastrointestinal cramping. It acts not by assisting in the peristaltic action, but rather by irritating the intestinal wall. It is therefore not recommended in inflammatory digestive disorders. It can be used safely and effectively in combination with other herbs to ameliorate the cramping. While nursing, it is best to go with another option unless it is unavoidable.

REPRODUCTIVE PHASE				GENERAL SAFETY RATING								

 Preconception Pregnancy Lactation No Contraindications Use with Caution Generally Avoid

Shatavari (*Asparagus racemosus*)

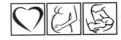

Part used:	Root
Main constituents:	Steroidal saponins; isoflavones; asparagamine; polysaccharides
Alternatives:	None

Shatavari is an ayurvedic reproductive tonic for women. It is called the "Indian ginseng" and is the female energetic counterpart to ashwaganda. Both a fertility enhancer and an aphrodisiac, it is used to balance estrogen levels, improve fertility, relieve vaginal dryness and alleviate pain that occurs during intercourse.

Shepherd's Purse (*Capsella bursa-pastoris*)

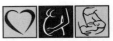

Part used:	Aerial portions
Main constituents:	Vitamin K; calcium; iron; magnesium; choline acetylcholine; tannin (tannic acid); essential oil; resin; diosmin; histamine; inositol; rutin; oxalates
Alternatives:	Plantain (*Plantago lanceolata; Plantago major*)
Notes for caution:	**During preconception:** Eat this herb only when it is cooked. High levels of oxalic acid bind to the body's supply of calcium and create deficiencies.
	During pregnancy: Shepherd's purse contains high amounts of oxalic acid, which can potentially be damaging to developing kidneys. It is also a known emmenagogue and abortifacient.
	During lactation: Eat this only when it is cooked. High levels of oxalic acid bind to the body's supply of calcium and create deficiencies.

Shepherd's purse is a great little weed to know. It is related to broccoli and tastes very similar, and is good enough to be a potherb. It is a very good styptic and can be helpful for minor outdoor injuries. It is commonly used by midwives to prevent hemorrhage, but can be just as effective for the common nosebleed.

Sichuan Lovage (chuan xiong)
(*Ligusticum chuanxiong*)

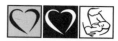

Part used:	Rhizome
Main constituents:	Volatile oils (ligustilide, sabinene, limonene, senkyunolide A-S); alkaloids (tetramethylpyrazine, perlolyrine, wallichilide, 3-butylidene-7-hydroxyphthalide, (3S)-3-butyl-4-hydroxyphthalide); organic acids (ferulic acid, sedanonic acid, folic acid, vanillic acid, caffeic acid, protocatechuic acid)[63]
Alternatives:	None
Notes for caution:	**During preconception:** Sichuan lovage is an emmenagogue.
	During pregnancy: Sichuan lovage is an emmenagogue. Pregnancy is not the time to move pelvic stagnation.

This herb is often used in traditional Chinese medicine for painful menstruation or lack of menstruation. It's also great for headaches and for relieving pain.

Skullcap (*Scutellaria lateriflora*)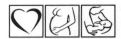

Part used:	Aerial portions
Main constituents:	Vitamins A, B₁, B₂, B₃, C; potassium; zinc; silicon; protein; phosphorus; manganese; iron; fiber; aluminum; scutellarin; salicyclic acid; chrysophanic acid; anthraquinones (aloe-emodin); flavonoids; saponins; fat; sugar
Alternatives:	None

This is my favorite herbal headache remedy. Skullcap is an antispasmodic and has been used to treat seizure disorders. It is also a sedative that can be very helpful to those who are having trouble getting to sleep or staying asleep. It has applications in all situations that are brought on by nervous stress or tension. Skullcap has traditionally been used to alleviate withdrawal symptoms and might be a good option for nursing through, to help a baby going through any sort of withdrawal.

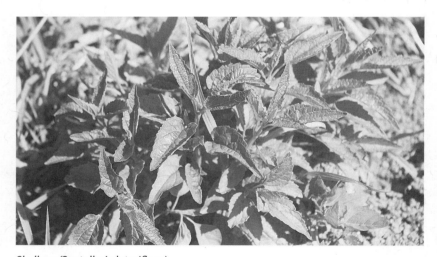

Skullcap (Scutellaria lateriflora)

REPRODUCTIVE PHASE   Preconception   Pregnancy   Lactation   GENERAL SAFETY RATING   No Contraindications   Use with Caution   Generally Avoid

Slippery Elm (*Ulmus rubra*)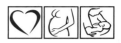

Part used:	Inner bark
Main constituents:	Vitamins A, B$_1$, B$_2$, B$_3$; tin; selenium; fiber; chromium; calcium; phosporus; mucilage; tannin; resin; volatile oil[35]
Alternatives:	None

This herb is best known for a high mucilage content that is highly nutritious. It is especially good for inflamed and irritated mucus membranes such as can be found in any type of digestive issue. I would turn to slippery elm if a family member were unable to take in nutrition in any way. Nutrition can be absorbed through a poultice or made into gruel.

Southernwood (*Artemesia abrotanum*)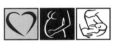

Part used:	Aerial portions
Main constituents:	Volatile oil; tannin; abrotanin
Alternatives:	Pumpkin seeds (*Cucurbita* spp.); garlic (*Allium sativum*); black walnut hull (*Juglans nigra*); cucumber (*Cucumis sativa*)
Notes for caution:	**During preconception:** Southernwood is an emmenagogue.
	During pregnancy: Southernwood is an emmenagogue.

Southernwood is very rarely added to food as it has a relatively strong flavor. It is known for its abilities to expel worms and as an emmenagogue.

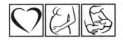

Spearmint (phudina) (*Mentha spicata*)

Part used:	Aerial portions
Main constituents:	Volatile oils (menthol, d-limonene, menthone, neomenthol); tannins
Alternatives:	None

Spearmint doesn't have as high a content of menthol as peppermint, but it has some similar applications when it comes to soothing digestive upsets. Spearmint tea also has been shown in recent studies to counteract the effects of hirsutism. It is also a mild diuretic and can therefore be helpful in removing toxins from the body.

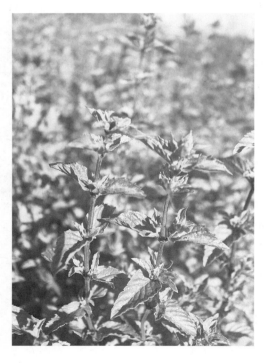

*Spearmint (*Mentha spicata*)*

REPRODUCTIVE PHASE   Preconception   Pregnancy   Lactation   GENERAL SAFETY RATING   No Contraindications   Use with Caution   Generally Avoid

Spikenard (*Aralia* spp.)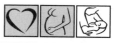

Part used:	Root
Main constituents:	Volatile oil; tannins; diterpene acids[41]
Alternatives:	Ginseng (*Panax ginseng*)
Notes for caution:	**During preconception and pregnancy:** Spikenard is a possible emmenagogue.

Spikenard is antifungal, expectorant, adaptogenic and antimicrobial. Herbalist Matthew Wood reports that it is the warm counterpart to eleuthero's cool energy.[60] Part of the ginseng family, spikenard improves the condition of the blood. It is also a favorite herb for strengthening a weakened, imbalanced female reproductive system, and is worth considering as a treatment for blocked milk ducts or mastitis.

Spirulina (*Arthrospira platensis*)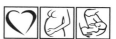

Part used:	Whole plant
Main constituents:	Vitamins A, B_1, B_2, B_3; zinc; selenium; protein; phosphorus; manganese; magnesium; iron; fat; chromium; phycocyanin; beta-carotene; zeaxanthin[35]
Alternatives:	None

Spirulina is an algae that is high in amino acids, vitamins and minerals. It is a nutritional supplement, but is also an immune system tonic. My favorite application for spirulina is for exhaustion following surgery or heavy blood loss. It is high in antioxidants and chlorophyll and helps to properly oxygenate our blood supply. It is absolutely specific for that type of postpartum exhaustion that leaves you feeling like you can't possibly get enough air or stay awake, and you have no energy at all.

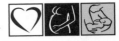

St. John's Wort (*Hypericum perforatum*)

Part used:	Aerial portions
Main constituents:	Hypericin; rutin; bitters
Alternatives:	**For anxiety and depression:** Lavender (*Lavendula angustifolia*); rose (*Rosa* spp.); lemon balm (*Melissa officinalis*); chamomile (*Matricaria recutita*)
Notes for caution:	**During pregnancy:** St. John's wort is an emmenagogue and abortifacient.
	During lactation: If a nursing child is undergoing treatment for jaundice, it is possible that the herb can increase sensitivity to UV light. Avoid using it until treatments are concluded.

St. John's wort has wonderful internal and external use. Internally, it is often used in formula to combat depression, anxiety and nervous tension. It is also important for relieving pain in nerve endings due either to blunt force trauma or nervous system disorder.

Externally, it can be made into an oil to help with that same type of pain and is also great for any kind of inflammation, bruising or burns. It is especially effective for treating sunburn. There is no reason to avoid the use of St. John's wort oil while building a baby.

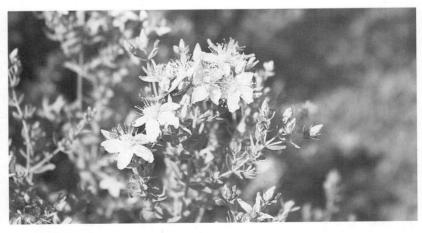

*St. John's Wort (*Hypericum perforatum*)*

Stillingia (*Stillingia sylvatica*)

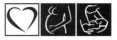

Part used:	Root
Main constituents:	Sylvacrol; alkaloids; fixed oil; diterpene esters; resins; calcium; oxalate; volatile oil; tannins[64]
Alternatives:	**For respiratory:** Elecampane (*Inula helenium*)
	For skin and blood cleansers: Dandelion root (*Taraxacum officinale*); burdock (*Arctium lappa*)
Notes for caution:	**During pregnancy and lactation:** Too much of this herb can lead quickly to toxicity that can involve racing heartbeat, vomiting, diarrhea and loss of muscular control.

Stillingia is a lymphatic cleanser that has many applications involving the respiratory system and general skin issues. Unfortunately, for stillingia to be effective, it must be relatively fresh. Only experienced practitioners should administer this herb, as too much can quickly result in toxicity.

Sunflower (*Helianthus anuus*)

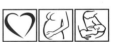

Part used:	Seed
Main constituents:	Vitamins B_1, B_2, B_5; potassium; magnesium; phosphorus; calcium; salicyclic acid; lipids; amino acids
Alternatives:	None

Because sunflower seeds (properly soaked and/or sprouted, of course) are a good source of vitamin B_5, they are supportive of the adrenal glands, with specific action in the case of adrenal exhaustion. Sunflower seeds are diuretic in nature and have applications in the respiratory system as well.

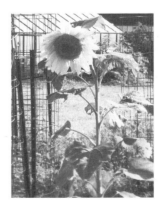

*Sunflower (*Helianthus annus*)*

PHOTO CREDIT © SCOTT WOOD

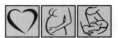

Sweet Flag (*Acorus calamus*)

Part used:	Rhizome
Main constituents:	Beta-asarone; volatile oil; terpenes (eugenol); ammines; tannins; resin; mucilage; gum starch; acorin[60]
Alternatives:	**For indigestion:** Bitter orange (*Citrus aurantium* spp.; *Citrus amara*); chamomile (*Matricaria recutita*)
Notes for caution:	**During preconception:** Sweet flag can be an emmenagogue.
	During pregnancy: The potential for toxicity is very slight unless sweet flag is used for long periods of time or in high doses. In these instances, it is believed that it can be an emmenagogue and abortifacient.
	During lactation: The potential for toxicity is very slight unless sweet flag is used for long periods of time or in high doses.

Sweet flag is banned for use in the United States because of the danger of confusing the original *A. calumnus* with introduced sweet flag cultivars. When the correct plant is used, it is helpful for acid indigestion, laryngitis and throat irritation, and congestion in the head that leads to confusion and memory loss.

   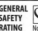

Tansy (*Tanacetum vulgar*)

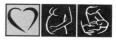

Part used:	Aerial portions
Main constituents:	Tanacetin; tannic acid; volatile oil (thujone); parthenolides; wax; resin; protein; sugar[41]
Alternatives:	Pumpkin seeds (*Cucurbita* spp.); garlic (*Allium sativum*); black walnut hull (*Juglans nigra*)
Notes for caution:	**During preconception:** Tansy is an emmenagogue.
	During pregnancy: While the essential oil of tansy is the most problematic, tansy itself is too variable in its constituent levels to say it is safe as a tea during pregnancy. It is best avoided in favor of another herb during this time. Empirical evidence shows tansy to be a uterine stimulant, emmenagogue and abortifacient with the potential to cause birth defects.
	During lactation: Thujone is a compound that, when taken in incorrect doses, can be toxic to mother and infant.

Both externally and internally, tansy is useful for repelling worms and pests. It also has a long history of use as an emmenagogue. In historical data, though, there is evidence of the toxicity that has more recently been identified as being caused by thujone. A woman who is intent on using tansy internally *must* work with an experienced practitioner, as an incorrect dose can be highly toxic.

REPRODUCTIVE PHASE				GENERAL SAFETY RATING							
Preconception	Pregnancy	Lactation		No Contraindications		Use with Caution		Generally Avoid			

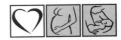

Tea (*Camellia sinensis; Thea sinensis*)

Part used:	Leaves
Main constituents:	Caffeine; tannin; boheic acid; volatile oil; theophylline; vitamin K
Alternatives:	Herbal tisanes (teas)
Notes for caution:	**During pregnancy:** Caffeine is known to cross the placenta and can contribute to low birth weight, preterm labor and birth defects.[44]
	During lactation: Caffeine has been found to appear in breast milk at half the level in the mother's plasma. It reduces the available iron supply in breast milk.

It's important to specify here that "tea" is anything made with a specific plant: *Camellia sinensis* or *Thea sinensis*. Usually found as red, black, white or green tea, this is not the same as an herbal tea. Many people use these teas medicinally, especially green tea. They can be very beneficial, but women who use tea therapeutically on a daily basis might consider changing to occasional use while nursing.

Thyme (*Thymus* spp.)

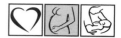

Part used:	Leaves
Main constituents:	Vitamins A, B$_1$, B$_2$, B$_3$, C; zinc; tin; sodium; silicon; iron; fat; fiber; cobalt; tannin; resin; pseudo-tannins;[35] alpha-linolenic acid; anethole; apigenin; borneol; caffeic acid; calcium; chromium; eugenol, ferulic acid; geraniol; kaempferol; limonene; lithium; luteolin; magnesium; manganese; methionine; coumaric acid; potassium; rosmarinic acid; selenium; thymol; tryptophan; ursolic acid[41]
Alternatives:	None
Notes for caution:	**During pregnancy:** This herb can be an emmenagogue in therapeutic doses. It is not an issue when used in the occasional herbal tea or in foods.

Thyme is best known for its culinary use, but is also very important for our health. It is high in volatile oils, so its inclusion in cooking gives us relief from upset stomach and slow digestion. It is also highly antiseptic, so its use in respiratory and digestive infections as well as sore throats, mouthwashes and externally on wounds is warranted. It is helpful in the relief of coughing and helps to break up mucus in the respiratory system. It is also a vermifuge. When used as a wash, thyme is a helpful for vaginal yeast infections.

REPRODUCTIVE PHASE
Preconception Pregnancy Lactation

GENERAL SAFETY RATING
No Contraindications Use with Caution Generally Avoid

Tobacco (*Nicotiana tabacum*)

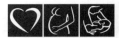

Part used:	Leaves
Main constituents:	Nicotine; nicotianin; nicotinine; nicoteine; nicoteline
	After smoking: Pyridine; furfurol; collidine; hydrocyanic acid; carbon monoxide
Alternatives:	None
Notes for caution:	**During preconception and pregnancy:** Tobacco is known to contribute to low birth weights, birth defects, miscarriage or preterm labor.
	During lactation: Avoid ingestion of tobacco in any form; it is known to result in a diminished milk supply. The excretion of nicotine in breast milk has been shown to cause immediate changes in respiration and oxygen saturation in the breast-feeding infant. It is also believed that it may alter a child's intelligence and behavioral development, and the inhalation of secondhand smoke is believed to increase future chances for lung cancer.
Male fertility:	Smoking tobacco is a major cause of impotence.

Historically, tobacco has been used as a heroic medicine internally for spasms in the digestive or urinary tract. The fresh plant has even been used externally in certain applications. It has gained its most notoriety, sadly, as a recreational drug that is smoked and abused by way of overuse.

REPRODUCTIVE PHASE	Preconception	Pregnancy	Lactation	GENERAL SAFETY RATING	No Contraindications	Use with Caution	Generally Avoid

Tree Peony (*Paeonia suffruticosa*)

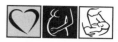

Part used:	Bark
Main constituents:	Paeonol; galloyl-paeoniflorin; galloyl-oxypaeoniflorin; suffruticoside A, B, C, D and E[65]
Alternatives:	**For pain:** Rosemary (*Rosemarinus officinalis*)
	For fever: Yarrow (*Achillea millefolium*); elder (*Sambucus nigra*)
	As an antispasmodic: Skullcap (*Scutellaria lateriflora*)
	As an anti-Inflammatory: Chamomile (*Matricaria recutita*)
Notes for caution:	**During preconception:** Tree peony is an emmenagogue.
	During pregnancy: Tree peony is an emmenagogue.

All parts of the tree peony are useful in the body in different ways. In the case of fertility, pregnancy and lactation, it is only the bark with which we need to be concerned. The bark is used for its ability to relieve pain and reduce fever. It is antispasmodic, anti-inflammatory and, like its relative the red peony, has some blood-moving abilities, often acting as a styptic.

Turmeric (haldi) (*Curcuma longa, Curcuma domestica, Curcuma aromatica*)

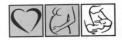

Galactagogue	
Part used:	Rhizome
Main constituents:	Vitamins A, B₃; zinc; sodium; silicon; selenium; protein; potassium; phosphorus; manganese; magnesium; iron; fat; fiber; curcumin; turmerone; atlantone; zingiberone; resin[35]
Alternatives:	Bitter orange (*Citrus aurantium* spp., *Citrus amara*); chamomile (*Matricaria recutita*); meadowsweet (*Filipendula ulmaria*); elder (*Sambucus nigra*)
Notes for caution:	**During preconception:** Avoid therapeutic doses while trying to become pregnant, as turmeric can act as an emmenagogue. **During pregnancy:** Although turmeric is an effective therapy for many imbalances, at therapeutic doses during pregnancy it can act as an emmenagogue or abortifacient. If used in food or in tea, it is relatively safe.

Turmeric is a yellow spice that is often used in Indian cuisine and in ayurvedic medicine. It is known as a powerful anti-inflammatory. Most recently, people are buying the synthesized or extracted curcumin because it is believed that this is the most active compound providing the anti-inflammatory benefits. The respected herbalists at Mountain Rose Herbs have found that, "although curcumin is available as a standardized extract, the whole herb may be more beneficial for you than the curcumin extract: Only very small amounts of curcumin are absorbed into the bloodstream. Turmeric as a whole herb stays in the digestive tract longer than curcumin, releasing antioxidant curcumin along with other beneficial substances."[66] Turmeric is helpful in fighting atherosclerosis and cancer.

Vetiver (*Vetiveria zizanoides*)

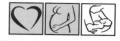

Part used:	Root; essential oil
Main constituents:	Alpha-vetivone; benzoic acid; beta vetivone; furfurol; vetiverol; vetivene; vetivenyl vetivenate[67]
Alternatives:	None
Notes for caution:	**During preconception and pregnancy:** Vetiver is an emmenagogue and abortifacient.

Internally, vetiver is often used for circulatory issues. This herb is also great to use externally for an outbreak of lice. Added to shampoos, baths and laundry wash water, it is effective at eradicating this pest. The essential oil, which is made from the root, is the more commonly used form. It is a known emmenagogue and is mentioned in some texts as being useful for balancing estrogen and progesterone. The essential oil has many health benefits. It is analgesic, antibacterial, antispasmodic, anti-inflammatory, cooling and sedative. Check labels to find vetiver virtually everywhere. It is used as a fixative and scent in soaps and skincare products, and is often added as a flavoring to food. You are more likely to come across vetiver in foods from outside the United States because inside the country it is allowable only as a flavoring in alcohol.

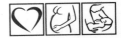

Valerian (*Valeriana officinalis*)

Part used:	Root
Main constituents:	Vitamin B₃; tin; sodium; selenium; potassium; iron; fat; fiber; cobalt; chromium; aluminum; volatile oils (valerianic acid, isovalerianic acid, borneol, pinene, camphine); alkaloids; calcium; tannins (acetic acid, ascorbic acid, caffeic acid); magnesium; manganese; flavonoids (quercitin, rutin); choline[35]
Alternatives:	None
Author's note:	Because of the number of volatile oils in this root, use the infusion, rather than the decoction, method when making a tea.

Valerian has a sedative action and is heavily used to treat insomnia. It doesn't work for everyone though. If you're a Type A personality, beware — a small percentage of folks might find they are stimulated by valerian rather than sedated. There isn't any danger with this herb, though, and its good qualities include its use as a muscle relaxant, heart toner, nerve sedative, antispasmodic and pain reliever.

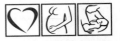

Violet (*Viola tricolor*)

Part used:	Flower; leaf
Main constituents:	Vitamins A, C; calcium; alpha-ionone; beta-ionone; beta-sitosterol; eugenol; ferulic acid; kaempferol; malic acid; methyl salicylate; palmitic acid; quercetin; rutin; scopoletin; vanillin
Alternatives:	None

Violets remind me of spring traditions. Many families gather the wild blooms to make syrups and jellies. Because violet is high in vitamins A and C, it is a very nutritious food source but, of course, it has many other benefits. One of its common names is "heartsease," because it really is a useful heart tonic. It is helpful for respiratory congestion or whenever a laxative is needed. It is an anti-inflammatory and also can be used to reduce a fever. It is a gentle medicine anyone can use — and it tastes good.

Watercress (*Nasturtium officinale*)

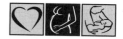

Part used:	Aerial portions
Main constituents:	Vitamins A , B_1, B_2, B_3, B_5, B_6, B_{17}, C, D, E, and K; calcium; phosphorus; potassium; iron; sodium; magnesium; copper; manganese; florine; sulfur; chlorine; iodine; germanium; silica; zinc; volatile oil; glycosides; fiber; protein with animo acids (arginine, histidine, isoleucine, leucine, lysine, threonine, phenyla-linine, methionine, tryptophan, valine); folic acid; coumarins[68]
Alternatives:	Wild mustard greens (*Brassica* spp.)
Notes for caution:	**During preconception:** Watercress is an emmenagogue.
	During pregnancy: Watercress is an emmenagogue and abortifacient.
	During lactation: It has been recorded that a mother eating watercress will often have a nursing baby with an upset stomach. It is best used sparingly. Be sure to monitor your baby's behavior accordingly.

Watercress is one of the salad greens we can turn to for extra flavor and a boost of iron. When used as an herbal treatment, it is most helpful for sore throats and stuffy noses, and is also showing some promise for oral cancers caused by smoking. Highly nutritive, it has a variety of uses that have been recorded over hundreds of years. Chief among these are its traditional uses in spring blood purifiers and digestive aids. It has been reported that watercress may act as a galactagogue.

White Oak (*Quercus alba*)

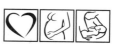

Part used:	Bark
Main constituents:	Zinc; selenium; manganese; fiber; calcium; tannins (plobotannin, egallitannin, gallic acid); flavonoids (quercitin); resin[35]
Alternatives:	None

White oak is mainly used externally to combat bacterial and viral infections. It can be used as a soaking bath or made into a wash for affected areas.

Wild Cherry (*Prunus serotina*)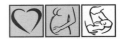

Part used:	Bark
Main constituents:	Volatile oil; resins; coumarins; acetylcholine; HCN; kaempferol; prunasin; quercetin; scopoletin; tannins
Alternatives:	Elecampane (*Inula helenium*); cramp bark (*Viburnum opulus*)
Notes for caution:	**During preconception and pregnancy:** The presence of a cyanogenic glycoside (prunasin) is believed to be teratogenic in nature when taken in excessive doses or for prolonged periods of time.

Wild cherry is most often found in cold and cough formulas. It is good for breaking up congestion and in relieving the urge to cough. It is also a bit of a sedative that helps the nervous system relax and rest so healing can take place. It has traditionally been associated with treating whooping cough.

Wild Ginger (*Asarum canadense*)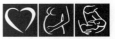

Part used:	Rhizome
Main constituents:	Beta-asarone; aristolochic acid; resin; mucilage
Alternatives:	None
Notes for caution:	**During preconception, pregnancy and lactation:** The potential for toxicity relating to beta-asarone is very slight, but aristolochic acid is strongly carcinogenic and nephrotoxic. Avoid it during preconception, pregnancy and lactation.

Wild ginger is not exactly the same as the true ginger (*Zingiber officinale*) used in food, although the root is somewhat spicy and has a similar smell. It has its best chance as a substitute only after having been dried. To further confuse the issue, Native populations in the United States used wild ginger in small amounts as flavoring for food, though they more often used it for chronic respiratory and stomach problems, contraception and much more. It is antiseptic and sedative and is being looked at, because of its aristolochic acid content, for its anti-tumor properties.

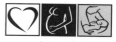

Wild Indigo (*Baptisia tinctoria*)

Part used:	Roots; leaves
Main constituents:	Alkaloids; glycosides; oleoresin[44]
Alternatives:	Elecampane (*Inula helenium*); mullein (*Verbascum thapsus*); elder (*Sambucus nigra*)
Notes for caution:	**During pregnancy:** Improper dosage can have a strong purgative effect. Use only with the guidance of an experienced practitioner.
	During lactation: Improper dosage can have a strong purgative effect. Use only with the guidance of an experienced practitioner.

Wild indigo is great for infections that involve phlegm, such as ear and sinus infections and laryngitis. Herbalist David Hoffman even suggests it as an external lotion to soothe sore nipples.[44] It is antiseptic and an immune stimulant, for which it is used in homeopathics. Any use other than as a homeopathic remedy *must* be undertaken only with the guidance of an experienced practitioner.

Wild Yam (*Dioscorea villosa*)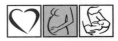

Galactagogue	
Part used:	Root
Main constituents:	Vitamins A, C; chromium; manganese; magnesium; aluminum; iron; fiber; zinc; tannin; saponins (diosgenin, sapogenin, yamogenin); ascorbic acid; beta-carotene; phosphorus; sodium; tin; cobalt[35]
Alternatives:	**For liver stagnation:** Dandelion root (*Taraxacum officinale*)
Notes for caution:	**During pregnancy:** It has been noted that wild yam can act as a uterine stimulant.
Male fertility:	Wild yam can be very important for men due to its ability to regulate hormones and to support a fully functional liver.

Wild yam has been used for centuries as a hormonal regulator. It is primarily known to support the progesterone part of a woman's cycle as well as the body's production of coritsone. Wild yam is helpful in cases of infertility, menstrual difficulties, miscarriage and endometriosis. In many cases, when the female hormone system is unbalanced, there is liver stagnation or congestion. Wild yam is specific for this condition. The roots of the plant contain steroidal saponins, as seen in the soapy bubbles the herb makes when it is boiled for tea. These saponins are required by the liver to synthesize sex hormones.

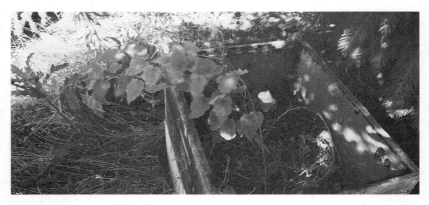

*Wild Yam (*Dioscorea villosa*)*

Wintergreen (*Gaulteria procumbens*)

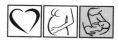

Galactagogue	
Part used:	Leaves
Main constituents:	Methyl salicylate; hydrocarbon; gaultherilene
Alternatives:	Meadowsweet (*Filipendula ulmaria*)
Notes for caution:	**During lactation:** Large, frequent doses of wintergreen can cause inflammation of the stomach. It is suspected that this same inflammation can be passed on to a nursing infant.

Wintergreen is a popular flavoring used in candies and breath mints. It is also used medicinally for rheumatism, but must be taken as a capsule to provide a buffer and avoid the irritation of the stomach that chronic use of the herb would cause. Wintergreen has a pain-relieving action and is indicated for back pain. It is also believed to be a galactagogue.

Witch Hazel (*Hamemelis virginiana*)

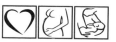

Part used:	Leaves
Main constituents:	Tannin; gallic acid; bitters; volatile oil; ascorbic acid; acetaldehyde; astragalin; beta-ionone; choline; hamamelidin; isoquercitrin; kaempferol; myricetin; phenol; quercitin; quercitrin; safrole; spiraeoside
Alternatives:	None

Witch hazel leaf is highly astringent, so it is often used both internally and externally to prevent hemorrhage, tighten pores and reduce the size and inflammation of hemorrhoids. It is also useful for varicose veins, bruises and swellings, and even in relieving diarrhea in children. Both the bark and leaves can be used interchangeably, although it is commonly the bark that is used for what we see in the store as witch hazel extract.

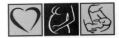

Wood Sorrel (*Oxalis acetosella*)

Part used:	Aerial portions
Main constituents:	Oxalic acid; potassium (potassium binoxalate)
Alternatives:	**For urinary tract:** Dandelion leaf (*Taraxacum officinale*); nettle (*Urtica dioica*)
	For fever: Elder (*Sambucus nigra*); yarrow (*Achillea millefolium*)
Notes for caution:	**During preconception:** Wood sorrel is an emmenagogue when used in high doses. High levels of oxalic acid bind to the body's supply of calcium and create deficiencies.
	During pregnancy: The herb contains high levels of oxalic acid, which can potentially be damaging to developing kidneys. In high doses, wood sorrel can act as an emmenagogue.
	During lactation: Eat wood sorrel only when it is cooked. High levels of oxalic acid bind to the body's supply of calcium and create deficiencies.

This herb was once used quite extensively as a potherb until common sorrel (*Rumex acetose*) came along. Steaming wood sorrel greatly reduces the oxalates. This herb has been used traditionally both fresh and dried for its diuretic and cooling properties. It has been helpful in fevers and urinary tract problems.

REPRODUCTIVE PHASE   Preconception Pregnancy Lactation **GENERAL SAFETY RATING** No Contraindications   Use with Caution   Generally Avoid

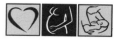

Wormseed (*Chenopodium ambrosioides*)

Part used:	Seed; volatile oil (chenopodium oil)
Main constituents:	Ascaridole; *p*-cymene; *a*-perpinene; betzine; choline, chenopodine
Alternatives:	Pumpkin seeds (*Curcurbita* spp.); garlic (*Allium sativa*)
Notes for caution:	**During preconception:** Wormseed is an emmenagogue.
	During pregnancy: Wormseed is an emmenagogue and abortifacient.
	During lactation: The quality of the oil used in the treatment of worms can vary greatly. If the oil is not of good quality, it can become a toxin. Wormseed must be used only with a qualified herbalist. A large dose or the use of the seed alone can pose a risk of potential liver toxicity.

As its name suggests, this herb has been most used for expelling round worms, especially in children. It is well suited for this purpose and can be very gentle in the hands of an experienced practitioner.

	Leaf/flower	Essential oil/ Alcoholic extract
Wormwood (*Artemisia absinthium*)	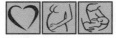	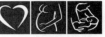

Part used:	Leaves; flowers
Main constituents:	Thujone; thujyl alcohol; acids; absinthin; tannins; resin; potash; starch
Alternatives:	Fennel (*Foeniculum vulgare*); bitter orange (*Citrus aurantium* spp., *Citrus amara*); artichoke (*Cynara scolymus*)
Notes for caution:	**Leaf/flower during preconception and pregnancy:** Due to the presence of thujone, it is not appropriate to take very high doses of tea or to use the herb excessively. If used in this way, it can be an emmenagogue or an abortifacient. **Leaf/flower during lactation:** The constituent thujone can have a negative effect through breast milk if the herb is taken improperly while breastfeeding. Do not take a very high dose of tea or use the herb excessively. **Essential oil/alcoholic extract during preconception and pregnancy:** Due to the presence of thujone, when taken nterni- ally wormwood can be an emmenagoge and abortifacient. **Essential oil/alcoholic extract during lactation:** Due to the presence of thujone, when taken internally wormwood can have a negative effect on a breastfeeding baby.

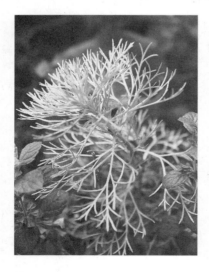

This herb is often used in formulas to make bitters to slow digestion and stimulate appetite. It is most commonly used for its abilities as a vermifuge and can be a safe way to get rid of roundworm and pinworm.

Note: If wormwood is used as a flavoring in a food substance in the United States, it is required to be thujone-free and is most likely safe to use.

*Wormwood (*Artemisia absinthium*)*

Leaf

Essential oil/
Alcoholic extract

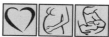

Yarrow (*Achillea millefolium*)

Part used:	Aerial portions; essential oil
Main constituents:	Vitamins B_1, B_2, C; calcium; chromium; fat; fiber; magnesium; manganese; phosphorus; potassium; protein; selenium; silicon; tin; terpenes (chamazulene, proazulene, thujone); saponins (sitosterol); tannins; salicyclic acid; fatty acids; alkaloids (achilleine, trigonelline, betonicine, stachydrine); resin[35]
Alternatives:	None
Notes for caution:	**Leaf during preconception and pregnancy:** Due to the presence of thujone, it is inappropriate to take very high doses of tea or to use the herb excessively. If used in this manner, it can be an emmenagogue or an abortifacient.
	Leaf during lactation: The constituent thujone can have a negative effect through breast milk if the herb is taken improperly while breastfeeding. Do not take a very high dose of tea or use the herb excessively.
	Essential oil/alcoholic extract during preconception and pregnancy: Due to the presence of thujone, when taken internally yarrow can be an emmenagoge and abortifacient.
	Essential oil/alcoholic extract during lactation: Due to the presence of thujone, when taken internally yarrow can have a negative effect on a breastfeeding baby.

Yarrow has an ancient history of use and can be found as battlefield medicine as far back as *The Iliad*. It is a styptic with strong abilities to staunch blood flow and hemorrhage. Topically, it is a blood and fluid "mover." It is this ability that makes it great for women. It can be a great aid in labor and childbirth, cramping or for moving old blood out of the uterus if a woman

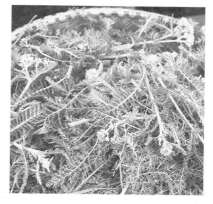

Yarrow (Achillea millefolium)

tends to have brown blood in her cycle. It is a highly effective poultice herb for bruising and swelling, especially associated with sprains and strains. It is also very useful in treating respiratory congestion and in lowering fever. Both internally and externally, it will help to expel mucus. Only the essential oil, alcoholic extract or exceedingly high dose of tea will contain thujone, so it is only these forms of the herb that are a threat.

Yellow Dock (*Rumex crispus*)

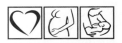

Part used:	Root
Main constituents:	Vitamins A, B_1, B_2, B_3, B_5, C; calcium; iron; magnesium; manganese; selenium; anthraquinone glycosides (emodin, nepodin); tannins (chrysophanic acid, oxalic acid); silicon; tin; protein; phosphorus; fat; fiber; aluminum[35]
Alternatives:	None

This herb is one of my favorites for anemia or constipation. Yellow dock is high in iron and tannins, which help it to act without laxative dependency or harsh griping. The action of this herb is not an irritant in the digestive tract but encourages appropriate peristalsis. It is important in the treatment of psoriasis and is an aid for cleansing the blood and improving the health of the liver. It is my choice of an iron supplement or laxative during pregnancy or nursing because it is gentle and nutritionally complete.

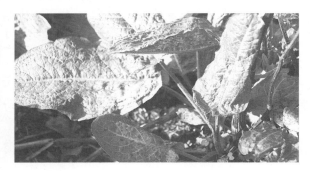

Yellow Dock
(Rumex crispus)

Yohimbe (*Pausinystalia yohimbe*)

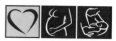

Part used:	Bark
Main constituents:	Ajmaline; corynantheine; corynanthene; quebrachin; tannins; yohimbine[41]
Alternatives:	Damiana (*Turnera diffusa*); horny goat weed (*Epimedium sagittatum; E. grandiflorum*)
Notes for caution:	**During preconception:** There are no studies to demonstrate the effects of yohimbine on a subsequent pregnancy.
	During pregnancy: There are no studies to demonstrate the effects of yohimbine during a pregnancy.
	During pregnancy: The alkaloid yohimbine is a potential toxin to the nursing infant.

While mainly taken by men to address impotence, this herb is popular in recreational use and has perceived effects as a sexual enhancer.

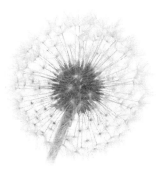

Foods and Supplements

THERE ARE SO MANY WAYS TO SUPPLEMENT FOR HEALTH THESE DAYS that it has become important to add a section on foods in a book like this. While it is encouraging that more people are working to heal their bodies with diet, it is worth sorting through those foods and supplements that can cause problems while we are building a baby, and those that are mistakenly avoided.

Acidophilus (*Lactobacillus acidophilus*)

Acidophilus, a common probiotic, is often recommended during pregnancy to support the health of the immune system or to support the digestive system while taking allopathic antibiotics. It is also a common supplement used to treat both mother and child for yeast overgrowth. When used as directed by manufacturers or your health care team, there are no negatives to using acidophilus at any time while you are building a baby. Do be aware of how the supplement is prepared if you have any specific food sensitivities. If you are lactose intolerant this is important, because most cultures are grown in milk. Dairy-free and lactose-free alternatives are available and are primarily grown on soy paste or garbanzo beans. Just remember that dairy-free means that there is absolutely no milk involved, while lactose-free means that some milk proteins could still be present (just not the milk sugar lactose).

Don't feel as though the only way to get probiotics is through a capsule or yogurt. There are other ways to get good bacteria into your system just by eating your dinner ... and some are dairy-free. Just be aware that fermented vegetable options (*) must be prepared the traditional way with sea salt and spring water, or lacto-fermented, rather than with vinegar. Good sources include

+ Sauerkraut *
+ Miso
+ Kimchi*
+ Kvass
+ Pickles*
+ Water kefir
+ Coconut kefir
+ Milk kefir
+ Raw milk yogurt
+ Traditional sourdough

Alcohol

In recent years alcohol has been proven to be non-impacting in occasional, small amounts and can potentially have some benefits. There is, of course, less cause to have a beer therapeutically during pregnancy, so it is always best to avoid doing so unless it can serve a purpose.[69] If an occasional specialty beer with strong hops is helpful for your milk production and letdown reflex, it won't cause a problem.[51] Studies have shown that alcohol will not help with letdown reflex, but there are many anecdotal experiences to the contrary. However, if you were a heavy drinker before your pregnancy and have returned to the habit, there is more chance that a high amount of alcohol is resident in your tissues and perhaps a greater chance of transmission in levels that are unacceptable to your child. Infants ingest up to 2 percent of your total alcohol consumption and have been shown to take less breast milk in subsequent feedings. Overburdening an infant's liver in this manner can lead to problems.

Artificial Sweeteners

Everyone should stay away from the chemical creations that fool our bodies into thinking we're eating something sweet. Every last one has side effects that are not worth the chemical taste they add to food. Our society has a sweet tooth, but we are much better off eating natural sugars than reaching for foods filled with these franken-sweeteners. If you are working to build a baby, you should be eating sweets in moderation and sticking to those that contain maple syrup, raw honey, sucanat or evaporated cane juice.

Aspartame — Sold around the world as NutraSweet, Equal, Spoonfuls, Canderel, Bienvia, NatraSweet and Miwon, this "is a neurotoxic substance that has been associated with numerous health problems including dizziness, visual impairment, severe muscle aches, numbing of extremities, pancreatitis, high blood pressure, retinal hemorrhaging, seizures and depression. It is suspected of causing birth defects and chemical disruptions in the brain."[70] The FDA recommends that pregnant and lactating women or people with advanced liver disease and phenylketonurics avoid products containing aspartame due to concern in regard to metabolizing phenylalanine. Heat or prolonged storage causes the sweetener to metabolize (think storage warehouses at the manufacturer or retailer), producing a known carcinogen.

Saccharin — This is found in numerous sodas and other processed foods and is usually listed by name on the ingredients panel. It is a neurotoxin and strong allergen. Those with sulfa allergies should be especially cautious. Saccharin is not recommended for anyone trying to build a baby.

Sucralose (Splenda) — This chemical by-product of chlorine and sugar has not been tested enough to show any kind of data on safety. The studies that have been done indicate an ability to cause mutation. They also show a negative effect on diabetes and blood sugar levels. In laboratory settings it has been shown to cause damage to the thymus gland, liver and kidneys of rats, mice and rabbits. It can also be linked to some effects on pregnancy and low birth weight.[71] It is best avoided at all times while building your baby.

Agave Nectar

I have seen agave nectar listed on sites giving advice on fertility! The intention is a good one. Agave nectar has a low glycemic index and therefore is believed to help keep blood sugar levels in check and thusly prevent fluctuations in hormones. Unfortunately, there are some very startling reasons to *avoid* agave nectar at any time while you are trying to get pregnant, carrying a child or nursing.

Agave nectar contains the highest fructose amount of any commercial sweetener … even *worse* than high-fructose corn syrup. High levels of fructose create insulin resistance, an even bigger problem than a temporary spike due to sugar intake. Further, agave nectar is mostly produced from *Agave americana* which is a known emmenagogue and abortifacient. Its contraceptive abilities have been noted in studies conducted in China and Sweden.[72] In fact, the saponins found in *Agave americana* are so strong that they can be "taken only once or twice instead of the 20 times per month necessary with the ordinary pill."[72]

Bee Pollen

Bee pollen is a complete protein and being high in nutrients is a great remedy for depression and lethargy. It is also a safe alternative to allergy medication. However, in rare cases the possibility exists for a reaction, so it is advisable to start with one little grain and watch to see if you have any itchy eyes, redness, etc. If you aren't that rare person, then one half to one teaspoon a day is a sufficient dose. Don't take bee pollen every day throughout the year. Instead take occasional breaks. It is possible to take it too often and build up an allergy-like reaction. For the best allergy protection, start to take your (local) pollen a month before you generally suffer from symptoms and continue on through allergy season.

On our farm we see many weightlifters, marathon runners and vegetarians who seek out pollen as a good protein source. You will typically find dried pollen in the store, and there is some disagreement

Main Constituents of Bee Pollen

Provitamin A; B_1 thiamin; B_2 riboflavin; B_3 nancin; B_5; B_6 pyridoxine; B_{12} (cyanocobalamine); pantothenic acid; vitamins C, F, D, E, H, K and PP; folic acid; choline; inositol; rutin; calcium; phosphorus; potassium; iron; copper; iodine; zinc; sulfur; sodium; chlorine; magnesium; manganese; molybdenum; selenium; boron; silica; titanium; amino acid; carbohydrates; fatty acids; enzymes; co-enzymes; fats.

on how best to prepare it for use. When dried, it loses the natural sugars and some of its delicate nutrition because of the heat treatment. We disagree with the need to dry for shelf stability. Instead we offer the pollen on our farm fresh from the hive. Pollen is best consumed raw but be sure to keep it refrigerated.

Borage Oil

Borage oil is one of the richest sources of the essential fatty acid gamma-linoleic acid (GLA), also known as omega-6. It should always be cold-pressed. The nutrition contained in borage oil is heat sensitive so you should never use it in a recipe that involves heating. While borage (*Borago officinalis*) carries with it some contraindications, note that there are no pyrrolizidine alkaloids found in the oil.

Because of its GLA content it is highly anti-inflammatory and gives rise in the body to prostaglandins. For this reason it is suggested for the following and much, much more: hot flashes, attention deficit disorder (ADD), high blood pressure, bone loss, diabetes, adrenal exhaustion, multiple sclerosis (MS), menstrual cramps, breast tenderness and for the regulation of metabolism.

Taken internally while trying to get pregnant, there are no contraindications. Borage oil, though, is part of a natural therapy to soften and open the cervix. It is typically recommended only during pregnancy in the last few weeks. At that time, it is taken in both an internal dose and a topical application directly to the cervix. Its action is only to aid in the easier opening of the Os, not to induce contractions. Borage is not contraindicated while nursing.

Brassica and Allium Plant Families

Many of the foods that are the most helpful in building our natural immune system can cause issues with nursing infants. Many nursing mothers have seen gassiness and refusal to nurse when they consume foods from the brassica (cabbage, broccoli) and allium (onions, garlic) families. Treat it on a case-by-case basis — do not assume that your baby will have the same problem with these foods that someone else's baby did. Instead, be aware and monitor your individual situation carefully. None of these foods are dangerous, but you may identify an allergy or food sensitivity and be able to head off a problem before it requires a visit to a doctor.

Brewer's Yeast (*Saccharomyces cervisiae*)

Brewer's yeast is a popular supplement because of its nutritional component. If you are having trouble with your milk supply, adding brewer's yeast to your food may help. It was important for me personally. At the time, lactation cookies were very popular as a nursing snack. (See Appendix G for a sample recipe.) I made mine with a heaping helping of brewer's yeast while having an occasional artisanal beer with a high hops content. The combination increased my milk on days I used either.

Cabbage Leaves

It has been suggested by some that the ability of cabbage leaves to reduce the pain and swelling of engorgement or mastitis is obvious when you look at the shape of the leaf itself. Removed from the cabbage, each leaf is the perfect shape to cup a sore breast — and fits nicely under your bra! Use these leaves just like you would a poultice, but don't re-use them!

Cheese

The Centers for Disease Control and Prevention (CDC) has amended their position on soft cheese for pregnant women. They now state that soft cheese is fine so long as you are sure it's pasteurized.[73] But they also say that processed cheese slices (which are made with nothing resembling dairy products) are perfectly safe for pregnant women!

Here in the United States, it is against the law to sell raw milk cheese unless it has aged for at least 60 days. During this time, the natural aging of the cheese prevents the growth of listeria, salmonella, E. coli and other harmful bacteria. More than the aging process, there is the consideration of how the milk was produced. Were the cows fed exclusively on grass? Were they raised without any growth hormones or antibiotics?

In short, exclusively grass-fed cows that are fed no growth hormones or antibiotics produce milk that is appropriate for raw milk consumption. If it fits all these criteria and then was handled properly during and after milking by both the farmer and the cheesemaker, it further qualifies for safety.

The bottom line is, pregnant women should definitely avoid raw milk cheese derived from grain-fed cattle. It is typically presumed to be safe to consume pasteurized milk soft cheese. If you are considering raw soft cheeses, grass-fed options can be healthful if you determine they are right for you.

Cod Liver Oil

Much has been made in the media about the toxicity of vitamin A and this has scared many away from this tried and true health aid. The truth of the matter is that synthetic vitamin A is dangerous in high dosages. However, vitamin A in food sources like cod liver oil is safe and necessary. (For recommended varieties, visit westonaprice. org/cod-liver-oil/cod-liver-oil-basics.) The recommended daily dose from the Weston Price Foundation for pregnant and nursing women is 20,000 IU (4 teaspoons regular cod liver oil or 2 teaspoons high vitamin fermented cod liver oil). There is some research that points to a higher level of vitamin A intake causing a higher need for vitamin E. If you are supplementing with higher than recommended levels of cod liver oil, it is best to ensure you are also adding extra vitamin E to your diet.

Should I buy fermented cod liver oil or just cod liver oil? There are some good options on both sides of the argument. Usually you will need to take less fermented cod liver oil at a time as it is more concentrated. There are various options, including the addition of butter oil. If you are taking cod liver oil or fermented cod liver oil alone, you will need to be sure to take it with a butterfat to make sure your body can properly absorb the vitamin A.

Henna (*Lawsonia inermis*)

This traditional skin and hair dye is completely safe when used externally from preconception through lactation. No need to watch your grey roots grow back in if you don't want to! Henna leaf powder is mixed into a paste and applied to the hair for thirty minutes to an hour. Henna is a hair conditioner, so it can be applied multiple times a month without damaging your hair. With the addition of other dye plants, you can get henna for all different colors. A common additive is indigo. Be careful that your henna contains just plants though, and do not buy "black henna." Some inferior brands of henna contain some of the very same dangerous chemicals you are trying to avoid from a salon. Another word of warning is that henna should only be used externally. There is a history of its use internally as an abortifacient in Africa.[34]

Evening Primrose Oil (*Oenothera biennis*)

Evening primrose oil is high in gamma-linoleic acid (GLA or omega-6). While trying to get pregnant there is no reason to avoid it. It should be cold-pressed because heating this oil damages its nutritional value. It benefits the immune, cardiovascular, reproductive and nervous system.

During pregnancy, it is generally used in the last few weeks to soften and ripen the cervix to prepare for labor. For this purpose it is taken internally as well as applied topically to the cervix. Evening primrose oil does not induce labor, it merely helps the cervix to prepare for opening.

Evening primrose oil is often suggested to nursing mothers to alleviate some of the negative symptoms associated with the first few weeks of nursing, namely cramping. It is also used to relieve symptoms associated with the monthly cycle and is fine for a nursing mother to use internally.

Fish

While fish can be a very nutritional choice, the location and habits of the fish species can have an impact on its tendencies to include heavy metals and other contaminants. In today's environment, one must also be aware of GMO fish that are up for approval for integration into the food supply. This included salmon at the time of writing.

You should definitely take mercury content into account while you are pregnant or nursing, but don't forget that mercury is a heavy metal and builds up concentration in our cells. Unless you are routinely using something to facilitate removal, such as chlorella, while you are trying to conceive, you will be stuck with heavy metals and their effects. You might agree that avoiding the species in the chart below at any time while you are building a baby is appropriate due to their mercury content.

The mainstream recommendations on canned tuna are not exactly appropriate. The average pregnant or nursing mother should eat no

Fish	Mercury (ppm)
Tilefish	1.45
Swordfish	1.00
Shark	0.96
King mackerel	0.73
Largemouth bass	0.52
Tuna (fresh or frozen)	0.32
Tuna (canned)	0.17

Sources: U.S. Food and Drug Administration U.S. Environmental Protection Agency

more than 1.5 (6 oz.) cans of tuna per week if it can't be avoided altogether.[74] There are other fish to avoid for various other reasons. It is
important to avoid many of the farmed fish because of what they are
fed (garbage, manure, soy, dyes, etc.). Be sure of where your fish have
been sourced. Also look at labeling for how the fish are caught. "Pole
and troll caught" or "wild" may be better choices over farm-raised, unless you know the farm's practices.

Pregnant women are still generally told to avoid eating raw fish,
but there is no evidence that it is unsafe. If you like sushi, enjoy it
while keeping in mind some guidelines. Keep your rolls confined to
low mercury fish and steer clear of tuna for now. Make sure you use
the pickled ginger. Ginger is not just a condiment — it acts as a vermifuge and can help guard against any possible parasite contamination.
Finally as with everything else, eat sushi in moderation. The upside
is that getting all that extra nori in your diet is boosting your calcium
levels!

Another great way to get your raw fish during pregnancy and
nursing is to buy a good brand of fermented raw fish, or make your
own. When used as a condiment along with a whole-foods diet, this
can really be a benefit to your digestion.

Kombucha

Kombucha is a liquid produced by a yeast in symbiosis with acetic
acid bacteria. There are many anecdotally reported health benefits,
but those that have been researched support its ability to increase the
liver's efficiency in detoxing the blood and in aiding digestion. When
kombucha is properly brewed, it is entirely safe. The small amount of
alcohol that it contains must be less than 0.5 percent if you are buying a commercially available non-alcoholic drink. Unless you have a
personal reason to avoid this amount of alcohol there is no reason to
do so. Kombucha is safe for pregnancy, but is generally recommended only if you have already been drinking it. Some people can have
reactions, including a potential healing crisis, when they first begin
drinking it. Pregnancy wouldn't be the time for that.

Lunchmeat

During all phases of building a baby it would be best to avoid conventional lunchmeats that are loaded with nitrites and nitrates. These substances are known carcinogens. As of 2006, lunchmeats may also contain any one of six different live viruses that were approved for protection against listeria.[75] While you'll hear most about eating raw lunchmeat during pregnancy because of the concerns over listeria contamination, it is wise to avoid conventional lunchmeats at all times while you are building a baby. Even during pregnancy, though, you don't have to pass up on a good panini or Italian sub! Choose organic, nitrite- and nitrate-free lunchmeat and heat it till steaming before eating.

"Natural Flavors" and MSG

In many cases your food producer is not required by law to actually list what is in your food. Because of our labeling laws, we do not always know what food has been genetically modified or irradiated unless it is certified organic in the United States. Be suspicious of anything you do not recognize. MSG (mono-sodium glutamate) is a great example here. It has been clear for more than 40 years that this additive in food was causing headaches, increased insulin production, liver inflammation, heart irregularities, brain abnormalities and much more. In short, it was identified as a harmful substance. However, MSG is still on the Generally Regarded as Safe (GRAS) list held at the FDA. Unfortunately, as the public became more aware of its toxicity, scientists developed more flavoring agents to get around the consumer. The new flavoring agents actually contain MSG, but have different names that most of us do not recognize:

+ MSG accent
+ Autolyzed plant protein
+ Autolyzed yeast
+ Aginomoto
+ Calcium caseinate
+ Citric acid (when processed from corn)

+ Gelatin
+ Glutamate
+ Glutamic acid
+ Hydrolized plant protein (HPP)
+ Hydrolized vegetable protein (HVP)
+ Monopotassium glutamate
+ Monosodium glutamate
+ Natural flavoring
+ Natural meat tenderizer
+ Sodium caseinate
+ Textured protein
+ Yeast food or nutrient
+ Yeast extract[76]

Beyond MSG, new flavoring agents are coming out all the time. They usually breeze through any approval processes for use in the food supply. A new maker of these flavoring agents is Senomyx, a company to keep your eye on. They create flavoring "experiences" rather than flavors, using technology that fools the human brain into thinking it is having the flavor experience designed to go with a product. A good rule of thumb is to eat real, whole food. Or eat food products that only list real, whole food in the ingredients. If it says "natural flavors," put it back on the shelf!

Nutritional Yeast (*Saccharomyces cerevisiae*)

Typically grown on beet or cane molasses, nutritional yeast is a bit different from brewer's yeast, which is part of the beer-making industry and typically grown with hops. Nutritional yeast is a common food additive especially for those who have decided to cut down on meat. It is safe to add to your food while you are building a baby, and as an added note, is gluten free.

Oscilococcinum

This is a popular homeopathic remedy for cold and flu. As with any other homeopathic remedy, there is no reason to avoid it during nursing.

Probiotics (*Lactobacillus plantarum; Bifidobacterium bifidum; and Bifidobacterium longum; Bididobacterium infantis,* etc.)

While acidophilus is the most common probiotic, there are others that are used routinely. All are intended to support a healthy digestive system, and thereby the immune system, and can be a popular adjunct therapy during allopathic treatment. They are all safe while you are building a baby so long as they are taken as directed by the manufacturer or by your health care team. They are grown on milk proteins, so keep that in mind with any individual food allergies.

Pumpkin (*Cucurbita* spp.)

The seeds of the pumpkin, when eaten roasted or made into tea, are helpful for expelling intestinal worms. The flesh is great for constipation. As mentioned earlier, these wonderful seeds are also a great supply for zinc, which is a great fertility boost for both partners.

Raw Honey

Raw honey is often withheld from infants under one year of age due to the potential presence of non-growing botulism spores. Until the age of one, children's digestive systems are not developed enough to handle this invader, but yours is. The spores cannot grow in honey and they produce their toxins only during the growth stage. While pregnant or nursing, a mother can safely ingest raw honey, as her digestive system will safely take care of any potential non-growing botulism spores before they pass across the placental or breast milk barrier.

Synthetic and Over-the-Counter Drugs

Always assume that any OTC or prescription drugs will cross the breast milk and placental boundary. Read all side effects of any medication you are considering and discuss this with your health care team before assuming that it will be safe for you and your baby.

Only the unbound portion of a drug is available for transmission through breast milk. If receptors (albumin and protein receptors) are full, this can increase the amount that is left unbound in the bloodstream. All of this gets quickly to a level not intended by the manufacturer because multiple drugs will use up receptors, leaving more unbound in the body. This increases the effects of drugs and their side effects and can happen just by mixing an OTC drug with a prescription or an antibiotic.

Sea Salt

Get rid of your iodized salt and replace it with sea salt to help avoid hypothyroidism. Sea salt contains iodine, but if you are concerned about needing more, add some seaweed to your diet as well.

Triphala

Triphala is an ayurvedic blend of three herbs that has been used for centuries for digestive balance, bowel regulation and body detoxification. It is extremely gentle and nurturing, but it exerts a downward energy and is not appropriate for pregnancy. At all other times, this is a great choice for daily use. For those who are trying to get pregnant, it is especially useful. Many women with fertility issues tend to have a congested liver. Triphala is a great first start in any work to rebalance hormones because of its detoxifying and tonic effect on the liver. While nursing, this is once again a great daily tonic. Removing the toxins that are built up in the system after pregnancy can be difficult otherwise.

Our farm, Mockingbird Meadows, makes a particularly nice blend of triphala and raw honey. The blend is delicious and easy to take, if I may say so. Until this blend came out, triphala was traditionally taken as a powder in water or as a capsule. Triphala Honey Spread also makes triphala more effective and sends it deeper in the body than is possible by taking the herb alone. The three "fruits" of triphala are:

Harada (haritaki), Terminalia chebula

Bitter in flavor, harada is primarily a laxative but is also astringent, lubricative, antiparasitical, alterative, antispasmodic and nervine. On its own it is used to treat chronic and acute constipation, nervousness and anxiety as well as feelings of heaviness.

Amla (amalaki), Emblica officinalis

Sour in flavor, amla is cooling, astringent, mildly laxative, alterative and antipyretic. On its own it is used to treat ulcers, digestive inflammation, constipation, liver congestion, pimples, infections and burning feelings in the body. Nutritionally, amla is a powerhouse, containing twenty times the vitamin C of an orange! And unlike the vitamin C in oranges, amla's vitamin C is heat stable so it does not get destroyed if you use it in cooking. As a side note ... guess what that pasteurized orange juice is lacking?

Bihara (bibhitaki), Terminalia belerica

Astringent, then sweet, bitter and pungent in taste, bihara is primarily a digestive and antispasmodic. On its own it is used to treat conditions of excess mucus such as asthma, bronchitis, allergies and hiccups.

Afterword

S O WHERE DO WE GO FROM HERE? It will take time for our society to shift its current baby-building paradigm. Those who are already married and trying to conceive have a chance to slow down and care for their bodies before they go any further. We need to get birthworkers involved in the conversation so that we can create a continuity of care from preconception all the way through to lactation.

Our food culture needs to change dramatically. Synthetic, genetically modified and chemically laden food may seem cheap. But the reality is that our government uses our tax dollars to subsidize this food. If those subsidies were ever to cease, modified, chemical-laden foods would be more expensive in most cases than food grown organically. We are all paying for the "cheap" food. The hidden costs are found not just in our tax dollars but in our rising health care needs. In a culture that celebrates the family that saves big money on food, this is a recipe for disaster. We need to decide as a culture that we would rather spend money on real food than pay for our health problems later. We need to begin to invest in our individual health, thereby investing in the future generation that we will produce in those bodies. Until we stand up as one voice and demand clean, whole and nutrient-dense food options as the norm, we have an uphill battle.

Without changes in our food supply, we will continue "de-selecting" for the human population at an alarming rate. I fear that those members of our population that continue to eat this food will no longer be able to reproduce naturally in the very near future. Unfortunately, the build-a-baby industry leaves couples powerless and voiceless while slowly robbing them of their hope. This is not the way to continue our species. Instead we need to be empowering people to take control of their health and take responsibility for themselves. In a society that vilifies the idea of outsourcing, I find it incredibly ironic that we are willing to outsource the responsibility for our own health and well-being to someone in a white coat.

We have given up control of our bodies and our reproductive health to the convenience of Western medicine. Taking back our health independence requires that we all know more about the plant allies that are all around us. We need to remember the basics of home health care and trust ourselves to carry them out. There are herbalists in almost every community that are great resources to learn these skills. We need to be growing our own medicine alongside our own food in our backyards. So many people are returning to a homesteading philosophy, but they forget that they need to grow medicine along with the carrots. There will always be someone growing herbs for sale, but we need to ensure that the threatened plants we all need are protected. This means buying sustainably grown herbs, growing your own and helping organizations like United Plant Savers to replant our nation's wild areas. The plants have evolved with us here on the planet, but they are much older. They are our teachers. They have so much they wish to share with us. They are waiting for us to mature out of our current disrespectful ways and begin to once again listen with reverance.

We have given up our power to the commercial food industry for a false sense of freedom. We have swallowed the idea that not having to "waste" time preparing food gives us more time to spend with ourselves and our families. This is shortsighted because the time it takes to prepare and eat our food with each other is the very intimacy that we crave. By removing ourselves from these traditional processes, we have become disconnected from our food and from nature's cycles. Our bodies are no longer grounded; our connections to ourselves and our community have been broken.

There is truth in the old adage "You are what you eat." Too many of us are eating "dead" or "synthetic" food. Irradiation is swiftly moving into view on the American food system horizon. We jokingly prepare for zombie apocalypse, but there is a scary reality here. When most of our society is eating "dead" food, they will become partly "dead" inside. Worse, the children we grow are made up of what we eat as well. The food we eat is what knits their bones ... with what building blocks will we choose to create our next generation?

Further Reading

AFP News. "You Are What Your Grandmother Ate, According to New Research." *New York Daily News*, 19 February 2014, nydailynews.com/life-style/health/grandmother-ate-new-research-suggests-article-1.1619988#ixzz30t7ZjVwF

Buhner, Stephen H. (2004). *The Secret Teachings of Plants*. Rochester, VT: Bear and Company.

Colbin, Annemarie. (1986). *Food and Healing*. New York: Ballantine Books.

Buhner, Stephen H. (2002). *The Lost Language of Plants*. White River Junction, VT: Chelsea Green Publishing.

Fallon, Sally, and Mary Enig. (2001). *Nourishing Traditions: The Cookbook that Challenges Politically Correct Nutrition and the Diet Dictocrats*, 2nd ed. Washington, DC: New Trends Publishing.

Gladstar, Rosemary. (1993). *Herbal Healing for Women*. New York: Fireside.

Gladstar, Rosemary. (2008). *Herbal Recipes for Vibrant Health*. North Adams, MA: Storey Publishing.

Gladstar, Rosemary. *Science and Art of Herbalism Home Study Course*. www.herbsandearthawareness.com

Green, James. (2000). *The Herbal Medicine-Maker's Handbook*. Berkeley: Crossing Press.

Green, James. (2007). *The Male Herbal: The Definitive Health Care Book for Men and Boys*. 2nd ed. Berkeley, CA: Crossing Press.

Grieve, Maud. (1971). *The Modern Herbal, Vols. I and II.* New York: Dover Publications.

Hoffman, David. (2003). *Holistic Herbal: A Safe and Practical Guide to Making and Using Herbal Remedies.* 4th ed. Hammersmith, London: Harper Collins.

Khalsa, Karta Purkh Singh, and Tierra, Michael. (2008). *The Way of Ayurvedic Herbs.* Twin Lakes, WI: Lotus Press.

Kim, Meeri. "Father's diet may affect offspring's development, study of mice suggests." *Washington Post*, 14 December 2013, washingtonpost.com/national/health-science/fathers-diet-may-affect-offsprings-development-study-of-mice-suggests/2013/12/14/006834a8-644e-11e3-91b3-f2bb96304e34_story.html?utm_content=buffer4cd46&utm_source=buffer&utm_medium=twitter&utm_campaign=Buffer

Phillips, Nancy, and Michael Tierra. (2005). *The Herbalist's Way, The Art and Practice of Healing with Plant Medicines.* White River Junction, VT: Chelsea Publishing.

Romm, Aviva. (2003). *Naturally Healthy Babies and Children: A Common Sense Guide to Herbal Remedies, Nutrition and Health.* Berkeley, CA: Celestial Arts.

Romm, Aviva. (2010). *Botanical Medicine for Women's Health.* St. Louis, MO: Churchill Livingstone.

Tierra, Michael. (1998). *The Way of Chinese Herbs.* New York: Pocket Books.

Tierra, Michael. (1998). *The Way of Herbs.* Riverside, NJ: Pocket Books.

Weed, Susun. (1986). *Wise Woman Herbal for the Childbearing Year.* Woodstock: Ash Tree Publishing.

Tompkins, Peter, and Christopher Bird. (2002). *Secrets of the Soil, New Solutions for Restoring Our Planet.* Anchorage, AK: Earthpulse Press.

Tompkins, Peter and Christopher Bird. (2002). *The Secret Life of Plants: A Fascinating Account of the Physical, Emotional and Spiritual Relations Between Plants and Man.* New York: Harper Perennial.

Weschler, Toni. (2002). *Taking Charge of Your Fertility.* New York: First Quill.

Wood, Matthew. (1997). *The Book of Herbal Wisdom.* Berkeley, CA: North Atlantic Books.

Wood, Matthew. (2008). *The Earthwise Herbal.* Berkeley, CA: North Atlantic Books.

Notes

1. J. M. Evans and R. Aronson (2005). *The Whole Pregnancy Handbook, An Obstetrician's Guide to Integrating Conventional and Alternative Medicine Before, During, and After Pregnancy.* New York: Gotham Books.

2. A. Ørgaard and L. Jensen (2008). The effects of soy isoflavones on obesity. *Experimental Biology and Medicine,* 233 (9), 1066–80. doi: 10.3181/0712-MR-347

3. L.F Palmer (2004). Formula Feeding Doubles Infant Deaths in America. Retrieved from thebabybond.com/InfantDeaths.html

4. S. Fallon and M. Enig (2001). *Nourishing Traditions: The Cookbook that Challenges Politically Correct Nutrition and the Diet Dictocrats.* Washington, DC: New Trends Publishing.

5. Centers for Disease Prevention and Control. (2010). Life expectancy. Retrieved from cdc.gov/nchs/fastats/lifexpec.htm

6. American Pregnancy Association (2012). What Is infertility? Retrieved from americanpregnancy.org/infertility/whatisinfertility.html

7. J. Green J. (2007). *The Male Herbal: The Definitive Health Care Book for Men and Boys.* Berkeley, CA: Crossing Press.

8. H. A. Feldman, I. Goldstein, D.G. Hatzichristou, R.J. Krane and J.B. McKinlay (1994). "Impotence and its medical and psychosocial correlates: Results of the Massachusetts Male Aging Study." *Journal of Urology,* 151, 54–61.

9. P.S. de Silva, A. Olsen, J. Christensen, E.B. Schmidt, K. Overvaad, A. Tjonneland and A.R. Hart (2010). "An Association between Dietary Arachidonic Acid, Measured in Adipose Tissue, and Ulcerative Colitis." *Gastroenterolgy*, 139(6), 1912–17. doi: 10.1053/j.gastro.2010.07.065 ncbi.nlm.nih.gov/pubmed/20950616

10. C. Shanahan and L. Shanahan (2008). *Deep Nutrition: Why Your Genes Need Traditional Food.* Lawai, HI: Big Box Books.

11. Autism Society (2006). Facts and statistics. Retrieved from autism-society. org/about-autism/aspergers-syndrome/facts-and-statistics.html

12. R. Kralmalnik-Brown (2010). "Human Intestinal Microbial Ecology and its Relationship to Autism." Biodesign Institute, Arizona State University, Tempe, AZ. Retrieved from autism.com/index.php/about_2011_funded

13. D. de Boissieu, M. Chaussain, J. Badoual, J. Raymond and C. Dupont (1996). "Small-Bowel Bacterial Overgrowth in Children with Chronic Diarrhea, Abdominal Pain, or Both." *Journal of Pediatrics*, 128(2), 203–07.

14. "Abstracts on the Effects of Pasteurization on the Nutritional Value of Milk" (2012). Retrieved from realmilk.com/health/abstracts-on-the-effect-of-pasteurization/

15. T. Siepmann, J. Roofeh, F.W. Kiefer and D.G. Edelson (2011). "Hypogonadism and Erectile Dysfunction Associated with Soy Product Consumption." *Nutrition*, 27, 859.

16. W.N. Jefferson, E. Padilla-Banks and R.R. Newbold (2005). "Adverse Effects on Female Development and Reproduction in CD-1 Mice Following Neonatal Exposure to the Phytoestrogen Genistein at Environmentally Relevant Doses." *Biology of Reproduction*, 73(4), 798–806.

17. W. Jefferson, E. Padilla-Banks, R. Newbold and M. Pepling (2006). "Neonatal Genistein Treatment Alters Ovarian Differentiation in the Mouse: Inhibition of Oocyte Nest Breakdown and Increased Oocyte Survival." *Biology of Reproduction*, 74(1), 161–8.

18. M. Domnitskaya (2010). "Russia Says Genetically Modified Foods are Harmful." Retrieved from english.ruvr.ru/2010/04/16/6524765.html

19. A. Nehlig and G. Debry (1994). "Consequences on the Newborn of Chronic Maternal Consumption of Coffee during Gestation and

Lactation: A Review." *Journal of the American College of Nutrition*, 13(1), 6–21.

20. B. Palmer (1998). "The Influence of Breastfeeding on the Development of the Oral Cavity: A Commentary." *Journal of Human Lactation*, 14(2), 93–8.

21. B. Palmer (1996). "The Significance of the Delivery System during Infant Feeding and Nurturing." *ALCA News*, 7(1), 26–9.

22. Universities of Fribourg, Lausanne and Bern (Switzerland). "The Physiology of the Placenta: Role of the Placenta in the Feto-Maternal Exchange Processes." *Human Embryology* (Fetal Membranes and Placenta). Retrieved from embryology.ch/anglais/fplacenta/physio03.html

23. R. Bowen (2001). "Transport across the Placenta." *Pathophysiology of the Reproductive System* (Implantation and Development of the Placenta). Retrieved from www.vivo.colostate.edu/hbooks/pathphys/reprod/placenta/transport.html

24. M. Neville (1998). "Milk Secretion: An Overview." National Institute of Health. Retrieved from mammary.nih.gov/reviews/lactation/Neville 001/

25. J.M. Marks and D.L. Spatz (2003). "Medications and Lactation: What PNPs Need to Know." *Journal of Pediatric Health Care*, 17(6).

26. R. A. Lawrence and R. M.Lawrence (2011). *Breastfeeding: A Guide for the Medical Profession* (7th Ed.), Maryland Heights, MO: Elsevier Mosby.

27. M. O'Connor (1998). "Breastfeeding and Drugs: Does the Medication Pass into Breastmilk?" Retrieved from breastfeedingbasics.org/cgi-bin/deliver.cgi/content/Drugs/pre_pass.html

28. N.G. Powers and W. Slusser (1997). "Breastfeeding Update. 2: Clinical Lactation Management." *Pediatrics in Review*, 18(5), 147–61.

29. S. Gardiner (2001). "Drug Safety in Lactation." Retrieved from medsafe.govt.nz/Profs/PUarticles/lactation.htm

30. C. Hobbs (1989). "*Taraxacum officinale*: A Monograph and Literature Review." *Eclectic Dispensatory of Botanical Therapeutics*. E. Alstat (ed.). Portland, OR: Eclectic Medical Publications.

31. E. Rácz-Kotilla, G. Rácz and A. Solomon (1974). "The Action of *Taraxacum officinale* Extracts on the Body Weight and Diuresis of Laboratory Animals." *Planta Medica*, 26(3), 212.

32. *The Harvard Medical School Family Health Guide* (2004). "Low Potassium Levels From Diuretics." Retrieved from health.harvard.edu/fhg/updates/update0704c.shtml

33. S.G. Sheps (2011). "Diuretics: A Cause of Low Potassium?" *Mayo Clinic.* Retrieved from mayoclinic.com/health/blood-pressure/an 00352

34. M. McGuffin, C. Hobbs and R. Upton (eds.) (1997). *Botanical Safety Handbook.* Boca Raton, FL: CRC Press.

35. M. Pederson (2012). *Nutritional Herbology: A Reference Guide to Herbs.* Warsaw, IN: Whitman Publications.

36. R. Gladstar (2001). *The Family Herbal: A Guide to Living Life with Energy, Health, and Vitality.* North Adams, MA: Storey Books.

37. R. Gladstar (1993). *Herbal Healing for Women.* New York: Simon and Schuster.

38. M. Tierra (1998). *The Way of Chinese Herbs.* New York: Pocket Books.

39. F.J. Brinker (1998). *Herb Contraindications and Drug Interactions* (2nd ed.). Sandy, OR: Eclectic Medical Publications.

40. S. Stohs and H. Preuss (2010). "The Safety of Bitter Orange (*Citrus aurantium*) and P-Synephrine." *HerbalGram*, 89, 34–39.

41. mountainroseherbs.com

42. S. Weed (1996). *Wise Woman Herbal for the Childbearing Year.* Woodstock, NY: Ash Tree Publishing.

43. M. Al-Balas, P. Bozzo and A. Einarson (2009). "Use of Diuretics During Pregnancy." *Canadian Family Physicians*, 55(1), 44–45.

44. D. Hoffman (1990). *Holistic Herbal: A Safe and Practical Guide to Making and Using Herbal Remedies.* Hammersmith, London, GB: Harper Collins.

45. X. Weng, R. Odouli and D.K. Li (2008). "Maternal Caffeine Consumption During Pregnancy and the Risk of Miscarriage: A Prospective Cohort Study." *American Journal of Obstetrics and Gynecology*, 198(3), 279.e 1–8. doi: 10.1016/j.ajog.2007.10.803

46. J. Chorostowska-Wynimko, E. Skopińska-Rózewska, E. Sommer, E. Rogala, P. Skopiński and E. Wojtasik (2004). "Multiple Effects of Theobromine on Fetus Development and Postnatal Status of the Immune System." *International Journal of Tissue Reactions*, 26(1-2), 53–60.

47. S. Weed (2002). *New Menopausal Years: The Wise Woman Way, Alternative Approaches for Women 30–90*. Woodstock, NY: Ash Tree Publishing.

48. Z. Zakay-Rones, N. Varsano, M. Zlotnik, O. Manor, L. Regev, M. Schlesinger and M. Mumcuoglu (1995). "Inhibition of Several Strains of Influenza Virus in vitro and Reduction of Symptoms by an Elderberry Extract (Sambucus nigra L.) during an Outbreak of Influenza B Panama." *Journal of Alternative and Complementary Medicine*, 1(4), 361–9.

49. V. Barak, T. Halperin and I. Kalickman (2001). "The Effect of Sambucol, a Black Elderberry-Based, Natural Product, on the Production of Human Cytokines: I. Inflammatory Cytokines." *European Cytokine Network*, 12(1), 290–6.

50. R.M. Bliss (2008). Study Shows Consuming Hibiscus Tea Lowers Blood Pressure." Retrieved from ars.usda.gov/is/pr/2008/081110. htm

51. La Leche League International (2013). "What about Drinking Alcohol and Breastfeeding?" Retrieved from lalecheleague.org/faq/alcohol. html

52. M. Grieve (1971). *A Modern Herbal: The Medicinal, Culinary, Cosmetic and Economic Properties, Cultivation and Folk-Lore of Herbs, Grasses, Fungi, Shrubs and Trees with Their Modern Scientific Uses* (vols 1–2). Mineola, NY: Dover Publications.

53. National Nutrient Database for Standard Reference. Nutrient Data for 09147 Jujube, Dried. Retrieved from ndb.nal.usda.gov/ndb/foods/show/2270

54. R. Teschke (2010). Assessment of clinical data on hepatotoxicity associated with kava use.

55. "Khella and Herbal Remedies." Retrieved from chinese-herbs.org/khella/

56. S. Dharmananda. "Safety Issues Affecting Chinese Herbs: Magnolia Alkaloids." Portland, OR: Institute for Traditional Medicine. Retrieved from itmonline.org/arts/magsafe.htm

57. J.P. Remington and H.C. Wood (eds.) (1918). "Ledum. Ledum palustre. Marsh tea." *The Dispensatory of the United States of America*. Retrieved from henriettesherbal.com/eclectic/usdisp/ledum.html

58. N. Martinez, V. Provencio and C. Jimenez (2002). "Medicinal Plants of the Southwest: Ocotillo." Retrieved from medplant.nmsu.edu/ocotillo.shtm

59. Peony, *Paeonia officinalis*. Retrieved from herbs2000.com/herbs/herbs_peony.htm

60. M. Wood (2009). *The Earthwise Herbal*. New York: North Atlantic Books.

61. Quassia tincture (tinctura Quassia amara). Retrieved from tropilab.com/quassiatincture.html

62. D. Jackson and K. Bergeron (2000). "Wild Carrot: *Daucus carotta.*" Alternative Nature Online Herbal. Retrieved from altnature.com/gallery/Wild_Carrot.htm

63. Rhizoma ligustici chuanxiong. Retrieved from shen-nong.com/eng/herbal/chuanxiong.html

64. Queen's delight: *Stillingia sylvatica*. Retrieved from herbs2000.com/herbs/herbs_queens_delight.htm

65. M. Yoshikawa, E. Uchida, A. Kawaguchi, I. Kitagawa and J. Yamahara (1992). "Galloyl-Oxypaeoniflorin, Suffruticosides A, B, C, and D, Five New Antioxidative Glycosides, and Suffruticoside E, a Paeonol Glycoside, from Chinese Moutan Cortex." *Chemical & Pharmaceutical Bulletin* 40 (8): 2248–50.

66. Mountain Rose Herbs. www.mountainroseherbs.com/products/tumeric-root-power/profile.

67. "Health Benefits of Vetiver Essential Oil." *Organic Facts*. Retrieved from organicfacts.net/health-benefits/essential-oils/health-benefits-of-vetiver-essential-oil.html

68. I. Shipard (2003). *How Can I Use Herbs In My Daily Life?: Over 500 Herbs, Spices and Edible Plants: An Australian Practical Guide to Growing Culinary and Medicinal Herbs* (5th ed.). Queensland, Australia: David Stewart.

69. C. O'Leary, N. Nassar, J. Kurinczuk and C. Bower (2009). "The Effect of Maternal Alcohol Consumption on Fetal Growth and Preterm Birth." *BJOG*, 116, 390–400.

70. R.L. Blaylock (1996). *Excitotoxins: The Taste that Kills*. Santa Fe, NM: Health Press.

71. J. Earles (2004). "Sugar-Free Blues: Everything You Wanted to Know about Artificial Sweeteners." The Weston A. Price Foundation for Wise Traditions in Food, Farming and the Healing Arts. Retrieved from westonaprice.org/modern-foods/sugar-free-blues?qh=YToxOntp OjA7czo3OiJzcGxlbmRhRhIjt9

72. P. Crabbe (1979). "Mexican Plants and Human Fertility." *Unesco Courier*, 7, 33–34. Retrieved from ncbi.nlm.nih.gov/pubmed/12309933

73. Centers for Disease Control and Prevention. (2012). "Prevent infections in pregnancy." Retrieved from cdc.gov/Features/pregnancy/

74. Environmental Working Group. (2013). "Focus Pocus: Table 1: The FDA Withholds Information from Pregnant Women on Mercury-Contaminated Fish, Citing 'Focus Groups' as Justification." Retrieved from heart-disease-bypass-surgery.com/data/articles/146.htm

75. Re: GRAS Notice 364 (Bacteriophages LAND12, OLB1, TSRW1, DSMP1, DP1). (2011). EAS Consulting Firm on behalf of OmniLytics. Retrieved from accessdata.fda.gov/scripts/fcn/gras_notices/GRN000 364.pdf

76. "Other Names for MSG." Retrieved from glutathionediseasecure. com/other-names for-MSG.html

Glossary

Abortifacient — Capable of causing the termination of a pregnancy.

Adaptogen — Capable of normalizing and restoring body functions and increasing the body's nonspecific resistance to stress.

Allopathic — A system of medical practice that treats disease by the use of remedies which produce effects different from those produced by the disease under treatment.

Alterative — A subtance that favorably improves the condition of the blood, restoring health and vitality. Alteratives often act by supporting the liver in cleansing the blood of impurities.

Anodyne — Capable of soothing or eliminating pain.

Amphoteric — An herb or other substance which promotes "balance" or homeostasis (normalcy) within the body. Usually this means that it is capable of equally opposite effects in the body depending on the need.

Antibacterial — Destroying or inhibiting the growth and reproduction of bacteria.

Anti-fungal — Destroying or inhibiting the growth and reproduction of fungi.

Antigalactagogue — Having properties that discourage the production of milk.

Anti-inflammatory — Capable of reducing inflammation.

Anti-parasitical — Having the ability to aid the body in removing parasite infestation.

Anti-pyretic — Having the ability to reduce fever.

Antispasmodic — Capable of preventing or relaxing muscle spasm.

Anti-viral — Destroying or inhibiting the growth and reproduction of viruses.

Astringent — Having the ability to constrict the proteins in our cells, often helping to reduce discharge or tighten pores.

Carminative — Having the ability to improve digestion, reduce gas and relieve intestinal cramping.

Catarrh — Inflammation of mucus membranes, particularly of the nose and throat, with free-flowing discharge.

Cathartic — A dramatic and complete purging of the bowels.

Decoction — The process of making an herbal tea of bark, roots, nuts and non-aromatic seeds. Add the herbs to water in a small saucepot (2–3 tsp herb per cup of water, 3–4 Tbsp herb per quart of water). Bring the mixture to a boil and reduce heat to a simmer. Simmer covered for 15–20 minutes.

Diaphoretic — A substance that can be used to reduce fever by inducing sweating.

Diuretic — A substance that increases the flow of urine and helps to flush toxins from the body through the kidneys.

Emetic — A substance that causes vomiting.

Emmenagogue — A substance that is helpful in bringing on a menstrual cycle. If a cycle is delayed during preconception because of fertility drugs, or during lactation because of fluctuating hormone levels, an emmenagogue tends to bring bleeding within days of steady chronic dosage.

Evacuant — see *Cathartic*

Galactagogue — A substance that encourages lactation

GMO (Genetically Modified Organisim) — Any plant or animal that has been altered on the genetic level in a laboratory or genetics facility. Not to be confused with a hybrid, which can occur in nature on its own or under the guidance of a human. GMOs are created by a combining of genetic material that would not otherwise occur in nature, such as a coming together of human and pig DNA or chemical herbicides and corn DNA.

GRAS (Generally Regarded as Safe) — A list maintained by the FDA by which they determine food and product safety and labeling requirements. Substances that do not find, or buy, their way onto the GRAS list are considered inappropriate to sell to the public.

Glycoside — An herbal carbohydrate that exerts a powerful effect on hormone-producing tissues. The glycoside breaks down into a sugar and a non-sugar component.

Healing Crisis — An acute crisis of symptoms that occurs as we begin to detoxify the body. Much long-term toxicity is deeply buried and entrenched, and the body has often adjusted to its presence in some ways. As the body begins to heal, the cells holding this toxicity either die off or cast off their toxic contents. This creates congestion and irritation in the eliminatory organs as everything is heading to the exits all at one time. Many of the symptoms that are felt at this time are similar to or even worse than the illnesses and imbalances that created the toxicity in the first place. Some experience rashes or headaches; if the original imbalance was part of menstrual cycle irregularities, the healing crisis may involve intense cramping or heavier than normal bleeding. Healing crises can also involve emotional imbalances.

Infusion — An herbal tea made from leaves, berries, aromatic seeds and/or flowers. A typical infusion is made by adding 2–3 tsp of herb per cup of water or 3–4 Tbsp of herb per quart of water and steeping it covered for 10–20 minutes.

Mastitis — Inflammation of the breast or milk ducts.

Mucilaginous — Being gelatinous, sticky or viscid.

Mutagenic — A substance that has the ability to encourage mutation.

Nephrotoxic — Toxic to the kidney.

Oxytocic — Bringing about birth by stimulating contractions of the uterus.

Purgative — see *Cathartic*

Poultice — A soft mass such as an herb mixture applied to an affected area. Be sure to change the herbs often if you are drawing out an infection.

Qi — (pronounced "chi") The concept of our circulating life force in traditional Chinese medicine. In ayurveda it is referred to as "prana."

Sedative — A substance that calms the nervous system.

Styptic — A substance that helps to induce clotting or stop the flow of blood.

Teratogenic — Of, relating to, or causing malformations of an embryo or fetus.

Thrush — An overgrowth of yeast found in the mouth characterized by a white tongue or patches of white inside the cheeks.

Tincture — A plant extract made by soaking herbs in a liquid (such as water, alcohol, vinegar, or glycerine) for a specified length of time, then straining and discarding the plant material. The remaining liquid is used therapeutically.

Tisane — A tea made entirely from one or more herbs.

Vermifuge — A substance that is helpful in the expulsion of intestinal worms.

Appendix A:
Whole-Food/Whole-Plant Resources

Acerola, bifidobacterium infantis, lactose and unrefined sunflower oil:
Radiant Life — radiantlifecatalog.com (888) 593-8333

At-risk native species and botanical sanctuaries:
United Plant Savers — unitedplantsavers.org
Mockingbird Meadows Herbal Health Farm — mockingbird meadows.com
Planting the Future. Edited by Rosemary Gladstar and Pamela Hirsch
Growing At-Risk Medicinal Herbs by Rich O. Cech

Breastfeeding and lactation resources:
Supplemental Nursing System — medelabreastfeedingus.com
Hygeia Transitional Supplementation Feeder — Hygeiainc.com
The HazelbakerTM Finger Feeder — fingerfeeder.com
La Leche League — llli.org

Cod liver oil (high quality):
Green Pastures — greenpasture.org

Couples Fertility Intensives/Retreats:
Mockingbird Meadows Eclectic Herbal Institute — mockingbird meadows.com

Cultures and fermentation supplies:

Cultures for Health — culturesforhealth.com

Fertility charts:

Taking Charge of Your Fertility — tcoyf.com/content/Master Charts.aspx

Flower essences:

Flower Essence Society — flowersociety.org

Food and farming associations and foundations:

Slow Food USA — slowfoodusa.org, slowfood.com

Biodynamic Farming and Gardening Association — biodynamics.com

Ohio Ecological Food and Farming Association — oeffa.org

Good work being done in ethnobotany:

Iamoe Center — iamoecenter.com

Herbal associations and foundations:

Herb Reseach Foundation — herbs.org/herbnews

American Botanical Council — herbalgram.org

International Herb Association — iherb.org/

American Herbalists Guild — americanherbalistsguild.com/

American Herbal Products — ahpa.org/

Northeast Herbal Association — northeastherbal.org/

American Herb Association — wildcrafting.com/american_herb_association.htm

American Spice Trade Association — astaspice.org

Herb Growing and Marketing Network — herbworld.com

Society for Economic Botany — econbot.org

United Plant Savers — unitedplantsavers.org

Herbal bodycare, honey spreads, herbal teas and health aids (chemical-free):

Mockingbird Meadows Herbal Health Farm — mockingbird meadows.com

Herbal education and apprenticeships:

Sage Mountain — sagemountain.com

Mockingbird Meadows Eclectic Herbal Institute — mockingbird meadows.com

Florida School of Holistic Living — holisticlivingschool.org

Vermont Center for Integrative Herbalism — vtherbcenter.org

United Plant Savers — unitedplantsavers.org

East West Herb Course — planetherbs.com

Herbal magazines and professional journals:

Herbal Gram — abc.herbalgram.org/site/PageServer

The Essential Herbal — essentialherbal.com/

Plant Healer Magazine — planthealermagazine.com/

Herb Quarterly — herbquarterly.com

Mother Earth Living — motherearthliving.com/

Medical Herbalism — medherb.com

Raw milk:

A Campaign for Real Milk — realmilk.com

Weston Price — westonaprice.org

Sustainably raised bulk dried herbs:

Mountain Rose Herbs — mountainroseherbs.com

Star West Botanicals — starwestbotanicals.com

Zack Woods — zackwoodsherbs.com

Pacific Botanicals — pacificbotanicals.com

Planetherbs Online (Chinese herbs and supplies) — planetherbs.com

Organic India (ayurvedic herbs) — organicindia.com

Sustainably raised herbal plants and seeds:

Horizon Herbs — horizonherbs.com

Companion Plants — companionplants.com/

Zack Woods — zackwoodsherbs.com

Seed Savers — seedsavers.org/

High Mowing Seeds — highmowingseeds.com

Traditional foods education and recipes:
GNOWFGLINS — gnowfglins.com

Mockingbird Meadows Eclectic Herbal Istitute — mockingbirdmeadows.com

Whole, nutrient-dense food research and education:
Weston Price — westonaprice.org

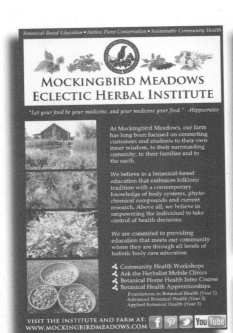

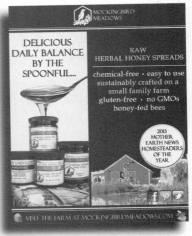

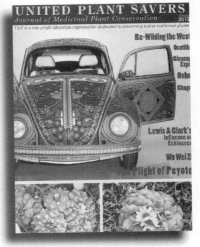

Appendix B: Baby Formulas

THE FOLLOWING BABY FORMULA RECIPES were written by Sally Fallon, author of *Nourishing Traditions: The Cookbook that Challenges Politically Correct Nutrition and the Diet Dictocrats*. She is also the founder of the Weston A. Price Foundation.

Raw Milk Baby Formula

(*Makes 36 ounces*)

Our milk-based formula takes account of the fact that human milk is richer in whey, lactose, vitamin C, niacin and long-chain polyunsaturated fatty acids than cow's milk but leaner in casein (milk protein). The addition of gelatin to cow's milk formula will make it more digestible for the infant. Use only truly expeller-expressed oils in the formula recipes; otherwise they may lack vitamin E.

The ideal milk for baby, if he cannot be breastfed, is clean, whole raw milk from old-fashioned cows, certified free of disease, that feed on green pasture. For sources of good-quality milk, see realmilk.com or contact a local chapter of the Weston A. Price Foundation.

If the only choice available to you is commercial milk, choose whole milk, preferably organic and unhomogenized, and culture it with a piima or kefir culture to restore enzymes (available from G.E.M. Cultures 253-588-2922 or gemcultures.com).

Ingredients:

- 2 cups whole raw cow's milk, preferably from pasture-fed cows
- ¼ cup homemade liquid whey. (See recipe for whey, below.) Note: Do NOT use powdered whey or whey from making cheese (which will cause the formula to curdle). Use only homemade whey made from yoghurt, kefir or separated raw milk.
- 4 tablespoons lactose[1]
- ¼ teaspoon bifidobacterium infantis[2]
- 2 or more tablespoons good quality cream (preferably not ultrapasteurized), more if you are using milk from Holstein cows
- ½ teaspoon unflavored high-vitamin or high-vitamin fermented cod liver oil or 1 teaspoon regular cod liver oil[3]
- ¼ teaspoon high-vitamin butter oil (optional)[1]
- 1 teaspoon expeller-expressed sunflower oil[1]
- 1 teaspoon extra virgin olive oil[1]
- 2 teaspoons coconut oil[1]
- 2 teaspoons Frontier brand nutritional yeast flakes[1]
- 2 teaspoons gelatin[1]
- 1⅞ cups filtered water
- ¼ teaspoon acerola powder[1, 2]

Instructions:

1. Put 2 cups filtered water into a Pyrex (glass) measuring pitcher and remove 2 tablespoons. (That will give you 1⅞ cups water.)
2. Pour about half of the water into a pan and place on a medium flame.
3. Add the gelatin and lactose to the pan and let dissolve, stirring occasionally.
4. When the gelatin and lactose are dissolved, remove from heat and add the remaining water to cool the mixture.
5. Stir in the coconut oil and optional high-vitamin butter oil and stir until melted.
6. Meanwhile, place remaining ingredients into a blender.
7. Add the water mixture and blend about three seconds.

8. Place in glass bottles or a glass jar and refrigerate.
9. Before giving to baby, warm bottles by placing in hot water or a bottle warmer. NEVER warm bottles in a microwave oven.

1. Available from Radiant Life 888-593-8333, radiantlifecatalog.com.
2. Earlier versions of this web page called for 1 tsp of bifidobacterium infantis and 1 tsp of acerola powder — these were typos.
3. Use only recommended brands of cod liver oil.

Appendix C: Breast Massage Techniques

Instructions on Breast Cleansing and Massage

For all of the massage techniques that follow, use a good massage oil that does not immediately absorb. Herbal infusions with an olive or sesame oil base are a nice choice. Have your partner lie down on their back with their torso bare. Straddle their body so that you can easily apply even, downward pressure. Apply oil to your hands and begin.

1. Using a firm continuous stroke with both hands, start at the base of the breastbone, move upward toward the collar bone and continue the stroke out to the shoulders and off the body. Repeat.
2. Using a firm continuous stroke with both hands, start at the base of the breastbone, move upward toward the collar bone and continue down both arms. When you reach the ends of the fingertips, be conscious that you are not only moving lymphatic fluid, you are also removing energy. A small shake at the end of the fingertips as you separate contact will "throw" the energy away. Repeat.
3. Using a firm continuous stroke with both hands, start at the base of the breastbone, move upward and follow the collar bone until you reach the arm pits, move downward along the sides of the body until you reach just the bottom of the breasts (you can alter this

stroke to follow the bottom of the rib cage for variety), completing the movement moving upward between the breasts, making a full circle. Repeat.

4. Using a firm continuous stroke with both hands, start at the base of the rib cage on the sides of the body and move upward into the arm pits. Use the heel of the hand to push up through the hollows, moving up over the shoulders and flinging away the energy. Repeat.

5. Using a cross-body movement, alternate your left hand to the right breast and the right hand to the left breast. Using an upward movement start at the opposite side lower rib cage, proceed across the nipple and finish with the breast side shoulder. The stroke you use here is less firm than others and needs to be completed with "throwing" the energy away. Repeat.

Manta Massage

This traditional massage involves a long, side manta (shawl) to invigorate and move tissues and fluid. I do not know what kind of cloth is used traditionally. A good-quality cotton sheet split along its length in at least two but no more than four sections would work fine. If this becomes a sacred ritual in your home between partners or among friends you may change the material to enhance the experience.

Front to Front:

Sitting on a firm surface, begin by facing one another with about a foot of space between you. You will most likely want to sit cross-legged, but you may also stretch out your legs if that is more comfortable.

1. Each partner will start by threading their cloth behind the back (concentrating across the bra strap area) and under both arms. You will need to stagger your holds to do this concurrently. For the warm-up, each partner will pull their cloth back and forth across the back of their partner. As you get going, it can be helpful for both to lean back against the resistance created by the other. This

is not a light stroke; you should be pulling firmly enough to move the skin and muscles of the back. Continue until the skin across your backs and on the sides of your body is warm and tingly.

2. Change the position of the cloth to be on the outside of the arms of your partner. Again, this will require staggering your holds as you do this for each other concurrently. This movement is up and down from the lower back to the top of the shoulder. Repeat as desired.

3. Change the position of the cloth again to be under the arms of your partner. This time as you pull the cloth back and forth, pull it in across the top of the breast and over the nipple as you complete each movement for each side. Repeat as desired.

Back to Front:

This time take turns with your partner. Sitting behind their back, thread your cloth to cover their breasts and go under the arms. Pulling the cloth left to right, ensure that the cloth stays over the breast and nipple area. Repeat until the breasts are warm and tingly.

Massage Technique Credit: Rocío Alarcón

Appendix D: Child Dosage Table

THIS DOSAGE TABLE IS INTENDED AS A GENERAL GUIDELINE ONLY. You should always take into account your child's age, weight, overall constitution, the nature of the illness and the strength of the herbs being used when deciding on dosage.

Chronic dosage (e.g., for eczema)

Teas (already steeped):	
Age	**Dosage (3x per day)**
1 year or younger	2 tsp
2–4 years	3 tsp
4–7 years	1 ½ Tbsp
7–11 years	2 ½ Tbsp
Adult	1 cup
Tinctures:	
Age	**Dosage (3x per day)**
3 months or younger	2 drops
3–6 months	3 drops
6–9 months	4 drops
9–12 months	5 drops
12–18 months	7 drops
18–24 months	8 drops

Chronic dosage (e.g., for eczema) *cont.*

Tinctures:	
Age	**Dosage (3x per day)**
2–3 years	10 drops
3–4 years	12 drops
4–6 years	15 drops
6–9 years	24 drops
9–12 years	30 drops
Adult	60 drops (1 tsp)

Acute dosage (e.g., for colic)

Teas (already steeped):	
Age	**Dosage (every 20–30 min.)**
1 year or younger	½ tsp
2–4 years	¾ tsp
4–7 years	⅜ Tbsp
7–11 years	⅝ Tbsp
Adult	¼ cup
Tinctures:	
Tinctures are not advised for acute situations as the dose required would be too small to measure in a home kitchen. Teas or homeopathics are better options instead.	

*Expanded from Rosemary Gladstar's Herbal Home Study Course.
(See Further reading page 317.)

Appendix E: United Plant Savers

Some of the plants in this Herbal are designated as either "At Risk" or "To Watch." These are plants that have been over-harvested or are in danger due to habitat destruction.

Rosemary Gladstar started United Plant Savers (UpS) because she and her colleagues in the world of herbalism saw a decline in the wild population of some of our most beloved native herbs. At the time, these plants had been overused in the wild because it was believed that they were more powerful than cultivated herbs. We have since learned that it is possible to raise many of these plants in a sustainable way while working to repopulate our wild areas. We have also learned that cultivated herbs are just as powerful as their wild counterparts.

Here in the West we have a tendency to romanticize the rainforest. There are many voices fighting against the destruction of that habitat and the loss of our herbal medicine heritage in that part of the world. What we need now is awareness that we have these same problems in our own back yard. It is the mission of United Plant Savers to replant our forests and support and encourage growers of the

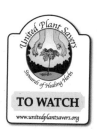 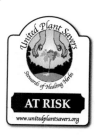

endangered plants. We can continue to partner with these endangered plants for the health of humanity, but we must do it in a way that ensures they are here for future generations.

For this purpose, United Plant Savers created the "At Risk" and "To Watch" designations. The "At Risk" herbs are most at risk of disappearing and the "To Watch" designees have declining populations.

As our culture begins to embrace our herbal heritage and take back its health independence, there is greater call for these herbs. This increasing demand could create a real problem. Many of the plants that are most at risk are the very herbs that are most helpful for women's health. The good news is that we can work in partnership with the plants in this herbal in the following ways:

+ Buy from ONLY sustainable suppliers. If you know that an herb is in danger from being over-harvested in the wild, be sure that you are not buying from someone who is selling plants they have clear-cut from a forest.
+ Plant as many of these herbs on your property as you can. If you are constantly using black cohosh capsules, deepen your relationship with the medicine by planting it in a shady area in your backyard. You may not harvest from this particular plant, but you have just contributed to its ability to have habitat.
+ If you harvest a threatened species yourself, be sure to replant, or take only enough so you don't threaten the local population. After all, if you wish to use a plant year after year, the best way to make sure it's available to you and your loved ones is to keep it growing successfully in its native environment. It's less work for you and healthier for the plant and the planet!
+ Use more abundant alternative herbs wherever possible.
+ Join UpS. Their organization works to establish botanical sanctuaries, move plants that are in the way of development, conduct research and much, much more.

Appendix F: Comfrey: Poison or Panacea?

comfrey-central.com/research/research_index.htm

THE ABOVE LINK IS THE BEST SOURCE of research information on comfrey, an herb used in organic gardening and as an herbal medicine. I include it here because as we get further into the idea of returning to natural medicines, we will continue to see plants like comfrey vilified by the Western medical establishment and drug companies. At times, these worries may be warranted, but let comfrey be an example of how to make a good decision when you see herbs in the news. When you read about a piece of research, always ask the following:

- Who funded the research and what was their motivation?
- What were the methods of the research?
- What are the applications to human use? Was this a trial on humans or animals?
- What are your own personal decisions after reading the research, and what are your individual health concerns that may be factored in to your decision?
- What is the historical information on the herb? Have there ever been any written indications of the same issue?

In the case of comfrey, here is what I have learned. Comfrey is a common name for plants in the genus *Symphytum*. Years ago, a study claimed to demonstrate that the plant had harmful effects, and as a result the herb has been classified as a poison in some countries. There are some varieties of comfrey that contain pyrrolizidine alkaloids (PAs), including *S. officinale*, though it is now probable that the most readily available variety here in the United States is *S. uplandica*, which does not.

At any rate, let's assume we are really getting *S. officinale* whenever we purchase dried comfrey for use. The study was done on 21-week-old rats, which do not have the same reaction to PAs as humans do. The rats were injected with a high dose of one of the isolated PAs (symphytine) rather than a dilution of the whole plant. When you isolate a compound within a plant you do not get the thousands of other chemicals that often act as a buffer for that compound. At any rate, we don't inject Comfrey, we eat it. When it is injected the effect of the compound is concentrated. A small number of the rats in the study subsequently developed liver cancer. Were we to duplicate the same level of PA consumption used in the study in our daily diet, we would need to consume anywhere between three-quarters of a pound and 114 pounds a day for at least 21 weeks. Given that the average amount in a therapeutic dose is a quarter of an ounce or less, this is possible but unreasonable. Finally, there is no information in the historic data of problems with the use of comfrey and there are no cases of veno-occlusive liver disease that can be definitively traced to its ingestion.

Many people continue to use comfrey internally without concern. In all such cases, you must balance the newer scientific findings on each herb with your own internal voice. If you feel that a "banned" herb is fine for you, be sure to let your health care team know of your decision so that they can offer you their perspectives and help you avoid any future negative interactions or overuse.

Appendix G: Gluten-Free Lactation Cookies

Ingredients:

1 cup organic gluten-free buckwheat flour
1 cup white rice flour
½ cup tapioca starch
4 Tbsp brewer's yeast
1½ tsp baking soda
1 tsp sea salt
1 cup butter (softened)
1½ cup firmly packed organic brown sugar
1 Tbsp vanilla
1–2 Tbsp maple syrup (to taste)
2 Tbsp freshly ground flax seed
2–4 Tbsp water
2 free-range organic eggs
2–5 Tbsp milk
3 cups gluten-free whole rolled oats
1 cup chocolate chips (can substitute dried fruit or carob chips here)

Instructions:

Preheat oven to 350 °F.

1. Whisk together the flours, tapioca starch, brewer's yeast, baking soda and sea salt in a big mixing bowl.
2. In a separate bowl, beat the butter, brown sugar, syrup and vanilla extract until combined.
3. Soak the flax seed in 2–4 Tbsp water for about 5 minutes, then add to the butter mix.
4. Beat in the eggs one at a time and stir to combine.
5. Add in the dry ingredients a little bit at a time and beat to combine until a dough forms, adding a tablespoon of milk at a time until you have a firm dough. Add in the oats.
6. Stir in chocolate chips. Cover the bowl with plastic wrap and chill the dough for an hour.
7. Preheat the oven to 350 °F. Scoop dough onto baking sheet, approximately 2 inches (5 cm) apart. Push down slightly to make flat, but keep a mounded shape in the center. This should make 20 good-sized cookies.
8. Bake in the center of the oven for 12–15 minutes, until the cookies are firm to the touch.
9. Let cookies set 5 minutes to cool and set, then transfer to a cooling rack, where they will continue to crisp.

Appendix H: Build a Baby Worksheet

Throughout your efforts to grow a healthy baby, providing relevant information to your health care team will help provide them with a better picture. Take this worksheet with you to each practitioner you see along the way, and keep track of lab results, general testing and diet throughout. Extra sheets may be necessary as this list is not intended to be all-inclusive, but rather to get you started. It includes key questions you should consider throughout this journey.

Preconception Phase

	Female	Male
Diet and supplements		
What are your sources for dietary fat?		
Do you eat organic or conventional foods?		
Do you choose grass-fed over conventional meats?		
What dietary supplements do you take?		
Are they food-derived? (You should see something like alfalfa, orange concentrate or raspberry leaf on the ingredient list.)		
NOTE: Complete a food journal for at least one week to identify your eating trends as they relate to conception.		
Lifestyle		
What is your general level of activity?		
What types of exercise or activity do you do each week?		
How do you solve problems?		
What is your basic belief system?		
General health		
Do you have any current health issues?		
Have you/are you addressing those prior to conception?		
Have you had any previous surgeries?		
Breast Assessment		
Is there any evidence of nipple inversion?		
Are there markers for insufficient glandular tissue or hypoplasia?		
Reproductive Health		
Do you have any identified reproductive issues?		

Preconception Phase *(continued)*

	Female	Male
Reproductive Health		
Male vitality sperm count		
Sperm mobility		
Estrogen level		
Testosterone level		
Insulin level		
Female cycles:		
Average cycle length		
Average luteal phase length		
Typical day of ovulation		
Cramping?		
Spotting?		
Brown blood during cycle?		
Emotional mood swings?		
Bleeding (light/average/heavy)?		
NOTE: Complete daily charts of your cycle as needed to help understand your body's rhythms and tendencies. It is valuable to have at least 3 cycles for an average.		
Blood		
Blood pressure (baseline when starting to attempt conception)		
Insulin level		
Blood type		
Hemoglobin count		
German measles immunization		
Progesterone		
Estradiol		
Magnesium		
Testosterone		
Calcium		
Allopathic medications		
What medications are you currently using or have you taken recently?		

Preconception Phase *(continued)*

	Female	Male
Birth control		
What type(s) of birth control have you used?		
For how long?		
When and why did you stop taking it?		
Herbs		
What herbs are you using currently or have you recently taken?		

Pregnancy Phase

	Female
Diet and supplements	
What are your sources for dietary fat?	
Do you eat organic or conventional foods?	
Do you choose grass-fed over conventional meats?	
What dietary supplements do you take?	
Are they food-derived? (You should see something like alfalfa, orange concentrate or raspberry leaf on the ingredient list.)	
NOTE: Complete a food journal for at least one week to identify your eating trends as they relate to your health and your baby's needs.	
Allopathic medications	
What medications are you currently using or have you taken recently?	
Herbs	
What herbs are you using currently using or have you taken recently?	

Pregnancy Phase *(continued)*

		Female		
Bloodwork averages	**1st Tri**	**2nd Tri**	**3rd Tri**	**Notes:**
Hemoglobin level				
Iron level				
Blood pressure readings				
Urinalysis				
Glucose				
Protein				

Birth Experience

	Mother	**Child**
WHEN did the birth take place?		
WHERE did the birth take place?		
Was any intervention required for you or your child?		
Did you have any issues passing the placenta?		
Estimated blood loss during birth?		
How long did labor last?		
How long was the pushing phase?		
What medications were given during the birthing process?		
What vaccinations were given?		
What were the baby's APGAR scores?		
What length of time passed before cutting the cord?		
Was the baby allowed to immediately latch?		
If there was delay in letting the baby nurse, why and for how long?		
Could you hear the baby swallowing while nursing?		
Were there any other identified issues not covered above?		
NOTE: You should write out and describe in detail your birth story (include emotional state, fears, concerns, etc.)		

Lactation Phase

	Mother	Child
Diet and supplements		
What are your sources of dietary fat?		
Do you eat organic or conventional foods?		
Do you choose grass-fed over conventional meats?		
What dietary supplements do you take?		
Are they food-derived? (You should see something like alfalfa, orange concentrate or raspberry leaf on the ingredient list)		
NOTE: Complete a food journal for at least one week to identify your eating trends as they relate to your health and your baby's needs.		
Allopathic medications		
What medications are you currently using or have you taken recently?		
Herbs		
What herbs are you currently using or have you taken recently?		
Baby's health		
Immunization records (date and type)		
Illness record		
Supplements given		
Allopathic drugs prescribed (date and type)		
NOTE: Describe your breastfeeding relationship prior to seeing a lactation consultant. Record the baby's actions (satisfied, sleeping, pulling away from the breast, fussy, crying, refusing to nurse, etc.).		
While Seeing a lactation consultant:		
Weights and dates (before and after nursing in office)		
Supplements needed? (Include how much, how often and date started.)		

Lactation Phase *(continued)*

	Mother	Child
Have there been any chiropractic adjustments? (Include dates and description.)		
Have there been any cranial–sacral adjustments? (Include dates and description.)		
Have there been any massage treatments? (Include dates and description.)		
Have there been any acupuncture treatments? (Include dates and description.)		
Record of meconium: Present at birth? For how many days? How many diapers per day?		
Record of wet diapers: How many per day? Color description of each?		
Record of soiled diapers: How many per day?		
Has there been any biting?		
Has there been any teething?		
Have there been any infections? (Include date and treatment protocol.)		
Have there been instances of breast lumps or mastitis? (Include dates and treatment protocol.)		
Have you experienced sore or cracked nipples? (Include dates and treatment protocol.)		

Index

PLANT INDEX

A

Acanthopanax senticosus, 119, 131, 168, 173, 206, 265
Achillea millefolium, 152, 160, 199, 243, 261, 281, 290, 293–294
Acidophilus, 297
Acorus calamus, 276
Actaea racemosa, 129
Agathosma betulina, 136
Agave americana, 300
Alchemilla vulgaris, 208
Alfalfa, 111
Allium sativum, 181, 211, 219, 250, 271, 277, 291
Aloe, 112
Aloe vera, 112
Althaea officinalis, 159, 222
Amalaki, 311

Amla, 311
Ammi visnaga, 207
Andrographis, 113
Andrographis paniculata, 113
Anemone pulsatilla, 251
Anethum graveolens, 118, 166, 177, 242, 254
Angelica, 114
Angelica archangelica, 114
Angelica sinensis, 167
Anise, 115, 118
Anthriscus cerefolium, 150
Apium graveolens, 146
Aralia spp., 273
Arborvitae, 116
Arctium lappa, 44, 138, 255, 264, 275
Arctostaphylos uva-ursi, 124, 148
Areca catechu, 125

Arisaema, 117, 180
Arisaema triphyllum, 117
Aristolochia clematis, 216
Arnica, 117
Arnica montana, 117
Artemesia abrotanum, 271
Artemesia cina, 211
Artemisia absinthium, 292
Artemisia vulgare, 230
Arthrospira platensis, 273
Artichoke, 118, 189, 230, 253, 292
Asarabacca, 119
Asarum canadense, 286
Asarum europaeum, 119
Asclepias tuberosa, 248
Asefetida, 118
Ashwaganda, 119, 226

Asparagus racemosus, 268
Astragalus, 120
Astragalus membranaceous, 120
Avena fatva, 236
Avena sativa, 131, 168, 197, 206, 236, 265

B
Bai guo, 184
Bai shao, 243
Bamboo shavings, 120, 180
Ban ixa, 246
Baptisia tinctoria, 287
Barberry, 121
Barley sprouts, 122
Barosma betulina, 136
Basil, 123
Bearberry, 124, 148
Bee balm, 125
Bee pollen, 300–301
Berberis aquifolium, 237
Berberis vulgaris, 121
Betel nut, 125
Bibhitaki, 311
Bihara, 311
Bilberry, 126, 216
Birth root, 126
Bitter apple, 157
Bitter cucumber, 157
Bitter melon, 127
Bitter orange, 114, 128, 132, 177, 253, 276, 282, 292
Blackberry, 130
Blackberry root, 208

Black cohosh, 22, 129
Blackhaw viburnum, 130
Black walnut hull, 131, 211, 219, 250, 271, 277
Bladderwrack, 131
Blessed thistle, 132
Bloodroot, 133
Blue cohosh, 22, 134
Blue vervain, 134
Boneset, 135
Borage, 135, 212, 301
Borago officinalis, 135, 212, 301
Brassica alba, 233
Brassica nigra, 233
Brassica spp., 285
Brewer's yeast, 302
Broom, 136
Buchu, 136
Buckthorn, 137, 179
Bugleweed, 137
Burdock root, 44, 138, 255, 264, 275
Butterbur, 139
Buttercup, 139

C
Cabbage, 302
Calendula, 140, 146, 148, 172
Calendula officinalis, 140, 146, 148, 172
California poppy, 141
Camellia sinensis, 125, 278
Camphor tree, 141

Cannibis sativa, 220
Capsella bursa-pastoris, 268
Capsicum annuum, 145, 250
Carduus marianus, 146, 227
Carthamus tinctorius, 261
Cascara segrada, 142
Cassia spp., 267
Castor bean, 143
Castor oil, 143
Cataria nepeta, 152, 192
Catnip, 144, 152, 192, 261
Caulis bambusae in taeniis, 120, 180
Caulophyllum thalictroides, 22, 134
Cayenne, 145, 250
Celandine, 146
Celery seeds, 146
Centella asiastica, 189
Cephalelis ipecacuanha, 198
Chaga, 228, 232
Chamaelirium luteum, 175
Chamaemelum nobile, 258
Chamomile, 129, 147, 166, 240, 263, 274, 276, 281, 282
Chandana, 263
Chaparral, 148
Chaste tree, 129, 149
Chelidonium majus, 146

*Chenopodium
   ambrosioides*, 291
Chervil, 150
Chickweed, 150
Chicory, 151
Chinese motherwort,
   152
*Chondrodendron
   tomentosum*, 238
*Chrysanthemum
   parthenium*, 177
Chuan bei mu, 180
Chuan xiong, 269
Cichorium intybus, 151
Cimicifuga racemosa, 22,
   129
Cinchona, 152
*Cinnamomum
   aromaticum*, 153
Cinnamomum camphora,
   141
Cinnamomum vernum,
   153
*Cinnamomum
   zeylanicum*, 153
Cinnamon, 153
Citrullus colocynthis, 157
Citrus amara, 114, 128,
   132, 177, 253, 276,
   282, 292
Citrus aurantium spp.,
   114, 128, 132, 177,
   253, 276, 282, 292
Clove, 200
Cnicus benedictus, 132
Cocoa, 154
Coffea arabica, 155
Coffee, 155

Coix lacryma-jobi, 202
Cola, 156
Cola acuminate, 156
Cola nitida, 156
Colchicum autumnale,
   226
Colocynth, 157
Coltsfoot, 158
Comfrey, 159, 347–349
Commiphora myrrha, 233
Coptis groenlandica, 189
Cordyceps, 232
Cordyceps sinensis, 232
Cornsilk, 124, 134, 160,
   174, 254
Corydalis, 160
Corydalis yanhusuo, 160
Cotton root, 161
Cow parsnip, 161
Cramp bark, 139, 162,
   200, 207, 210, 214,
   215, 219, 251, 266,
   286
Cranberry, 124, 163
Crataegus spp., 122, 191
Crocus sativus, 261
Cucumber, 163, 219,
   271
Cucumis sativa, 163,
   219, 271
Cucurbita spp., 250,
   271, 277
Curare, 238
*Curcuma aromatica/
   domestica/longa*, 226,
   249, 282
Curcurbita spp., 211,
   219, 291, 309

Cymbopogon citratus,
   210
Cynara scolymus, 118,
   189, 230, 253, 292
Cytisus scoparius, 136

D
Damiana, 164, 295
Dandelion, 44, 112, 124,
   136, 137, 142, 143,
   146, 148, 157, 165,
   169, 179, 192, 197,
   199, 202, 211, 213,
   225, 226, 230, 236,
   238, 252, 255, 257,
   267, 275, 288, 290
Daucus carota, 254–255
Da zao, 203
Devil's claw, 166
Dill, 118, 166, 177, 242,
   254
Dioscorea villosa, 17
Dong quai, 19, 167
Dryopteris felx-mas, 219
Dulse, 168
Dyers broom, 169

E
Echinacea, 135, 170
Echinacea purpurea, 135
Echinacea spp., 170
Elder, 121, 135, 144,
   152, 166, 171, 178,
   188, 192, 199, 215,
   237, 242, 261, 281,
   287, 290
Elecampane, 119, 133,
   139, 172, 196, 197,

200, 207, 214, 215, 219, 246, 248, 251, 266, 275, 282, 286, 287
Eleuthero, 119, 131, 168, 173, 206, 265
Eleutherococcus senticosus, 119, 131, 168, 173, 206, 265
Emblica officinalis, 311
Ephedra sinica/vulgaris, 219
Epimedium sagittatum/ grandiflorum, 196, 295
Equisetum spp., 197
Escholtzia californica, 141
Eucalyptus, 173, 210
Eupatorium cannabinum, 192
Eupatorium grandiflorum, 196, 295
Eupatorium perfoliatum, 135
Eupatorium purpureum, 203
Euphrasia officinalis, 174
European vervain, 174
Evening primrose oil, 304–305
Eyebright, 174

F
False unicorn root, 175
Fennel, 104, 118, 132, 176, 253, 292

Fenugreek, 177
Ferula assa-foetida, 118
Feverfew, 177
Filipendula ulmaria, 227, 282, 289
Flax, 178
Foeniculum vulgare, 104, 118, 132, 176, 253, 292
Forsythia, 178
Forsythia suspense, 178
Fo ti, 179
Fouquieria splendens, 236
Frangula, 179
Fritillaria spp., 180
Fritillary, 180
Fucus vesiculosus, 131

G
Galega officinalis, 72, 186
Ganoderma lucidum, 232
Garlic, 181, 211, 219, 231, 250, 271, 277, 291
Gaulteria procumbens, 289
Genista tinctoria, 169
Gentian, 146, 182, 211, 213, 225, 230, 236
Gentiana lutea, 146, 182, 211, 213, 225, 230, 236
German chamomile, 258
Ginger, 160, 183, 226, 306

Ginkgo, 184, 189
Ginkgo biloba, 184
Ginseng, 119, 173, 185, 273
Glycyrrhiza glabra, 212
Goat's rue, 72, 186
Goji berry, 216
Gokshura, 186
Goldenrod, 124, 134, 174, 187, 203, 204, 254
Goldenseal, 121, 170, 172, 188, 237
Goldthread, 189
Gossypium herbaceum, 161
Gotu kola, 184, 189
Grifola frondosa, 232
Groundsel, 213
Guarana, 190
Gymnema, 190
Gymnema sylvestre, 190

H
Haldi, 282
Hamamelis virginiana, 22, 289
Harada, 310
Haritaki, 310
Harpagophytum procumbens, 166
Hawthorn, 191
Hawthorn berry, 122
Heartsease, 284
Hedeoma pulegoides, 242
Helianthus annuus, 135, 202, 217, 275
Helianthus tuberosus, 127

Hemp agrimony, 192
Hemp seed oil, 220
Hepatica nobilis, 213
Heracleum lanatum, 161
Hibiscus, 193
Hibiscus sabdariffa, 193
Hing, 118
Holy basil, 194
Honeysuckle, 178
Hops, 189, 195
Hordeum vulgare, 122
Horehound, 196, 197
Horny goad weed, 196, 295
Horsetail, 197
Ho shou wu, 179
Hou po, 218
Huang bai, 245
Humulus lupulus, 189, 195
Hydrastis canadensis, 172, 188
Hypericum perforatum, 274
Hyssop, 197
Hyssopus officinalis, 197

I

Ilex paraguayensis, 224
Indian ginseng, 268
Inonotus obliquus, 228, 232
Inula helenium, 119, 139, 172, 196, 197, 200, 207, 214, 215, 219, 246, 248, 251, 266, 275, 286, 287
Ipecac, 198

J

Jaborandi, 199
Jamaica dogwood, 200
Jasmine, 201
Jasminum officinale, 201
Jatamansi, 201
Jerusalem artichoke, 127, 202, 217
Job's tears, 202
Joe pye weed, 203
Juglans nigra, 131, 211, 219, 250, 271, 277
Jujube seeds, 203
Juniper, 204
Juniperus communis, |204
Juniperus sabina, 265

K

Kava kava, 205
Kelp, 206
Khella, 207
Knot grass, 207
Kombucha, 306

L

Lactobacillus acidophilus, 297
Lactuca virosa, 111
Lady's mantle, 208
Laminaria spp., 265
Larrea divaricate, 148
Larrea tridentata, 148
Lavender, 205, 208, 274
Lavendula angustifolia, 205, 208, 274
L. barbarum, 216
L. chinensis, 216

Ledum palustre, 121, 188, 237
Ledum paulstre, 223
Lemon balm, 137, 205, 209, 274
Lemongrass, 210
Lentinula edodes, 113, 121, 178, 188, 232, 245
Lentinuus edodes, 237
Leonardus cardiaca, 137
Leonurus cardiaca, 229
Leonurus heterophyllus, 152
Leonurus sibiricus, 152
Lepidium meyenii/ peruvianum, 217
Leptandra, 211
Lettuce, wild, 162
Levant wormseed, 211
Levisticum officinale, 215
Lian qiao, 178
Licorice, 212
Life root, 213
Ligusticum chuanxiong, 269
Ligusticum porter, 237
Linum usitatissimum, 178
Liverwort, 213
Lobelia, 214
Lobelia inflate, 214
Lomatium, 215
Lomatium dissectum, 215
Long birthroot, 216
Lovage, 215
Lycium, 216

Lycopus europaeus, 137
Lycopus virginicus, 137

M
Maca, 217
Ma chi xiang, 252
Madagascar periwinkle, 217
Madder, 218
Magnolia, 218
Magnolia officinalis, 218
Mahonia aquifolium, 237
Ma huang, 219
Maitake, 232
Mai ya, 122
Male fern, 219
Marijuana, 220
Marjoram, 221
Marrubium vulgare, 196
Marshmallow, 159, 222
Marsh tea homeopathic, 121, 188, 223, 237
Mate, 224
Matricaria recutita, 129, 147, 166, 240, 258, 263, 274, 276, 281, 282
Mayapple, 225
Meadow saffron, 226
Meadowsweet, 227, 282, 289
Medicago sativa, 111
Melissa officinalis, 137, 205, 209, 274
Mentha piperita, 192, 244
Mentha pulegium, 213, 242

Mentha spicata, 272
Milk thistle, 146, 227
Milky oats, 236
Mistletoe, 228
Mitchella repens, 240
Momordica charantia, 127
Monarda spp., 125
Motherwort, 22, 137, 229
Mo yao, 233
Mugwort, 230
Muira puama, 231
Mullein, 133, 158, 196, 197, 231, 246, 248, 287
Mushroom, 232
Mustard, 233
Mustard greens, wild, 285
Myristica fragrans, 235
Myrrh, 233

N
Nardostachys jatamansi, 201
Nasturtium officinale, 285
Nepeta cataria, 144, 261
Nereocystis luetkeana, 206
Nettle, 44, 124, 139, 234–235, 290
Nicotiana tabacum, 280
Niu ban zi, 138
Nutmeg, 235
Nutritional yeast, 308

O
Oats, 236
Oatstraw, 168, 197, 206, 236, 265
Oat tops, 236
Ocimum basilicum, 123
Ocimum sanctum, 194
Ocotillo, 236
Onions, 181
Oregon grape root, 237
Origanum marjorana, 221
Oscilococcinum, 131, 308–309
Osha, 237
Oxalis acetosella, 290

P
Paeonia officinalis, 243
Paeonia suffruticosa, 281
Panax ginseng, 119, 185, 273
Panax quinquefolius, 119, 185
Pareira, 238
Parsley, 238
Partridgeberry, 239
Pasque flower, 251
Passiflora incarnata, 240
Passionflower, 240
Pau d'arco, 240, 262
Paullinia cupana, 190
Pausinystalia yohimbe, 295
P. chinense, 245
Peach, 241
Pennyroyal, 213, 242
Peony, 243

Peppermint, 144, 192, 244
Petasites hybridus/ officinalis, 139
Petroselinum crispum, 238
Phellodendron, 245
Phellodendron amurense, 245
Phudina, 272
Phytolacca americana, 249
Pilocarpus spp., 199
Pimpinella anisum, 115, 118
Pine, 246
Pinellia, 246
Pinellia ternate, 246
Pinus spp., 246
Piper methysticum, 205
Piscidia erythrina, 200
Plantago lanceolata, 207, 268
Plantago major, 207, 268
Plantago spp., 247
Plantain, 207, 247, 268
Pleurisy root, 248
Podophyllum hexandrum/peltatum, 225
Poison ivy, 247
Poke root, 249
Polygala senega, 266
Polygoniun multiflorum, 179
Polygonum aviculare, 207
Pomegranate, 250
Portulaca oleracea, 252

Prickly ash, 250
Prunus persica, 241
Prunus serotina, 139, 200, 207, 214, 215, 219, 251, 266, 286
Ptychopetalum olacoides, 231
Pulsatilla, 251
Pulsatilla vulgaris, 251
Pumpkin seeds, 211, 219, 250, 271, 277, 291, 309
Punica granatum, 250
Purslane, 252

Q
Quassia, 253
Quassia amara, 253
Queen Anne's lace, 254–255
Quercus alba, 285

R
Ranunculus spp., 139
Raspberry leaf, 239
Red clover, 148, 255, 264
Red raspberry, 131, 168, 206, 256, 265
Reishi, 232
Rhamnus cathartica, 137
Rhamnus frangula, 179
Rhamnus purshiana, 142
Rheum officinale/ palmatum, 257
Rhodymenia palmetto, 168
Rhubarb, 72, 257

Ricinus communis, 143
Roman chamomile, 258
Rosa spp., 144, 205, 209, 259, 274
Rose, 144, 205, 209, 259, 274
Rosemary, 114, 129, 162, 173, 223, 243, 260, 281
Rosmarinus officinalis, 114, 129, 173, 223, 243, 260, 281
Rubia tinctorum, 218
Rubus fruticosus, 130, 208
Rubus ideaus, 131, 168, 206, 239, 256, 265
Rubus villosus, 130, 208
Rue, 260
Rumex acetose, 290
Rumex crispus, 44, 112, 137, 142, 143, 157, 169, 179, 192, 211, 213, 225, 226, 236, 238, 257, 261, 267, 294
Ruta graveolens, 260

S
Saccharomyces cervisiae, 302
Safflower, 261
Saffron, 261
Sage, 262–263
Salvia officinalis, 262
Sambucus nigra, 121, 135, 152, 166, 171, 178, 188, 192, 199,

215, 237, 242, 261, 281, 282, 287, 290
Sandalwood, 263
Sanguinaria canadensis, 133
Santalum album, 263
Sassafrass, 44, 264
Sassafrass albidum/ officinale, 44, 264
Savin, 265
Scutellaria lateriflora, 22, 129, 141, 144, 177, 203, 240, 270, 281
Seaweed, 168, 206, 265
Senecio aureus, 213
Senega, 266
Senna, 267
Senna spp., 267
Shatavari, 268
Shepherd's purse, 268
Shiitake, 113, 121, 178, 188, 232, 237, 245
Sichuan lovage, 269
Silybum marianum, 146, 227
Skullcap, 22, 129, 141, 144, 177, 203, 240, 270, 281
Slippery elm, 271
Solidago virgaurea, 124, 134, 174, 187, 203, 204, 254
Somnifera, 119
Sopari, 125
Southernwood, 271
Spearmint, 272
Spikenard, 273
Spirulina, 273

Stellaria media, 150
Stillingia, 275
Stillingia sylvatica, 275
St. John's wort, 274
Sunflower, 135, 275
Sweet flag, 276
Symphytum, 347
Symphytum officinale, 159, 348
Symphytum uplandica, 348

T
Tabebuia impetiginosa, 240, 262
Tanacetum parthenium, 177
Tanacetum vulgar, 277
Tansy, 277
Tao ren, 241
Taraxacum officinale, 44, 112, 124, 133, 136, 137, 142, 143, 146, 148, 157, 165, 169, 179, 192, 197, 199, 202, 211, 213, 225, 226, 230, 236, 238, 252, 255, 257, 267, 275, 288, 290
Tea, 278
Terminalia belerica, 311
Terminalia chebula, 310
Thea sinensis, 278
Theobroma cacao, 154
Thuja occidentalis, 116
Thyme, 148, 172, 173, 213, 223, 262, 279
Thymus spp., 279

Thymus vulgaris, 148, 172, 173, 213, 223, 262
Tian nan xing, 117
Tobacco, 280
Trametes versicolor, 232
Tree peony, 281
Tribulus terrestris, 186
Trifolium pratense, 148, 255, 264
Trigonella foenum-graecum, 177
Triphala, 157
Tulsi, 194
Turkey tail, 232
Turmeric, 226, 249, 282
Turnera aphrodisiaca, 164
Turnera diffusa, 295
Tussilago farfara, 158
Twak, 153

U
Ulmus rubra, 271
Urtica dioica, 44, 124, 139, 234–235, 290
Uva ursi, 124

V
Vaccinium myrtillus, 216
Vaccinium vitis-idaea, 124, 163
Valerian, 22, 141, 177, 201, 229, 284
Valeriana officinalis, 141, 201, 229, 284

Verbascum thapsus, 133, 158, 196, 197, 231, 246, 248, 287
Verbena hastate, 134
Verbena officinalis, 174
Veronica virginica, 211
Vetiver, 283
Vetiveria zizanoides, 283
Viburnum opulus, 139, 162, 200, 207, 210, 214, 215, 219, 251, 266, 286
Viburnum prunifolium, 130
Vinca rosea, 217
Viola tricolor, 284
Violet, 284
Viscum album, 228
Vitex agnus-castus, 129, 149

W
Watercress, 285
White oak, 285
Wild cherry bark, 139, 200, 207, 214, 215, 219, 251, 266, 286

Wild ginger, 286
Wild indigo, 287
Wild lettuce, 162
Wild mustard greens, 285
Wild yam root, 17, 288
Wintergreen, 289
Witch hazel, 22, 289
Withania somnifera, 119, 226
Wolf berry, 216
Wood sorrel, 290
Wormseed, 291
Wormwood, 292

X
Xanthoxylum americanum, 250

Y
Yan hu suo, 160
Yarrow, 144, 152, 160, 199, 243, 261, 281, 290, 293–294
Yellow dock root, 44, 112, 137, 142, 143, 157, 169, 179, 192,

211, 213, 225, 226, 236, 238, 257, 261, 267, 294
Yi mu cao, 152
Yohimbe, 295

Z
Zanthoxylum americanum, 250
Zea mays, 124, 134, 160, 174, 254
Zingiber officinale, 160, 183, 226, 286
Ziziphus spinosa, 203

GENERAL INDEX

A

Acidophilus, 297–298
Acne, 138, 311
Acupuncture, 55
Adaptogenic, 119, 273
Adoption, xx, 9
Adrenal health, 17, 119, 173, 234, 301
Agave nectar, 300
Aging, 179, 184
Alcohol, 298
Alkaloids, 95–96, 139
Allergies, 139, 215, 218, 235, 311
Allium, 302
Alternative therapies, 54–56
Analgesic, 283
Anemia, 127, 154, 294
Antacid, 166
Anthraquinones, 96, 120, 137, 142, 179, 257
Antibacterial, 125, 128, 140, 153, 170, 173, 181, 207, 215, 233, 237, 245, 283
Antibiotic, 188
Antifungal, 128, 131, 140, 148, 153, 181, 237, 273
Antigalactagogue, 122, 137, 201, 219, 238, 262
Antihistamines, 103
Anti-inflammatory, 113,
121, 128, 140, 147, 148, 153, 166, 171, 174, 177, 202, 220, 223, 227, 237, 241, 245, 252, 260, 281, 282, 283, 284
Antimicrobial, 121, 136, 170, 181, 273
Antirheumatic, 166
Antiseptic, 125, 136, 221, 279, 286, 287
Antispasmodic, 201, 207, 215, 219, 221, 240, 270, 281, 283, 284, 311
Antiviral, 113, 170, 171, 181, 183, 209, 215, 237
Anxiety, 144, 205, 209, 259, 274, 311
Aphrodisiac, 164, 181, 185, 268, 295
Appetite, 114, 128, 176, 220, 253, 292
Aristolochic acid, 96
Aromatherapy, 176
Arthritis, 129, 139, 145, 146, 166, 173, 202, 204, 223, 249
Artificial sweeteners, 299–300
Aspartame, 299
Aspirin, 227
Asthma, 133, 139, 200, 214, 215, 240, 251, 265, 311
Astringent, 207, 208, 213, 227, 259, 289

Atherosclerosis, 282
Attention deficit spectrum, 209, 301
Ayurvedic, 119, 120, 186, 201, 259, 268, 282, 310

B

Balance. see Hormonal balance
Barky Rooty Tea, 17, 18
Bedwetting, 159
Bee pollen, 300–301
Berberine, 97
Beta-asarone, 96
Bididobacterium infantis, 309
Bifidobacterium bifidum, 309
Bifidobacterium longum, 309
Birth kit, 22
Bitters, 48–49, 114, 118, 132, 182, 189, 208, 253, 292
Bladder, 124, 159, 187, 203, 245
Bleeding, 11, 19, 22, 43, 167, 184, 207, 246
Bloating, 218
Blood
  brown, 12, 294
  cleansing, 255, 264, 273, 275, 285, 294
  stagnation of, 161
  supply, 235
  thinners, 255

Blood pressure, 130, 136, 181, 191, 193, 212, 301

Blood sugar, 127, 153, 177, 186, 190, 202, 227

Blunt force trauma, 241

Bone broths, 51

Bone loss, 301

Bone marrow, 120

Borage oil, 301–302

Brain, 184, 189

Brassica, 302

Breast cancer, 57

Breastfeeding. *see* Nursing

Breast health, 56–60, 186, 301

Breast massage, 59–60, 249, 339–341

Breast milk bank, 27–28

Brewer's yeast, 302

Bronchitis, 133, 215, 248, 251, 265, 311

Bruising, 117, 140, 234, 274, 289, 294

Burns, 140, 274

C

Cabbage, 302

Caffeine, 70, 154, 155, 156, 190, 224, 278

Calcium, 50, 111, 131, 159, 168, 197, 206, 265

Cancer, 146, 217, 228, 232, 249, 282, 285

Cardiac glycosides, 97

Castor oil, 143

Cathartics, 96, 169, 192, 249

Charting, 41–42

Cheese, 302–303

Chicken pox, 209

Children's dosage, 343–344

Chiropractic, 55, 70–71

Chlorophyll, 235, 273

Cholesterol, 111, 181, 193

Circulatory system, 145, 184, 186, 193, 250

Cleansing, 98–103

Clomid, 6, 8

Coconut oil, 261

Cod liver oil, 48, 65, 303–304

Cognitive function, 189

Colic, 141, 144, 166, 238, 242

Comfrey, 347–349

Common cold, 117, 171, 172, 178, 181, 183, 193, 215, 221, 231, 240, 242, 286, 308

Comprehensive approach, xiv–xv, 3

Congestion, 116, 117, 119, 172, 173, 174, 231, 236, 242, 246, 276

Constipation, 128, 157, 226, 294, 311

Contraception, 286

Contractions, 114, 124, 129, 175, 180, 199, 242, 256, 260

Convulsions, 220

Copper, 43

Corn syrup, 68, 300

Cortisol, 119

Cough, 114, 115, 158, 159, 176, 178, 180, 196, 219, 251, 286

Cramps, 114, 130, 162, 176, 210, 218, 257, 267, 293, 301

C-section, 189

Cuts, 140

Cyanogenic glycosides, 97

Cysts, 143

D

Dandruff, 138

Decongestants, 103, 173

Dental health, 35

Depression, 161, 185, 205, 208, 209, 216, 236, 259, 274

Detoxing, 98–103

Diabetes, 127, 186, 202, 217

Diaphoretic, 199, 215, 221

Diarrhea, 128, 130, 207, 208, 289

Diet foods, 69

Digestion. *see also* Indigestion absorption, 52, 145

digestive unrest, 118
herbal therapies for,
118, 122, 125, 132,
145, 150, 156, 161,
177, 182, 189, 197,
204, 206, 208, 210,
215, 218, 225, 230,
237, 242, 246, 250,
254, 257, 272, 279,
285, 292, 311
and lacto-fermented
foods, 66
Diuretics, 136, 146,
150, 163, 169, 197,
199, 202, 204, 207,
215, 222, 227, 233,
238, 241, 252, 254,
272, 275
Dizziness, 191
Dosage
children's, 343–344
nursing through, 78

E
Ear infections, 231, 287
Earthing, 56
Eating disorders, 132
E. coli, 210, 303
Eczema, 138, 150, 255,
264
Edema, 136, 163.
see also Swelling
Emetics, 169, 174, 198,
226
Emphysema, 265
Endometriosis,
138, 288
Energy level, 120, 185

Engorgement, 262, 302
Ephedra, 219
Erectile dysfunction, 45.
see also Impotence
Estragole, 98, 123
Estrogen, 41, 43, 148,
175, 268, 283
Evacuants, 112, 137,
142, 179
Evening primrose oil,
304–305
Exhaustion, 236, 273
Expectorant, 116, 133,
215, 221, 237, 273
Eye irritations, 147, 174

F
Fainting, 127
Fats, 47–48, 68, 69,
99–100
Fatty acids, 48
Fatty lumps, 143
Favism, 127
Fermentation, 31
Fertility.
see also Infertility
and charting,
41–42
herbal therapies for,
39–44, 191, 217,
255, 268
and male partner,
44–47, 212, 256
mental component,
53–54
and nutrition, xv–xvi
personal journey,
6–19

Fertility Awareness
Method, 11
Fevers, 135, 144, 152,
192, 197, 224, 250,
281, 284, 290, 294
Fibrocystic breast
lumps, 57–58
Fibroids, 138
Finger feeder, 27, 31, 72
Fish, 305–306
Flatulence, 115, 176,
238, 242
Flower essences, 95
Flu, 135, 171, 178, 181,
183, 193, 221, 240,
248, 308
Follicles, 217
Food.
see also Nutrition
appropriate diet,
34–35
changes required,
313–315
foods to avoid, 68–70
importance of, 36–37
ingredients to
eliminate, 14
for preconception,
47–53
for pregnancy and
lactation, 64–70
processed foods,
99–100
Formula.
see Supplemental
feeding
Fructose, 68, 300
Fungus, 128, 131

G

Galactagogues, 72, 137, 166, 227

Gallbladder, 118, 140, 146, 182, 211, 213, 225, 227, 236, 253

Gas pains, 176

Genetically modified organisms (GMO), 69–70, 305

Genotoxins, 96

Glandular tissue, 57, 72, 186

Glaucoma, 199

Goiter, 131, 168, 206

Gout, 139, 146, 223, 254, 264

Grains, 50–53

Gripe water, 166

H

Headaches, 119, 127, 147, 177, 190, 208, 210, 221, 240, 269, 270

Heart, 137, 145, 191, 193, 228, 229, 246, 259, 284

Heartburn, 227, 276

Heart palpitations, 71, 191

Heat, 163

Hemorrhages, 159, 207, 234, 268, 289, 293

Hemorrhoids, 234, 289

Henna, 303

Herbal usage guide, 107–110

Herbs.
see also Plant Index
asking herbs for help, 16–18
and breast milk, 77–79
general use, 81–82
quality of, 83–85, 86
standardized method versus simplers method, 87–88
sustainable suppliers, 85–87
whole form, 2
whole versus isolated constituents, 89–91

Herpes, 209

Hiccups, 311

High fructose corn syrup, 68, 300

Hippocrates, xxii, 82

Hirsutism, 272

Home birth, 20–24, 33–36

Homeopathics, 93–94

Honey, raw, 309

Hormonal balance
versus cure, 36
herbal therapies for, 175, 236, 288
importance of, 39–40, 53
for male partner, 45
understanding, 42–43

Hot flashes, 134, 174, 301

Hypoplastic breasts, 57

Hypothyroidism, 131, 206, 209, 265

I

Immune system, 170, 173, 232, 249, 259, 273, 287

Immunostimulant, 113

Impotence, 45, 103, 184, 186, 196, 231, 236, 280, 295

Incontinence, 187

Indigestion, 128, 147, 177, 207, 276.
see also Digestion

Infections, 121, 159, 170, 223, 232, 247, 279, 285, 311

Infertility.
see also Fertility
causes of, 41
herbal therapies for, 239, 288

Inflammation, 111, 113, 174, 177, 249, 263, 274, 311

Insomnia, 141, 195, 203, 208, 220, 240, 284

Insufficient glandular tissue, 58

Insulin, 51

Intestines, 245

Iodine, 131, 168, 206, 265, 310

Iron, 43, 47, 48, 111, 278, 285, 294

J

Jaundice, 121, 227, 245, 250

Joint irritation, 241

K

Kefir, 14, 31, 67, 335

Kidneys

danger to, 173, 216, 218, 252, 257

herbal therapies for, 17, 124, 134, 165, 174, 179, 187, 197, 203, 204, 216, 224, 234, 245

Kombucha, 306

L

Labor

delivery of placenta, 114, 256

facilitation of, 213, 293

herbal therapies for, 239

restorative after, 208

stalled labor, 126, 134, 242

Lactation, 64–70, 72

Lactation consultant, 26–27, 30

Lactation cookies, 349–350

Lactobacillus acidophilus, 297–298

Lactobacillus plantarum, 309

Lacto-fermented foods, 66

La Leche League, 73

Laryngitis, 276, 287

Lavender oil, 94

Lawsonia inermis, 303

Laxatives, 112, 137, 142, 143, 178, 179, 192, 238, 249, 257, 261, 267, 294

Leaky gut syndrome, 76

Libido, 186, 231

Lice, 253, 283

Liver

danger to, 124, 139, 148, 158, 159, 192, 203, 205, 213

herbal therapies for, 17, 113, 138, 165, 179, 182, 189, 211, 213, 216, 225, 227, 236, 253, 255, 288, 294, 311

nutritional value, 48

role of, 43–44, 62–63

Lunchmeat, 307

Lungs, 117, 197, 200, 213, 216, 246, 248

Luteinizing hormone, 148, 186

Lymphatic cleanser, 275

M

Magnesium, 48, 65

Malaria, 152

Male partner and fertility, 44–47

Manta massage, 340–341

Massage, 55, 339–341

Mastitis, 262, 273, 302

Meat, 34–35, 47, 48, 307

Memory, 218, 276

Menopause, 129, 234

Menstruation

bringing on, 215, 269

cramping, 210, 218, 242, 269, 301

delayed, 114, 130, 213, 229, 242

hormonal levels, 236

lack of, 201

PMS, 148, 234

regulation of, 114, 140, 152, 167, 186, 196, 208, 230, 241, 242, 288

Mental component, 53–54, 73–75

Menthol, 272

Mercury, 305

Migraines, 177

Milk

blocked ducts, 273

increasing supply, 135, 148, 186

raw, 30, 31, 33, 34, 66, 303

reduction of, 137, 143, 201, 263

stimulation of, 72, 111

Miscarriage, 19–20, 175, 223, 239, 288

Morning sickness, 120, 175, 244

MSG, 307–308

Mucus, 159, 172, 188, 231, 237, 271, 279, 294, 311

Multiple sclerosis, 301

Muscle relaxant, 284

Muscle soreness, 141, 145

N

Natural flavors, 307–308

Nausea, 127, 153, 220, 227, 241, 244

Nerve pain, 166, 220

Nervous debility, 236

Nervous system, 195, 199, 209, 218, 258, 259, 274, 286

Niacin, 335

Nipples
  cracked, 140, 222, 287
  inverted, 57–58

Nosebleeds, 268

Nursing.
  see also Lactation
  detoxification during, 102–203
  individual needs, 3–4, 30
  mental component, 73–75
  nursing through, 75–79
  personal journey, 24–29

Nutrition. *see* Food

Nutritional yeast, 308

O

Oenothera biennis, 304–305

Oils
  essential, 94–95
  hydrogenated, 68, 99

Omega-3, 48, 65

Omega-6, 48, 65, 301–302, 304

Organ meats, 48

Orthostatic hypotension, 191

Oscilococcinum, 308

Over-the-counter (OTC) drugs, 103–104, 309–310

Ovulation, 41

Oxalates, 97

P

Pain relief, 160, 166, 213, 220, 240, 243, 254, 260, 268, 269, 274, 281, 284, 289

Palpitations, 71, 191

Parasites, 163, 181

Pelvic floor, 187

Performance anxiety, 231

Personal journey, xvii–xxiii, 5–37

Phlegm, 120, 246, 287

Pituitary gland, 148

Placenta expulsion, 114, 152, 256

Pleurisy, 248

Pneumonia, 248

Poison ivy, 247

Preconception
  detoxification during, 102
  foods for, 47–53
  health during, 60–64

Pregnancy
  detoxification during, 102
  foods for, 64–70
  personal journey, 19–20

Premarin, 6

Premature ejaculation, 179, 196

Premenstrual syndrome, 148, 234

Prescription drugs, 45, 63, 103–104, 309–310

Probiotics, 297–298, 309

Progesterone, 41–42, 43, 148, 283, 288

Prostate, 159

Protein, 66

Psoriasis, 138, 150, 237, 255, 264, 294

Psychological distress, 201

P-Synephrine, 126

Pumpkin, 309

Purgatives, 267

Pyrrolizidine alkaloids, 96, 135, 139, 158,

159, 192, 203, 213, 348

Q
Qi, 55, 246
Quinidine, 152
Quinine, 152

R
Rashes, 112
Raw honey, 309
Reiki, 55
Reproductive structures, 46
Respiratory system, 133, 141, 148, 207, 213, 215, 237, 246, 248, 265, 275, 279, 286, 294
Rheumatism, 141, 146, 166, 196, 202, 223, 226, 249, 289

S
Saccharin, 299
Saccharomyces cerevisiae, 308
Safrole, 98, 123
Sciatica, 166
Sea salt, 131, 168, 206, 265, 310
Seasonal affective disorder, 209
Sedatives, 141, 144, 201, 203, 258, 270, 283, 284, 286
Seizures, 270
Sex hormones, 119

Shingles, 209
Side effects, 91
Simplers method, 87–88
Sinus infections, 287
Sitz baths, 56, 140
Skin conditions, 138, 150, 172, 236, 241, 246, 247, 255, 264, 275
Skin tags, 133
Sleep problems. *see* Insomnia
Smoking, 45
Soil depletion, 92
Sore throat, 240, 262, 276, 285
Soy, 68–69
Spasms, 201, 280
Sperm
count, 179, 196
motility, 44, 120, 179
quality of, 44, 179
survival time, 186
Splenda, 299
Sprains, 260, 294
Stagnation
blood, 161, 241
pelvic, 152
Stamina, 173
Standardized method, 87–88
Stapylococcus aureus, 210
Stimulants
appetite, 114, 132, 176
general, 125, 145, 154, 156, 173, 190, 224, 233, 250

immune, 287
respiratory, 246
uterine, 121, 126, 133, 134, 141, 146, 167, 177, 178, 188, 189, 198, 204, 207, 208, 230, 233, 237, 238, 240, 245, 248, 250, 254, 257, 264, 277, 288
Stress, 119, 173, 194, 236, 270, 274
"Stuck" energy, 55–56, 60
Styptic, 268, 281, 293
Subluxation, 71
Sucralose, 299
Sugars, 69
Sunburn, 274
Sunscreen, 112
Superfoods, 47
Supplemental feeding
equipment for, 71–73
formulas, 335–337
personal journey, 27–33
Supplements
probiotics, 297–298
vitamins, 92–93
Swelling, 243, 289, 294

T
Tapeworms, 250
Teas, 16–18, 78, 79
Teething, 147
Tennis elbow, 143
Theobromine, 154
Thiamine, 197

Thrush, 181
Thujone, 98
Thyroid, 131, 137, 168, 206, 209, 265
Tinctures, 22, 78, 79
Tinnitus, 129
Tonic emetic, 134
Tonic Tea, 17
Toothache, 200
Topical treatments
  after C-sections, 189
  antibacterial, 233
  antiseptic, 173
  as blood and fluid mover, 293
  for bruises, 159
  in labor, 301, 304
  for lice, 253
  for pain, 139, 141
  for skin problems, 150
Toxin clearing, 148
Traditional Chinese Medicine, 87
Trans fats, 68, 99–100
Tremors, 240
Triphala, 310–311
Tumors, 114, 143, 217, 228, 286
Tuna, 305–306

U
Ulcers, 140, 159, 311

United Plant Savers, 90, 345–346
Urinary incontinence, 187
Urinary stones, 254
Urinary tract, 114, 124, 136, 148, 159, 163, 187, 227, 280, 290
Uterine fibroids, 138
Uterus, 239

V
Vaccinations, 31–32, 63
Varicose veins, 234, 289
Varicosities, 207
Vermifuge, 237, 253, 279, 306
Vision, 126, 216
Vitamin A, 43, 65, 284, 303
Vitamin B, 111
Vitamin B1 (thiamine), 197
Vitamin B3 (niacin), 335
Vitamin B5 (pantothenic acid), 275
Vitamin B6 (pyridoxine), 67
Vitamin B12, 43, 47, 48
Vitamin C, 193, 238, 284, 311

Vitamin D, 43, 65
Vitamin E, 43, 303
Vitamin K, 43, 234
Vomiting, 224. *see also* Nausea

W
Water retention, 234
Weaning, 122
Weight loss, 150
Weston Price Foundation, 303
Whole foods
  as detoxification, 101
  preparation of, 14–16
Whole grains, 50–53
Whooping cough, 251, 286
Withdrawal, 270
Worksheet, 351–357
Worms, 163, 183, 219, 250, 271, 277, 291, 292

Y
Yeast, 297, 302, 306
Yeast infections, 131, 240, 279

Z
Zinc, 47, 48

About the Author

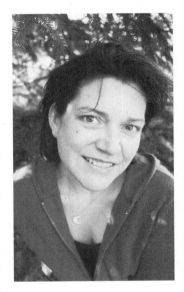

Dawn Combs is an ethnobotanist with over 20 years' experience in women's health issues. She began her career with a B.A. in Botany and Humanities/Classics, and later apprenticed with Rosemary Gladstar. After resolving her own infertility diagnosis through whole foods and natural herbal remedies, she chose to specialize in helping women rebalance their bodies for fertility. Dawn is an educator, a contributor to several national magazines, co-owner of Mockingbird Meadows and director of its Eclectic Herbal Institute. She lives in central Ohio with her husband Carson and her children, Aidan and Jacy. Her family was recently recognized by *Mother Earth News* as one of their 2013 Homesteaders of the Year.

If you have enjoyed *Conceiving Healthy Babies* you might also enjoy other

BOOKS TO BUILD A NEW SOCIETY

Our books provide positive solutions for people who want to make a difference. We specialize in:

**Sustainable Living • Green Building • Peak Oil
Renewable Energy • Environment & Economy
Natural Building & Appropriate Technology
Progressive Leadership • Resistance and Community
Educational & Parenting Resources**

For a full list of NSP's titles, please call 1-800-567-6772 *or check out our website* at:

www.newsociety.com

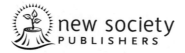